Physical Assessment

A Guide for Evaluating Drug Therapy

R. Leon Longe, Pharm.D.
Professor
College of Pharmacy
The University of Georgia
Athens, Georgia
and
Clinical Professor
Department of Family Medicine
Medical College of Georgia
Augusta, Georgia

Jon C. Calvert, M.D., Ph.D.
FAAFP, JrFACOG
Professor, Department of Family Practice
University of Oklahoma College of Medicine, Tulsa
Tulsa, Oklahoma

Fellow, American Academy Family Physicians
Junior Fellow, American College Obstetrics and Gynecology

Edited by:
Lloyd Yee Young, Pharm.D.
Director of Pharmacy/IV Therapy
Southwest Washington Medical Center
Vancouver, Washington
and
Adjunct Associate Professor of Clinical Pharmacy
College of Pharmacy
Washington State University
Spokane/Vancouver, Washington

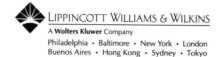

LIPPINCOTT WILLIAMS & WILKINS
A **Wolters Kluwer** Company
Philadelphia · Baltimore · New York · London
Buenos Aires · Hong Kong · Sydney · Tokyo

Printing and Binding: Edwards Brothers, Ann Arbor, Michigan
Typesetting: Impressions, Madison, Wisconsin
Page and Cover Design: Rick Walsh

Lippincott Williams & Wilkins
351 West Camden Street
Baltimore, MD 21201-2436 USA

ISBN: 0-915486-20-2
Library of Congress Catalog Card Number: 94-76859

First Printing, June 1994
Second Printing, August 1995
Third Printing, October 1996
Fourth Printing, August 1997
Fifth Printing, January 1999
Sixth Printing, October 1999

Acknowledgments

The creation of this book has been a labor of love and a commitment that began more than a decade ago as a series of articles that were published in *Drug Intelligence and Clinical Pharamcy* under the guidance, mentorship, and editorial support of Dr. Donald Francke. After the death of Dr. Francke, Harvey A.K. Whitney, Jr. continued the support first proffered by Dr. Francke. To these men, we are indebted.

This series of articles has been completely refocused, revised, and rewritten to form this new book, **Physical Assessment: A Guide for Evaluating Drug Therapy.** This new publication reflects the input from a decade of doctor of pharmacy candidates from the University of Georgia, insights and clinical experiences of Dr. A Thomas Taylor, editorial contributions of Lloyd Y. Young, Pharm.D., encouragement of Linda L. Young, and the dedication of the Applied Therapeutics staff, especially Rick Walsh and Nannette Naught. We are grateful to these individuals.

To my wife, Linda and my children, Kim, Bob, and Michael for encouragement, support and keeping the dream alive, I (RLL) am most grateful above all.

Throughout the years of development of this text, my (JCC) family has provided understanding and support. To my wife, Lynnette, and our sons, Stephen and Joshua, my love and my gratitude.

To our Creator and Touchstone, we are eternally grateful.

R. Leon Longe

Jon C. Calvert

Notice to Reader

Drug therapy information is constantly evolving. Our ever-changing knowledge and experience with drugs and the continual development of new drugs necessitates changes in treatment and drug therapy. The editors, authors, and the publisher of this work have made every effort to ensure the information provided herein was accurate at the time of publication. *It remains the responsibility of every practitioner to evaluate the appropriateness of a particular opinion or therapy in the context of the actual clinical situation and with due consideration of any new developments in the field.* Although the authors have been careful to recommend dosages that are in agreement with current standards and responsible literature, the student or practitioner should consult with several appropriate information sources when dealing with new and unfamiliar drugs.

Contents

Preface

The past several years have introduced us to new visions of health care delivery as America grapples with the reform of its health care system. During this period of time, physicians have revitalized the importance of primary care and pharmacists have embraced the philosophy of pharmaceutical care. According to the Commission to Implement Change in Pharmaceutical Education, "It is the concept of pharmaceutical care, in all of its ramifications, that is revolutionary. It envisions pharmacists as activists on behalf of patients, working before dispensing to assist prescribers in appropriate drug choices, and working after dispensing to help patients achieve the desired outcomes of their therapy. It envisions pharmacists as competent, caring, and committed to the well-being of their patients. The educational revolution that must be implemented to reach these challenges will be significant. . . ." In light of these changes, it seems especially pertinent for a pharmacist (Dr. Longe) to collaborate with a physician (Dr. Calvert) in the publication of a book to assist pharmacists in the implementation of pharmaceutical care. This book is entitled **Physical Assessment: A Guide for Evaluating Drug Therapy.**

The primary purpose of this textbook is to introduce the art and science of the physical examination of a patient and to provide the reader with examples of application of physical assessment to therapeutics. The first chapter of this book introduces general concepts in physical assessments and teaches the student how to obtain a medical history by interviewing the patient. The second chapter approaches the evaluation of the whole patient by describing the four fundamental physical examination techniques of inspection, palpation, percussion, and auscultation.

The remaining 15 chapters utilize a body systems approach and contain sections on anatomy and physiology; methods of physical assessment along with selected normal and abnormal physical findings; a pharmacotherapeutic case illustration; and several examples for the monitoring of drug therapy. The presentation of the physical assessment of the patient in conjunction with a case and examples for monitoring the pharmacotherapy of a patient provide the student insight into the inter-relationship of these components. As a result, this book attempts only to provide a broad overview of the physical assessment process and does not attempt to be encyclopedic in either the breadth or depth for physical examinations.

The content of this book comes alive when the student applies the information to the care of patients and to the evaluation of clinical outcomes. The proper application of knowledge to develop skills, however, requires coaching, mentoring, and considerable ongoing practice.

As with all first editions, this is just a beginning. We welcome your comments and suggestions as to how we might continue to improve this first effort.

Physical Assessment

A Guide for Evaluating Drug Therapy

Clinical Assessment and Interviewing the Patient

Clinical assessment is an orderly process and is completed in seven distinct steps with each step building on information gathered during the previous one. The steps are: 1) history taking; 2) physical examination; 3) developing a working diagnosis; 4) obtaining supportive or differentiating laboratory studies or procedures; 5) developing a final diagnosis; 6) initiating treatment; and 7) ongoing evaluation of effectiveness of treatment and potential side effects of medications.

The clinician assembles the medical history by gathering subjective information while talking with the patient. This history reflects the patient's perspective of his or her medical condition and is obtained by posing a series of questions to the patient. Of all the steps in the assessment of drug therapy, this is the most important and often accurately points to the eventual diagnosis after substantiation in steps two and three. This first step also is the one that requires the greatest amount of skill. Questions must be asked in such a way that they are not leading and yet uncover as much of an in-depth history as possible. Questions also must be carefully related to each other so that the answer to one question triggers another set of questions which follow specific protocols. For example, if a patient complains of pain, a series of seven specific questions should then be asked (see Table 1.1).

The patient history gathered by the clinician directs or focuses the physical assessment to more fully examine specific organ systems. For example, if the subjective data suggest the possibility of respiratory illness, the clinician should examine the chest, lungs, and upper respiratory tract to either support or refute this suggestion. It is not uncommon for seasoned clinicians to "uncover" other medical concerns during a focused examination for a given problem. In this case, for example, while evaluating the respiratory system and the neck for lymph node enlargement, the examiner may well find an enlarged thyroid gland indicative of thyroid disease.

The clinician then brings together the subjective information of the history with the objective data from the physical exam to formulate a working diagnosis. This working diagnosis may point to laboratory studies or diagnostic procedures needed to support or refute the diagnosis. Further confirmation or differentiation for a patient with respiratory symptoms could be obtained with specific laboratory studies (e.g., complete blood count

Medical History Example: Clarification of Pain

Table 1.1

Location of Pain	Patient is asked to describe and point with 1 finger to where the pain begins or is located.
Onset/Duration of Pain	At what point in time was the pain first noted? (e.g., It began 3 months ago; last Wednesday; last night about 1 hour after eating dinner.) How long did the pain last? (e.g., It lasted for an hour and gradually went away; it has not gone away since it started and it is just as intense now as when it started; the pain comes and goes, gets real bad then it almost goes away before it starts to come back again.)
Character of Pain	How does the patient describe the pain? (e.g., It is sharp like pins and needles sticking me; it is dull like a tooth ache only worse; it is throbbing, feels like my heart pounding in my head.)
Frequency of Pain	Since the pain first began, has it recurred and if so, has it remained the same, improved, or worsened? (e.g., The pain has occurred about once a week for the past 2 years and has not changed in intensity; at first the pain was not very frequent, about once every 2 to 3 weeks, but now it occurs every day and even awakens me at night.)
Aggravation of Pain	Is there anything the patient does or does not do that makes the pain worse or that brings it on? (e.g., About 1/2 hour after I eat spicy foods I begin to hurt in the pit of my stomach; whenever I feel stressed to the max I get this headache in the back of my head/neck that moves to my forehead.)
Relief of Pain	Is there anything the patient does that relieves the pain? (e.g., When my stomach starts to hurt, if I curl up in a ball, it feels much better; when I am working and my chest starts to hurt, I stop and sit down and in a few minutes the pain goes away.)
Radiation of Pain	Does the pain move anywhere after it begins? (e.g., When I am working and get that tight chest pain, sometimes it also hurts in my neck and down my left arm; the severe pain in my left flank keeps coming and going and now it hurts at the base of my penis also.)

looking for an elevated white blood cell count associated with infection) and/or procedures (e.g., a chest x-ray which might demonstrate a pneumonia).

Once the final diagnosis is determined, a treatment plan is developed and implemented; however, a treatment plan sometimes must be initiated before a "final diagnosis" has been determined. The clinician should monitor the patient closely after initiating a treatment plan to observe the effectiveness of the plan and be aware of any adverse effects of the prescribed medication. In evaluating responses to drug treatments, the clinician monitors both subjective and objective data in light of the expected clinical outcomes. Clinical parameters that reflect the efficacy and safety of each drug should be monitored while maintaining an awareness that drugs can positively or negatively affect these parameters.

The predictive power of a monitoring parameter (e.g., symptom, sign, or laboratory test) depends upon the parameter's association with the clinical observation. As the prevalence of this association increases, the predictive power of the clinical parameter increases. For example, a patient on digoxin therapy complains of nausea, a slow irregular pulse, and dizziness. Since these symptoms are parameters used to monitor the safety of the drug, they are likely to be the result of digoxin toxicity.

Monitoring parameters should be selected based upon specificity, sensitivity, and selectivity. When evaluating drug response, the specificity of the parameter is important to estimate the likelihood of false negatives. For example, the clinician must determine how prevalent the association of this parameter is to the outcome being monitored. The sensitivity of the monitoring parameter for a certain drug also is important in the estimation of false positives. Unfortunately, the literature often fails to quantify monitoring parameters for a particular patient population. These judgments are, therefore, qualitative assessments that improve with clinical experience over many years.

Clinical assessments should be undertaken with careful thought and thoroughness. Snap judgments are often wrong because they fail to consider all other possibilities that are associated with a clinical observation. Data should be collected and facts reported without bias toward any preconceived judgments. Furthermore, the total

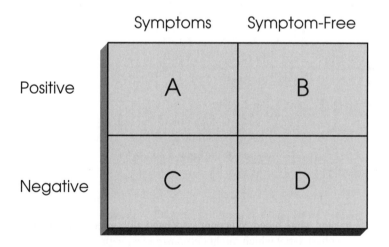

Fig. 1.1 The letters in the box indicate the presence or absence of symptoms associated with the treatment of a patient with a specific medication. A is the number of true positives; the patient's symptoms are caused by the medication. B is the number of false positives; the patient's symptoms are the same as those caused by the medication, but are not a result of the medication. C is the number of false negatives; the patient does not have symptoms but should. D is the number of true negatives; the patient does not have symptoms and should not have symptoms. Sensitivity = A/(A+C); specificity = D/(B+D).

patient should be considered and not just one specific monitoring parameter for a particular problem. For example, clinicians should not focus solely on blood pressure reduction while ignoring a medication's effect on brain perfusion. Too often, the specialist sees only the broken rib in the x-ray and not the tuberculous cavity in the lung. Remember to treat the total patient.

The clinician also must use technology appropriately. The clinical laboratory, diagnostic procedures, computerized calculations, and pharmacokinetic formulas employed in the calculation of serum drug concentrations often mesmerize junior clinicians. The experienced clinician recognizes the limits of mathematical formulas and the possibility of errors in laboratory results, and evaluates the whole patient. When confronted at the bedside with a clinically improved patient and either an abnormal laboratory result or an abnormal physical finding, the clinician should consider the overall condition of the patient to guide management decisions.

The pharmacist is professionally responsible for the management of drug therapy. The societal application of pharmacy is to manage the drug use process. With this responsibility, the pharmacist must always serve as an advocate for the patient, utilizing all resources available to ensure appropriate, economical, safe, and effective drug management.

INTERVIEWING THE PATIENT

The patient interview uncovers the data which form the foundation for subsequent treatment evaluations and decisions. When properly conducted, the interview process focuses the clinician's attention on specific problems and can lead to therapeutic decisions without the need for an extensive physical examination of the patient. Also, the interview begins a professional relationship in which the clinician and patient can learn about, and develop confidence in, each other. The clinician uses the data gleaned from the interview to identify problems and develop therapeutic goals; the patient uses the interview to judge the clinician's professional competence.

The interview has either a limited goal of evaluating major symptoms or a more comprehensive goal of evaluating a patient's past and present health problems. In most cases, the clinician determines the goal of a particular interview session with a patient. The type of interview depends upon the needs of the patient, the time available, and the patient's physical or mental condition. This chapter focuses on two types of interviews: the medication history interview and the treatment evaluation interview.

The Interview Process

Regardless of whether you need to obtain a medication history or a more comprehensive overview of the patient's medical condition, the basic principles for conducting an interview are the same. Although interviewing a patient appears to be a deceptively simple process, considerable practice is required before gaining proficiency in this skill. However, as with all skills, interviewing can be improved with routine use of proper techniques.

Preparation. Review information from existing records (e.g., charts, office medical records, transfer files, or medication profiles) before you interview a patient. Even a brief review of the files can provide valuable background information on previous medical problems and treatments. Also, you can gather biographical information about the patient to facilitate greetings and initial interactions. This preparation before the interview can help reassure the patient of your professional involvement and concern.

Nonverbal Communication. In any interaction, we express ourselves through nonverbal actions. During an interview, you should use body language to convey an unhurried, interested, sympathetic, professional, and self-confident image to the patient. The following are some nonverbal techniques to enhance communication with a patient and improve data collection:

- Squarely face the patient and maintain eye contact 60% to 70% of the time.

- Use hand gestures when you speak.

- Sit or stand comfortably; do not appear anxious to leave the room or disinterested in what the patient has to say.

- Position yourself at the patient's eye level when possible.

- Create an open body posture by leaning toward the patient and uncrossing your arms and legs.

- Wear clean, neat, comfortable professional clothing.

- Use silence to allow the patient to compose his or her story.

- Relax.

The environment in which you conduct the interview can also hinder or foster communication. If possible, interview the patient in a private, quiet area free from interruption. The television or radio should either be turned off or the volume decreased, and visitors should be asked to leave with the permission of the patient. Although spouses or relatives can be helpful in confirming information, they can lead the interview astray by focusing on details that contribute only marginally to the overall understanding of the patient's condition. The presence of relatives, however, is important when interviewing a mentally incompetent patient or a child. Physical barriers such as a desk in an office or flowers on a table over a hospital bed, can impede patient communication and should be rearranged to enhance the interview process. If the patient is lying down, sit or stand next to the bed. (Do not sit *on* the bed.) Position yourself about two to four feet away from the patient (not too close and not too far). Your position often will depend upon how well you know the patient; however, always maintain an attitude, posture, and position that reflects professionalism.

Your appearance can help convey interest, respect, and professionalism. You should be neat, well groomed, and comfortably dressed. A lab coat and professional attire are usually appropriate when talking with most adults; however, pediatric or psychiatric patients may feel threatened by a white coat. When in doubt as to appropriate attire, base your decision upon other health care workers in your patient care area, or make inquiries of your supervisor.

Verbal Communication. Effective communication during an interview depends upon your ability to engage in active listening. This involves the use of several verbal and nonverbal techniques including: interpretation, reflection, clarification, empathy, facilitation, and confrontation. **Interpretation** is an inference from the interviewer's perspective of a possible problem. An example of an interpretative approach would be: "You are asking a lot of questions about your medicine. Is something bothering you?" **Reflection** means repeating the patient's words to invite the patient to expand in more detail. It helps you guide the interview without breaking continuity. If a patient says, "When I stand up quickly I get dizzy," you can then reflect this statement by saying, "You say you get dizzy?" When a patient makes ambiguous statements, use **clarification** to get a proper response. For example, you can clarify by saying, "I do not understand, please tell me again what you mean." **Empathetic** statements show understanding and acceptance of a patient's feelings. You can communicate empathy with a statement such as, "You must have felt very sick." Be sure that your nonverbal behavior agrees with an empathetic response. **Facilitation** involves the use of body movements, facial expressions, or short statements to encourage talking. For example, while leaning forward you can say, "Please continue." **Confrontation** refers to making an objective observation about the patient's behavior. This can be an effective method of dealing with patients who withhold information. For instance you can say, "You look more upset than you are saying."

Beginning the Interview. On first contact with a patient, introduce yourself, even if the patient appears to be confused or comatose. Some patients can recall information they heard while in a comatose state. Your introduction should include your name and your role on the health care team (e.g., "My name is John Smith, I am a pharmacist."). Ask the patient for a few minutes of his or her time to conduct the interview. If the present time is inappropriate, arrange for another time. Be sure to address adult patients with respectful titles. Do not act flippant, and do not use first names or colloquialisms (e.g., "darling"). Children and adolescents, however, may be less frightened if you use their first names. After greeting the patient, state the reason for the interview (e.g., "I need to understand how you think your medicines are working.").

Open-Ended and Closed-Ended Questions. Use a combination of open- and closed-ended questions to gather information from the patient. Open-ended questions encourage talking. They begin with *who, what, where, when,* or *why* and require more than a "yes" or "no" response from the patient. Closed-ended questions, on the other hand, prompt short responses such as a "yes" or "no" answer. Although closed-ended questions are often necessary for obtaining certain details, they are generally not as effective as open-ended questions in obtaining information from the patient. A closed-ended question such as, "Have you used any drugs for indigestion?" tends to exclude information; whereas the open-ended question, "Can you tell me about the drugs you have used for indigestion?" tends to elicit more information. Closed-ended questions limit the patient's response, resulting in potentially incomplete or inaccurate information.

Your goal is to obtain accurate information from the patient by stimulating conversation. Permit patients to respond to open-ended questions in their own way, as long as they do not ramble incoherently. Actively listen as you gently, but firmly, guide the interview to focus on the patient's problems.

While the interviewer should limit direct questioning, direct questions sometimes are necessary to uncover details. As a rule, proceed from general questions to more specific questions. For example, begin your questions with "Do you take anything for stomach problems?" and proceed to "When you do, what do you take?" and "Does this particular antacid work best for you?"

The Medication History

The traditional medical history (see Table 1.2) is most often obtained by a physician. The pharmacist generally reads and interprets this medical history. Then, by integrating pharmaceutical knowledge with interviewing skills, the pharmacist questions the patient about specific problems that are associated with the use of medications.

Many drug history forms are available to guide practitioners.[1-3] A word of caution: While filling out these forms, do not allow the process of recording data to detract from the interview itself. Sit back, listen, and only write down key information; add details to your notes after you leave the patient. The review-of-systems approach organizes the medical history according to major body systems.[3] This methodical approach provides a guide for the discovery of symptoms related to known problems as well as previously unidentified conditions. Symptoms commonly associated with specific organ systems and various categories of drugs are listed in Table 1.3.

The Medication History Interview. Table 1.4 on page 1–11 lists common medical abbreviations that may be used in the patient medical history.

The medication history interview gathers information on prescription and nonprescription drugs. It should include: the identification of all pertinent unlabeled medications; information about known drug allergies and previous adverse reactions; therapeutic responses; drug abuse behavior; and medication compliance. A medication history form using the review-of-systems approach is presented in Table 1.5 on page 1–12.

Table 1.2

The Medical History

Section	Contents
Patient Profile	Age, race, sex, date of birth, marital status
Chief Complaint (CC)	The reason for seeking medical attention
Present Illness (PI)	A chronological account of events and symptoms of the chief complaint; laboratory/diagnostic procedures as well as negative findings
Past Medical History (PMH)	General state of health Childhood illnesses Immunizations Medical illnesses Psychiatric illnesses Surgical procedures Hospitalizations Injuries Medications Allergies
Family History (FH)	Age and health of living relatives Age and cause of death of relatives Occurrence and relation of family members with diabetes mellitus, high blood pressure, cancer, mental illness, tuberculosis, and other serious or hereditary illnesses
Social History (SH)	Financial situation, health habits (sleeping, diet, recreation, use of tobacco, alcohol, or other drugs of abuse), education, religion, and family dynamics
Review of Systems (ROS)	Common symptoms by body system; the body areas reviewed are: general, skin, head, eyes, ears, nose and sinuses, mouth and throat, neck, breasts, chest and lungs, heart, vascular, gastrointestinal, urinary, reproductive, musculoskeletal, neurologic, psychiatric, endocrine, and hematologic

The Opening. Identify yourself and the reason for the interview. Determine whether the patient has any medications on hand. If the patient's medications are available, examine the labeling and contents of the medications and record the data. Following identification of medications, continue with the medication interview.

Review of Systems. An organ system approach that proceeds from head to toe is often helpful in organizing and standardizing the medication history interview. Standardization of the interview process minimizes the possibility of overlooking review of a particular organ system.

Drug History: A Review of Systems Approach

Table 1.3

Organ System	Symptoms	Drugs[a]
General	Fever, fatigue, weight change, pain	Narcotic and non-narcotic analgesics, antibiotics, antipyretics
Mental Status	Nervousness, sadness, insomnia, hallucinations, irritability, tension	Antidepressants, antipsychotics, hypnotics, anxiolytics, stimulants
Integument	Rashes, dryness, itching, hair loss, dandruff	Antibiotics, antifungals, corticosteroids, antidandruff-antiseborrheics, anesthetics/antipruritics, cytotoxics, antivirals, anti-infestation agents, antiseptics/disinfectants
Head/Face	Dizziness, fainting, seizures, headache	Antivertigo drugs, analgesics, anticonvulsants
Eyes	Redness, poor eyesight, pain, blurring, discharge, glaucoma, cataracts	Glaucoma drugs, mydriatics, cycloplegics, topical antibiotics, corticosteroids
Ears	Hearing loss, tinnitus, earache, discharge, excessive wax	Topical anti-infectives, ceruminolytics
Nose/Sinuses	Colds, runny nose, hay fever, sinus problems	Antihistamines, cough and cold medicines, antiallergy drugs, nasal decongestants, topical corticosteroids
Mouth/Pharynx	Sore throat, gum soreness or bleeding, dental problems, mouth ulcers, hoarseness	Antibiotics, cough and cold medicines, antihistamines, local anesthetics, decongestants, antiallergy drugs
Neck	Swollen lymph nodes, goiter, swollen glands, neck pain	Antithyroid drugs, thyroid hormones, antibiotics, analgesics
Chest/Lungs	Dyspnea, wheezing, cough, asthma, bronchitis, emphysema, pneumonia, tuberculosis, hemoptysis	Beta-adrenergics, antibiotics, bronchodilators, corticosteroids, antihistamines, anticholinergics, antimycobacterial drugs, antitussives, expectorants
Cardiovascular	Chest pain, hypertension, heart attacks, heart murmur, paroxysmal nocturnal dyspnea, orthopnea, palpitations, intermittent claudication, orthostatic hypotension	Beta-adrenergic blocking drugs, calcium channel blockers, angiotensin-converting enzyme inhibitors, antianginal drugs, antiarrhythmic drugs, cardiac glycosides, antihypertensives, antihyperlipidemic agents, diuretics, anticoagulants, hemorheologic agents, antiplatelets, thrombolytics

Table 1.3

Drug History: A Review of Systems Approach (Continued)

Organ System	Symptoms	Drugs[a]
Abdomen	Swallowing problem, heartburn, diarrhea, constipation, nausea/vomiting, pain, vomiting blood, blood in stool, hemorrhoids, ascites, change in bowel habits	Antacids, H_2-blockers, laxatives, hemorrhoidal preparations, sucralfate, proton pump inhibitors, cholinergic drugs, antidiarrheal agents, anticholinergic/ antispasmodic drugs
Urinary	Dysuria, frequency, urgency, pain, nocturia, dribbling, incontinence, polydipsia, bleeding, urinary retention, stones	Diuretics, antidiuretic hormone, potassium supplements, electrolyte supplements, anticholinergics, tricyclic antidepressant drugs, alpha-adrenergic drugs, cholinergic drugs, urolithiasic drugs
Genital-Reproductive	*Female:* vaginal discharge, itching, menstrual problems, venereal diseases, hot flashes, premenstrual tension	Anticandidial products, birth control pills, hormone shots, estrogen replacement, progestins, topical antifungal agents, nonsteroidal anti-inflammatory drugs
	Male: itching, discharge, sores, testicular pain/swelling, poor libido	Antibiotics, hormones
Musculoskeletal	Joint swelling, pain, deformities, redness, stiffness, limit of movement, gout, arthritis, backache, muscle cramps	Nonsteroidal anti-inflammatory drugs, immunosuppressants, hypouricemics
Neurologic	Fainting, blackouts, seizures, local weakness, numbness, tremors, tingling, walking problems, muscle wasting, spasm, stiffness, vertigo	Anticonvulsants, muscle relaxants, anticoagulants, antiparkinson agents, anticholinergics, antihistamines, antivertigo, antiemetics
Endocrine	Thyroid problems, diabetes mellitus, diabetes insipidus, Addison/Cushing disease	Adrenocortical hormones, thyroid hormones, insulin, oral hypoglycemic drugs, androgenic agents, estrogens

[a] If unfamiliar with frequently prescribed legend drugs, consult the "Top 200 Drugs" list published in *Pharmacy Times* annually. For over-the-counter (OTC) preparations, consult the latest edition of the *Handbook of Nonprescription Drugs*.

Using open-ended questions, ask the patient for a history of any health problems and treatments. Begin with questions focusing on the head (e.g., "What do you use when you have a headache?"); then continue with questions focusing on medications for eyes, ears, nose, throat, lungs, heart, abdomen, gastrointestinal system, and urinary tract until the head to toe approach is completed.

Common Abbreviations Used in Medical Histories

Table 1.4

Adm	Admission	P	Plan
ADR	Adverse drug reaction	PE	Physical examination
AFVSS	Afebrile, vital signs stable	PH	Past history
BF	Black female	PHx	Past history
BM	Black male	PI	Present illness
C/O	Complains of	PMH	Past medical history
CC	Chief complaint	PN	Progress note
CF	Caucasian female	POMR	Problem-oriented medical record
CM	Caucasian male	Prog	Prognosis
DOB	Date of birth	Px	Prognosis
Dx	Diagnosis	PTA	Prior to admission
FH	Family history	RAN	Resident's admission note
H&P	History and physical	ROS	Review of systems
H/O	History of	Rx	Therapy
HPI	History of present illness	RXN	Reaction
Hx	History	S	Subjective
IMP	Impression	S/P	Status post
IPPA	Inspection, palpation, percussion, auscultation	SOAP	Subjective, objective, assessment, and plan
L&W	Living and well	SOB	Shortness of breath
L	Left	Sx	Symptoms
LAT	Lateral	Tx	Therapy
Med Hx	Medication history	WD	Well developed
NAD	No apparent distress	WF	White female
NKA	No known allergies	WM	White male
O	Objective	WN	Well nourished

As you review each body system, assume that the patient uses medications. For example, ask, "When you have eye problems, what do you take?" The patient will either deny any problems in the body system or quickly acknowledge drug usage. Give special attention to questions about an organ system with known disease or drug treatments. Use direct, closed-ended questioning for each drug mentioned. Obtain the drug name (if known), indication (if known), dose, frequency, and any adverse effects the patient has experienced. In many instances the patient will only be able to give a vague physical description of the medication. If the identity of the drug must be more accurately known, return later with product samples for the patient to identify.

For each identified medication, assess therapeutic response to determine the probable indication for use. Patients often use a drug without knowing the desired effect.

Medication History

Table 1.5

Patient Name: _____ Age: _____ Gender: _____ DOB: _____

Drug Allergies/Adverse Reactions: _____

Organ System	**Symptom**	**Treatment**
General		
Mental Status		
Head/Face		
Eyes		
Ears		
Nose/Sinuses		
Neck		
Chest/Lungs		
Cardiovascular		
Abdomen		
Urinary		
Genital-Reproductive		
Integument		
Musculoskeleton		
Neurologic		
Endocrine		

Active Medications

Name	Strength	Frequency	Indication/Outcome

Assessment (Reliability of data and significant issues)

_____

_____

_____

_____

Interviewer: _____ Date: _____

The response of a patient to a medication can be reflected by the continuation or discontinuation of the medication. Drugs are usually discontinued when desired effects have been achieved or when side effects are unacceptable.

Past Drug Allergies and Adverse Reactions. After surveying the history of health problems and associated drug usage, ask about past known drug allergies or adverse reactions that the patient has not already mentioned. If an adverse drug event is noted, inquire further as to the approximate dates of the event, a description of events, and management. The approximate date of occurrence of a drug allergy is important because drug manufacturing processes have improved considerably over time, resulting in formulations with fewer impurities that might have provoked the allergy (e.g., penicillins, insulin). It might also be beneficial to ask if the patient has taken the medication since the adverse event and to inquire specifically about exposure to similar drugs (e.g., ampicillin or amoxicillin in a purportedly penicillin-allergic patient). The description of events and management often provides insights into the severity of the drug reaction and of other exposure to concurrent drugs (e.g., drug combination products or preservatives in parenteral formulations).

Many patients confuse allergies with adverse reactions. Make every effort to separate true allergic reactions from reactions that are merely the pharmacological extension of a drug's action. For example, a patient may say, "Ampicillin makes me sick to my stomach and gives me diarrhea." If you misinterpret this adverse reaction as an allergic reaction, the patient's medical record may then be inaccurately labeled as "allergic to ampicillin." An incorrect allergy notation can prompt future use of a less than optimal medication because of concerns for an allergy that are unknowingly based upon misinformation.

Drug Abuse Behavior. Ask the patient to describe his or her social drug habits including the use of tobacco, recreational drugs, and alcohol. Remember that this can be a sensitive issue.

Social drug abuse is a frequent problem to which patients do not readily confess and often underestimate. Information on drug abuse is difficult to obtain unless the patient is secure and confident in the interview relationship. Carefully maintain a professional attitude and never express moral judgment on a patient's actions or behavior. Remember, judgments can be communicated to a patient both verbally and nonverbally. Take care to control your words, your facial expressions, and body language.

Compliance measures the patient's understanding of the appropriate use of medications. Ask the patient to describe a routine day of medication usage. This question identifies which drugs are regularly used by the patient and also helps to identify the patient's understanding of prescribed medications. If the patient uses medications in a manner that differs from the labeling, then question further to determine his or her reasons.

Closing the Interview. After you complete your prepared questions, ask if there is anything else that the patient needs to tell you about his or her history of medication use. Thank the patient and extend an offer to be available to answer any questions the patient may have about drugs before leaving. The student-examiner should only provide answers to patients on pharmacotherapeutic topics and should refer specific care issues to the patient's physician.

Confidentiality of the Record. Patient information is confidential and protected by law. The release of patient information is limited to persons involved in the patient's care; however, insurance companies and some governmental agencies can access the information with due process. When admitted to a healthcare facility, the patient, or a legal designee, generally signs a waiver consenting to treatment and the sharing of information with persons of a "need to know" status. The student-examiner must confine discussion of patient information to other health providers directly caring for the patient. Avoid discussions about patients in public areas (e.g., elevator, hallway, or cafeteria).

Information obtained from the medication history or pharmacists' consults and opinions should not be written into the medical record without prior authorization from the medical staff (e.g., the medical record committee) because of legal ramifications and the potential for civil tort action. When writing patient-specific notes into the medical record, use a black ball-point pen and date and time each entry on the day of the event; do not pre- or postdate an entry. Information should be focused on the patient's drug therapy rather than on the disease state. Subjective information as stated by the patient may be recorded. For example, "Mr. Smith states he has experienced difficulty breathing resulting from past penicillin therapy." Such subjective patient comments are of interest to physicians and documentation of such comments *per se* seldom increases vulnerability to medicolegal entanglements. Objective data such as physical findings (e.g., rash), laboratory data (e.g., eosinophilia), consultant notes, and radiographic reports are usually already in the medical record and can be used to support the purpose of your note. Always avoid recording anything that reflects negatively upon the patient, another healthcare provider, or clinical results (e.g., "lab error"). If you write in the wrong medical record or wrong section, or write in error, draw a single line through the entry, sign the entry, and write "error." Never deface or cover your mistake; be honest. Efforts to hide mistakes merely draw unnecessary attention. Documentation in the paperless or computerized medical chart should follow these same basic guidelines.

Treatment Evaluation Interview

During follow-up visits to a clinic or a pharmacy, the pharmacist may need to interview the patient to evaluate the patient's response to the prescribed treatment and to evaluate whether the patient has experienced any difficulty or adverse effects from the medications. To evaluate the safe and effective use of drugs, confront the patient with specific questions. For example, begin the dialog with, "Tell me how your blood pressure medicine is doing," and follow up with specific questions such as, "Have you had any problems with dizziness?" Use your understanding of therapeutics and pathophysiology to ask key questions that illuminate desirable and undesirable responses to medications. For example, if a patient reports a fall, question the patient about drugs known to increase the risk of falling (e.g., antihypertensive or psychoactive agents). As part of routine monthly visits for prescription renewals or nursing home drug reviews, focus your questions on subjective and objective indicators of effectiveness and safety.

If the patient has a specific drug-related complaint, obtain the following information: onset (when was the problem first noted), interval events (from time of onset to present), status, and reason for seeking help. To elicit a response, open the conversation by asking, "How may I help you?" Listen and record the specific complaint as voiced by the patient. Next, determine the duration and historical accounting of intervening events. Ask, "When did this start troubling you?" and "What has happened since the problem began?" Next, ask the patient why he or she is seeking help today, rather than at an earlier date. This will help detect any events which have changed (or not changed) the patient's condition.

CONCLUSION

Before examining a patient, the skillful clinician uses the patient interview to identify potential problems and decide upon a course of action. Physical assessment, laboratory, and other tests further define the suspected problem. By obtaining a careful historical account of the patient's problem, clinicians may avoid misdiagnoses, wrong impressions, and impaired decisions. The patient interview is often the most important component of clinical assessment.

REFERENCES

1. McKenzie MW. How to conduct a patient medication history interview. In: Ray M, ed. Basic Skills in Clinical Pharmacy Practice. Chapel Hill: American Society of Hospital Pharmacists,1983:79–127.

2. Anon. Pharmacy Health Questionnaire. Amer Pharm. 1980:20:35–37.

3. Truitt CA et al. An evaluation of a medication history method. Drug Intel Clin Pharm. 1982:16:592.

Physical Examination and Techniques

2

APPROACH TO PHYSICAL EXAMINATION

*P*atients are often anxious about a physical examination and need to be reassured by a confident, caring clinician who always attempts to make the patient comfortable. The room temperature should be comfortable (i.e., not too cool and not too warm), and the room should be adequately lighted. The patient should have a private place to undress and should be given a gown or sheet to cover his body for both comfort and modesty. When you first enter the examining room, wash your hands and begin conversing with the patient to establish the needed rapport for a trusting relationship.

Ask the patient to have a seat on the examining table. When conducting an exam in a hospital room, adjust the height of the bed or use pillows to support the patient in an appropriate position. Be sure the examining room door is closed, or the curtain drawn around the patient's bed, to assure privacy. Explain what you will be doing during all components of the physical examination. This helps reassure the patient and also provides some sense of dignity, along with a sense of "being in control." Then, begin your examination confidently without wasting effort and with a clear purpose.

PHYSICAL ASSESSMENT TECHNIQUES

Observational skills are important to physical assessment and the development of these skills is not an easy task. They require a sound knowledge base, clinical experience, and keen senses of sight, hearing, smell, and touch. The careful use of these senses forms the basis of the four primary physical examination techniques: **inspection, palpation, percussion**, and **auscultation**. The order in which these four techniques are applied to physical assessment varies depending upon the area of the body being examined. The proper order for examining the chest or heart is: inspection, palpation, percussion, and auscultation. However, the proper order for examining the abdomen should always be: inspection, auscultation, percussion, and palpation. If auscultation of the abdomen follows percussion and/or palpation, the patient's bowel activity may be falsely altered by your manipulation, leading you to a false conclusion. For example, you may think you detect hyperactive bowel sounds when, in fact, the bowel sounds are normo-active.

Inspection

Inspection refers to the observation of physical signs displayed by the patient and depends to a large extent upon the knowledge of the examiner. The examiner's understanding of the significance of a visual, olfactory, or auditory observation is based more upon knowing what to look *for* than what to look *at*. In order to identify a problem, you must first know how it would be manifested in the patient; otherwise, you may not even detect the presence of the condition. With heightened awareness, you will learn to identify signs such as the shuffling gait of a patient with suspected parkinsonism or the drooping eyelid and dilated pupil of a person presenting with possible third cranial nerve palsy. Thus, successful inspection depends upon a solid grounding in the clinical sciences, an alert mind, disciplined eyes, and of course, adequate lighting and exposure of the inspected area.

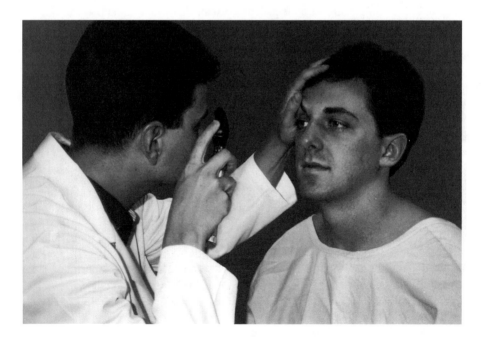

Fig 2.1 Inspection is the primary physical assessment technique employed during the ophthalmoscopic exam (see Chapter 5: Eye).

Palpation

Palpation encompasses the various ways of perceiving by the sense of touch. Use your fingertips to distinguish hard and soft areas (e.g., when evaluating a breast mass). The palm of the hand is used to detect the presence or absence of vibration (e.g., when lobar pneumonia is suspected). Evaluate temperature variation with the back side of your fingers when demarcating the limits of a superficial cellulitis or identifying mastitis deep within the breast. To prevent a dulling of tactile sensation and to enhance the sense of touch, superficial intermittent palpation is preferred to deep, intermittent palpation. For example, use the fingertips to palpate the skin to evaluate texture; however, use the palm to palpate the chest to detect the vibrations of a cardiac thrill which resonates like the purr of a cat.

Percussion

Percussion is a procedure used to evaluate structures lying no deeper than 4 to 5 cm under the skin. Using the fingers or a plessor, indirectly strike the body surface to elicit sounds that vary in quality according to the density of the underlying tissues. Do not directly strike the body surface to elicit sound, but rather strike the pleximeter finger with a plexor instrument or plexor finger. Transmitting the impact through the pleximeter finger not only protects the patient from unnecessary trauma (e.g., bruising), but, of equal importance, allows the pleximeter finger to sense the vibrations generated with each tap. The experienced clinician can perform percussion in a noise filled room because he or she is sensing the "waves" generated (a more refined and accurate method than listening with the ear). Percussional sounds are described as tympanitic, hyperresonant, resonant, dull, or flat and correspond to the density of the

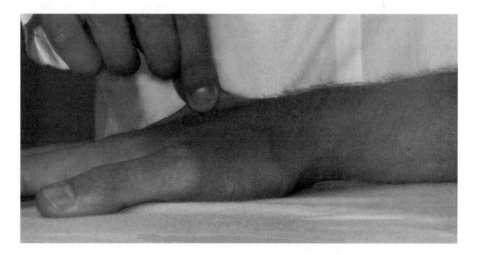

Fig 2.2   Palpation over a bony area of the body is used to assess skin mobility and turgor (see Chapter 4: Skin).

underlying structures progressing from least dense to most dense. Percussion of the thigh results in a **flat sound**, while the lung produces a **resonant sound**. The **dull sound** of a dense structure (i.e., the liver), the **hyperresonant sound** of an over-expanded lung, and the **tympanitic sound** of a hollow structure (i.e., air-filled stomach or bowel) are commonly encountered percussional notes.

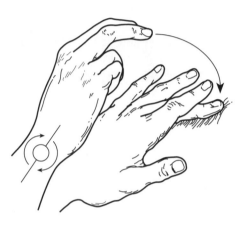

Fig 2.3   During percussion, the examiner strikes the pleximeter finger with the plexor finger of the opposite hand. Indirectly transmitting the impact through the pleximeter finger protects and patient and allows the pleximeter finger to sense the vibrations generated with each tap.

Auscultation

Auscultation is the process of listening to sounds originating within an organ or body cavity and is usually augmented by use of an acoustically well-built, personally-fitted stethoscope. The quality of the stethoscope and skill of the person using it determine the effectiveness of the auscultatory exam.

In general, auscultatory findings are generated by substances moving through body systems. For example, various sounds, normal and abnormal, will be generated as air moves through the airways of the lung; blood moves through the blood vessels and across the heart valves; or bowel contents traverse the stomach, small intestine, and large intestine. The ability to recognize the presence or absence of normal or abnormal sounds assists in physical assessment.

The examiner uses the techniques of inspection, palpation, percussion, and auscultation to gather the sensory data that serve as the core of physical assessment. Although these four techniques are relatively straightforward and easily learned, they must be honed through careful study and frequent repetition before you gain mastery of their use. Even then, the sensory data collected with these techniques must be correlated with sound clinical knowledge and experience before the adept technician develops into a competent clinician.

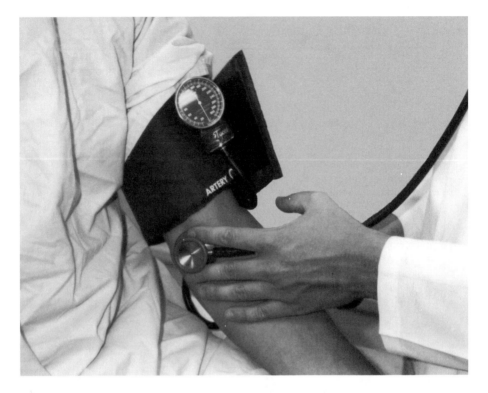

Fig 2.4   The examiner auscultates the sounds generated by blood moving through the brachial artery when assessing blood pressure (see Chapter 10: Blood Vessels).

OVERVIEW OF THE
PHYSICAL EXAMINATION

Physical diagnosis is an art and a skill learned after much study and practice. For most physicians, two years in medical school and three years in residency training provide the basis for life-long learning, daily application, and continuous refinement of these skills. For most pharmacists, a general understanding of physical examination findings of the physician is adequate. However, for some pharmacists, more extensive knowledge and the ability to apply some physical examination skills are necessary to monitor the effects of medications on specific organs.

Table 2.1 provides a general outline of the format commonly used to record the results of a physical examination. Subsequent chapters in this book describe the individual components of this outline in further detail.

Physical Examination Outline

Table 2.1

General Survey (Observe the general state of health and note the following throughout the physical exam.)

Age:

Race:

Gender:

Stature/Build:

Signs of Distress:

Measurements

Height:

Weight:

Vital Signs

Respiratory (rate, rhythm):

Temperature (rectal, oral, or other method should be documented):

Pulse (rate, rhythm):

Blood Pressure (sitting, standing):

Mental Status   Chapter 3

Appearance/Behavior (hygiene, facial expression, dress, posture):

Level of Consciousness (alert, confusion, stupor, delirium, coma):

Orientation (person, place, time):

Affect/Mood (happy, sad):

Memory (past, present):

Judgment ("burning building"):

Abstract Reasoning (proverb or analogy):

Thought Content/Processing (hallucination, delusion, illusions, sadness, guilt, euphoria):

Integument   (Observe throughout the exam.)   Chapter 4

Skin [color, texture, temperature, mobility, turgor, lesions (type/location)]:

Nails (color, attachment, angle, clubbing, lesions):

Hair (color, distribution, texture):

Head/Face   Chapter 5

Head/Face (size, shape, scars, bumps):

Skin (scars, lesions, color):

Table 2.1

Physical Examination Outline (continued)

Nose/Sinuses	Chapter 7

Nasal Patency:

External Nose (lesions, symmetry):

Internal Nose

    Mucosa (moist, color, bleeding, swelling):

    Turbinates (polyp):

    Septum (perforation, deviation):

Sinuses

    Frontal (tenderness, light glow):

    Maxillary (tenderness, light glow):

Mouth/Pharynx:	Chapter 7

Lips (moist, color, lesions):

Buccal Mucosa (moist, color, lesions):

Gums (moist, color, lesions):

Hard/Soft Palate (moist, color, lesions):

Teeth (condition, missing, caries):

Tongue (color, lesions):

Project Tongue to evaluate CN12 (tongue in midline):

Salivary Glands (inspect and palpate):

Oropharynx (color, moist, odor, lesions):

"Ah" test to evaluate CN9/10 (soft palate retracts symmetrically):

Neck	Chapter 8

Trachea (midline):

Skin (supple, mass, tender, lesions):

Thyroid (mass, tenderness, bruit):

Jugular Vein (30° angle, neck vein distention):

Carotid Artery [pulse (rate, rhythm), bruit]:

Lymph Nodes (enlarged, tender, nontender, mobile, fixed, matted):

Eyes	Chapter 5

Visual Acuity

    Newspaper to evaluate near vision:

    Snellen Chart to evaluate far vision (read all letters on 20/20 line at 20 ft):

Physical Examination Outline (continued)

Table 2.1

Eyes (continued)	Chapter 5

External Structures

Eyelids, Eyelashes, Eyebrows (symmetry, lesions):

Sclera (color, lesions):

Conjunctivae (inflamed):

Irides (color, lesions):

Pupils (size, symmetry):

Lacrimal Glands/Ducts:

Function

Pupillary Light Response (size, symmetry):

Accommodation/Convergence to evaluate CN2:

Visual Fields by Confrontation to evaluate CN2:

Extraocular Movements to evaluate CN3, CN4, and CN6 (eyes show

full range of motion in all four visual quadrants and diagonals;

see Chapter 5: Eye):

Ophthalmologic Exam

Cornea and Lens (opacities):

Disc, Cup-Disc Ratio, Vessels, Retina, Macula:

Ears	Chapter 6

Screen Hearing (whisper or finger snap):

Auricles (symmetry, lesions):

Otoscopic Exam

External Canal (cerumen, swelling, discharge, lesions):

Tympanic Membrane (landmarks, perforation, inflammation):

Chest/Lungs	Chapter 9

Signs of Respiratory Distress (labored breathing):

Lung Expansion: Tactile/Vocal Fremitus (muffled):

Percussion (resonance):

Breath Sounds (vesicular/bronchial, wheeze/crackle/rub):

Table 2.1

Physical Examination Outline (continued)

Heart/Anterior Chest	Chapter 11

    Palpation of Chest (heaves, pulsation, thrills):

    PMI Location:

    Apical Pulse (rate, rhythm):

    Aortic Area: Pulmonic Area (physical split):

    Tricuspid Area: Mitral Area:

Leg/Foot Pulses	Chapter 10

    Popliteal Artery (left, right):

    Dorsalis Pedis (left, right):

    Posterior Tibial (left, right):

Veins/Legs	Chapter 10

    Varicose Veins:

    Edema:

Abdomen (Patient supine: flex hips and knees at 45° angle.)	Chapter 12

    Skin (scars, lesions, mass, pulsations, contour, peristalsis):

    Bowel Sounds (absent, hypoactive, active, hyperactive):

    Arteries (bruits in aorta, renal, iliac):

    Percuss/Palpate (soft, tenderness, mass, fluid, gas, edema, aortic pulse,

      hepatojugular reflux; see Chapter 12: Abdomen):

    Liver Border/Span/Contour:

Musculoskeletal (Range of Motion) Strength	Chapter 13

    (5/5 = normal; compare symmetrically)

    Neck:

    Shoulder:

    Elbow:

    Wrist:

    Fingers:

    Spine:

    Hip:

    Knee:

    Ankle:

Table 2.1

Physical Examination Outline (continued)

Joint Findings	Chapter 13

Inspect/Palpate/Auscultate (skin temperature, swelling, nodules, crepitus):

Neurological	Chapter 14

Motor Function

    Coordination/Balance:

    Walk (normal and heal-to-toe):

    Finger to Nose:

    Romberg:

Sensory Function

    Pain:

    Light Touch:

Reflexes

Cranial Nerves (remaining)

    Test of Smell to evaluate CN 1:

    Palpate Temporomandibular Joint to evaluate CN 5-motor (open/closed mouth):

    Light Touch/Pain/Temperature of Forehead, Cheek, Chin to evaluate CN 5-sensory:

    Clench Teeth, Frown, Close Eyes Tightly and Resist Opening, Smile,

      Whistle to evaluate CN 7-motor:

    Taste Test to evaluate CN7-sensory:

    Shoulder Shrug to evaluate CN 9:

Reproductive System: Breast	Chapter 15

Inspection

    Abnormal Discoloration of Skin:

    Nipple or Skin Retraction:

    Nipple Discharge:

    Nodular Areas of Fullness:

    Orange Peel Appearance of Skin:

Palpation

    Nipple Discharge:

    Abnormal Nodularity of Breast Tissue:

    Lymph Node Enlargement (supraclavicular, axillary):

    Areas of Warmth or Marked Tenderness:

Table 2.1

Physical Examination Outline (continued)

Reproductive System: Female	Chapter 16

External Genitalia (perineum, vulva, perianal)

Inspection of Skin

    Abnormal Discoloration:

    Nodular or Raised Areas:

    Condition of Hymenal Ring:

Palpation

    Glands of Vulva (enlargement, tenderness, secretions):

Internal Genitalia (vagina, uterus, fallopian tubes, ovaries)

Inspection

    Cystocele, Urethrocele, Rectocele, Enterocele, Prolapse of Uterus and Cervix:

Speculum Examination

    Vaginal Wall Discoloration, Ulceration, Cystic or Nodular Areas:

    Vaginal Discharge:

    Cervix (appearance external os, discoloration, ulceration, raised, cystic or nodular areas, bleeding):

    PAP Smear:

Palpation

    Bimanual Examination:

        Uterus (size, shape, consistency, position, mobility):

        Ovaries (size, shape, consistency, position, mobility):

        Fallopian Tubes (size, shape, consistency):

    Recto-Vaginal Examination:

        Recto-Vaginal Septum Defects:

        Rectal Mucosa (thickening or masses):

        Condition of Uterosacral Ligament:

        Confirm Position of Uterus:

        Contour of Posterior Uterine Surface:

        Presence of Abnormal Contents Posterior Cul de Sac:

Reproductive System: Male	Chapter 17

Extragenital Inspection/Palpation

    Lymphatic System (neck, supraclavicular area, inguinal area):

    Breast (gynecomastia):

Table 2.1

Physical Examination Outline (continued)

Reproductive System: Male (continued)	Chapter 17

Inspection

    Skin of Mons Pubis, Penis, Scrotum (color, raised or nodular areas, ulcerated areas, hair distribution):

    Retracted Foreskin and Glands (uncircumcised male):

    Urethra (site of opening, stricture, discharge):

Palpation

    External

        Scrotum (cystocele, varicocele):

        Epididymis (enlargement, nodularity, tenderness):

        Testicle (size, shape, consistency, nodularity):

        Inguinal Canal (inguinal hernia):

    Internal

        Prostate (size, shape, consistency, nodularity, tenderness):

        Seminal Vesicle (size, shape, consistency, nodularity, tenderness):

Muscle Strength Rating	Chapter 13

  0 no movement

  1 slight contraction without joint motion

  2 muscle and joint movement with gravity

  3 slight movement against gravity

  4 movement against gravity and slight resistance

  5 movement against gravity and full resistance (normal)

Deep Tendon Reflex Rating	Chapter 14

  0 no response

  1 slight response

  2 normal response

  3 exaggerated response

  4 hyperactive response (with or without clonus)

Pulse Rating	Chapter 10

  0 absent

  1 weak

  2 normal

  3 strong

  4 bounding

Mental Status Examination

*T*he mental status examination (MSE) is a basic part of the physical examination. It begins the collection of patient data and is valuable in the assessment and management of both mental and physical illnesses. Some parts of the MSE are used in every patient encounter. For example, assessment of a patient's mental competence helps the clinician determine the accuracy and reliability of the medical history. This chapter describes the basic knowledge needed to conduct the MSE and presents a general screening approach to detecting and measuring mental health problems. If a possible psychiatric problem is detected during this screening, a more extensive psychiatric examination should be completed.

MENTAL STATUS EXAMINATION

The mental status examination, conducted through a series of questions and observations, uncovers information about the patient's overall mental and physical health. The interviewer evaluates both the content of the patient's responses and the behavior of the patient during the interview through careful listening and observation of the patient's appearance, behavior, emotional state, and cognitive functions.

This examination, like all patient interviews, should be conducted in a quiet, private setting. The patient should feel secure, be willing to speak freely and honestly, and be assured of confidentiality. The MSE is usually conducted informally while taking the patient's medical history. As the patient tells his story, pursue leads indicating unusual behavior, history of drug abuse, psychiatric hospitalizations, or other clues of mental health problems. Listen for responses showing intellectual deficits, affective disturbances, thought disorders, symptoms of delusions, hallucinations, manic or depressive behaviors, disorientation, or other indicators of possible mental health problems.

Direct the topics of the conversation, but allow the patient considerable freedom in responding to open-ended questions. Encourage the patient to keep talking with both verbal and nonverbal cues. Be careful, however, not to let the patient control the focus of the interview. If the patient experiences emotional outbursts (e.g., crying), provide the patient time to recover composure. Avoid using psychiatric or medical terminology (e.g., "arms and legs" are preferred over "upper and lower extremities").

Use words commensurate with the patient's level of intelligence and understanding; try not to talk down to, or over the head of, the patient. Value judgments about the patient are not appropriate and may stifle the interview. Remember, judgments can be communicated to a patient both verbally and non-verbally.

Direct, closed-ended questions usually elicit more meaningful information when evaluating certain mental health problems. For example, to evaluate the progression of Senile Dementia of the Alzheimer Type (SDAT), use direct questions to assess the patient's intellectual function, ability to make judgments, and ability to recall information (i.e., memory). Although an alert and intelligent patient may resent what appears to be a nonsensical question (e.g., "What is the name of this place?"), direct questioning of this type is sometimes unavoidable.

Evaluation: Appearance and Behavior

Appearance refers to an individual's outward look (i.e., dress, hygiene, and grooming) in relation to age, environment, culture, and activity. Appearances commonly reflect how individuals view their role in society, in activities, and in their immediate surroundings. Outward appearances, therefore, can sometimes provide valuable clues about the mental health of an individual. For example, when an individual who usually is well-groomed appears for work poorly groomed, disheveled, and wearing dirty clothes, the mental status of that individual could be in question. Less than expected grooming and/or appearance is often observed in patients with schizophrenia, organic brain syndromes, or depression. Likewise, excessive grooming is sometimes a sign of anxiety or obsessive-compulsive disorders.

Behavior refers to the way an individual acts in the presence of others and includes both verbal and nonverbal responses. Facial expression, posture, speech, and motor activity are components of behavior. Disturbances of behavior can sometimes reflect a change in mental status. During the interview, carefully watch the patient's face for expressions of anxiety, depression, anger, apathy, euphoria, or flat affect (i.e., lack of expression). A person's posture or body language commonly changes as topics of conversation change. The presence or absence of such changes can also serve as an indication of mental status. Note other nonverbal expressions of behavior, including the frequency of voluntary and involuntary movements, postures, pace, and movement characteristics. Also, listen to speech characteristics such as clarity, rate, volume, and rhythm.

Evaluation: Emotional State

Affect and mood are two components of the emotional state. **Affect** refers to immediate feelings associated with a particular thought, manifested by the patient in outward emotional responses. An affect inappropriate to a stimulus can suggest a disturbance of mental health. For example, a patient who cries while describing favorite hobbies could be described as having an inappropriate affect. Watch and listen carefully for responses showing inappropriate hostility, suspicion, happiness, or sadness. Normally, affect also varies with the situation and subject of discussion. Thus, unchanging affect can also be an indication of a mental health problem. For example, if a patient remains sad beyond an expected period, ask about feelings of discouragement, thoughts of self-harm, and crying spells.

Mood refers to a prevailing state of mind over an extended period of time that is influenced by emotion (e.g., to be in the mood for work). Clear alterations in mood are best evaluated over long periods of observation. As part of the MSE, ask about the patient's mood (i.e., "Are you happy or sad about your life?") in order to determine whether these long-term emotions appear appropriate in light of events in the patient's life. Affect and mood disorders are often noted in patients with schizophrenia, paranoia, mania, anxiety, and depression.

In addition to affect and mood, thought content and thought processing are measurements of a patient's emotional state. **Thought content** refers to what a person thinks about. **Thought processing** refers to how a person thinks. Thought processing should be logical, coherent, relevant to the individual, and should lead to reasonable conclusions or goals. In severe mental illness, thought processing and content can degenerate into ramblings or strings of tangential ideas. Abnormal thought processing and content are the primary symptoms used to diagnose psychotic diseases. Paranoia, delusions, obsessions, hallucinations, illusions, and other abnormal ideations often become more evident when you evaluate thought content and thought processing.

Evaluation: Cognitive Functions

Alertness and orientation describe a patient's **state of consciousness**. **Alertness** refers to a patient's awareness of his or her environment and situation. Abnormal states of alertness or consciousness include confusion, lethargy, delirium, stupor, and coma. **Orientation** refers to a person's knowledge of person, place, and time. Orientation can be evaluated by asking the patient to state his name, the day of the week, season or year, and the name of the facility or city where he currently resides. Disorientation is frequently associated with organic brain syndromes (e.g., dementia).

Memory tests assess a patient's ability to recall both past and present information. Defects in memory are reflected in failure to recall, inattentiveness to questioning, or inability to hear, retain, and recite back information. Questions about date of birth, education, family history, and other past factual information measure **past (distant) memory**. Asking the patient to describe the history of present illness or a recent meal tests **present memory**. To test present memory, give the patient three unrelated facts such as an address, a color, and a person's name. Have the patient immediately repeat the information. Then ask the patient to repeat the facts later in the interview. Delirium, dementias, amnesia, Korsakoff's psychosis, and anxiety are conditions associated with an impaired memory.

Attention span and the ability to concentrate are additional components of cognitive function. To measure sustained attention and concentration, instruct the patient to sequentially subtract seven from 100 (i.e., 100, 93, 86, 79, . . .); stop the patient after five tries. However, remember that a patient's performance in this test can also be hindered by anxiety. **Insight** tests determine whether patients understand the importance of their illness or situation. Questions should evaluate the patient's degree of awareness of her problem or the patient's inability to recognize the presence of a problem.

Evaluation: Higher Intelligence

In addition to the basic cognitive functions of alertness, orientation, memory, attention span, and insight, higher intellectual function tests evaluate the patient's command of language, fund of knowledge, abstract reasoning, and judgment. These tests are not routinely performed unless indicated. Begin testing **language** skills by asking the patient to describe a familiar object, such as a pencil. The patient's ability to understand written language can be determined by writing a simple command and instructing the patient to read and perform the task (e.g., "Touch your nose with your right hand."). To determine written language skills, ask the patient to write a sentence. The written sentence should have at least a subject and a verb. Lastly, show the patient a drawing of a circle, a cross, a cube, and two overlapping pentagons, and ask the patient to copy these figures. "Language" testing is a very broad term used in psychiatry for various mental tests of complex cognitive functions (i.e., to copy a drawing requires coordination of psychomotor skills). For example, a deterioration of a patient's language functions is a measure of Senile Dementia of the Alzheimer's Type (SDAT).

Reading skills, culture, education, environment, and pathologic conditions all influence language skills. Mental retardation, organic brain syndromes (e.g., dementia), or cortical damage (e.g., a cerebral infarction to the language center causing aphasia or dysphasia) impair language skills. Poor vision or hearing, impaired motor skills, anxiety, or depression can also impair performance in language testing.

Evaluate the patient's **fund of knowledge** by asking questions about general topics (e.g., "What is the Capitol of the United States?"). Be careful not to confuse fund of knowledge testing with memory testing. If the patient's education and cultural circumstances are taken into consideration, responses to such questions can be used as an indicator of the patient's general knowledge base. Mental retardation and psychoses adversely affect a patient's fund of knowledge.

Abstract reasoning can be examined by asking the patient to interpret proverbs and analogies. Abstract reasoning refers to the ability to think logically or to grasp similarities and/or differences between words or ideas (e.g., "A bird in the hand is worth two in the bush"). Use several different proverbial phrases because the patient may not be familiar with a particular proverb. Analogies can be used to evaluate abstract reasoning by asking the patient to explain the similarities between two words (e.g., a peach and an apple, a dog and a cat, a bathtub and a swimming pool). Carefully appraise each answer for abstract reasoning, not concrete thinking. Also, remember that the patient's educational and cultural backgrounds influence abstract reasoning. Mental retardation, disorientation, dementia, or schizophrenia may be associated with inappropriate abstract reasoning.

Judgment tests are used to evaluate the patient's ability to decide on a course of action based upon accepted social behavior. Evaluate a patient's judgment by asking "If you saw your house on fire, what would you do?" or "What would you do if a police officer tried to stop you for speeding?" Determine if the patient's decisions are based on reality- or nonreality-based information. Use of poor judgment may be seen in patients with mental retardation, psychoses, or organic brain diseases.

The key components of a mental status evaluation (i.e., appearance and behavior, emotional state, cognitive functions, and higher intelligence) are summarized in Table 3.1. Common medical abbreviations that might accompany a mental status examination are listed in Table 3.2 on page 3–8.

PHARMACOTHERAPEUTIC CASE ILLUSTRATION

History

R.L., a 66-year-old male nursing home patient, was reported as having poor hygiene, dirty clothes, and poor grooming. Upon questioning, he denied any problems. With an expressionless face and low voice he said, "I'm okay. Don't bother with an old man like me. Take care of people who are sick." He appeared calm and relaxed. Yet, the nursing staff insisted he was much less physically active than usual, would not participate in group activities, and stayed in his room. R.L. had difficulty responding to questions. He said he suffered from many physical ailments including backaches and other somatic problems. He also complained about constipation and said he wanted "something for it" and "something to give me some energy." He admitted to a poor appetite and frequent nocturnal urination. He stated that his roommate kept the heater "too low" and said, "I can't sleep good at night. I wake up a lot of times and can't go back to sleep." These problems have appeared in the last month.

Social history (SH) revealed that R.L.'s elderly wife visited him frequently, but he seldom saw his children. His wife has a heart condition and depends upon neighbors for transportation. Financially, Mr. and Mrs. R.L. have Social Security benefits and a small pension.

Table 3.1

Mental Status Examination

Appearance and Behavior

Appearance

Describe the patient's dress and grooming.

Behavior

Observe the manner of speech, unusual body/facial movements, and posture.

Emotional State

Affect and Mood

Describe the patient's affect. How does the patient make you feel? Is he or she sad or euphoric? Does the patient respond appropriately? Is he or she excited, agitated, aggressive, crying, or excessively talkative?

Thought Content and Thought Processing

Are the patient's thoughts logical, relevant, organized, and coherent? Is he or she expressing thoughts of compulsion, obsession, phobias, anxieties, feelings of unreality, depersonalization, delusions, illusions, or hallucinations?

Cognitive Functions

State of Consciousness

Alertness: How aware is the patient of his or her surroundings? Are responses inappropriate? Does the patient appear drowsy? Does the patient fall asleep during questioning? Is the patient's attention span or ability to concentrate diminished? Is the patient reactive or excited, with rambling comments? Describe the patient as alert, confused, delirious, stuporous, or comatose.

Orientation: Determine the patient's awareness of name, name of location, and the day, month, season, or year (i.e., oriented to person, place, and time).

Memory

Past Memory: Ask the patient about birthdays, wedding anniversaries and other events from the patient's past.

Present Memory: Question the patient about his or her current illness; instruct the patient to repeat and remember 3 unrelated words for recall later in the interview.

Table 3.1

Mental Status Examination (continued)

Cognitive Functions (continued)

Attention/Concentration

Ask the patient to repeatedly subtract 7 from 100 (e.g., 93, 86, 79, 72, 65); or ask the patient to spell a word backwards (e.g., "noitnetta").

Insight

Ask the patient to explain his or her reasons for seeking medical attention.

Cognitive Functions: Higher Intelligence

Language

Naming: Show the patient a familiar object and ask him or her to name it.

Writing: Ask the patient to write a sentence containing a subject and a verb.

Reading: Ask the patient to read a sentence and do what it says
(e.g., "Touch your nose with your right hand.").

Copying: Ask the patient to copy drawings of a circle, cross, cube, and overlapping pentagon.

Fund of Knowledge

Test the patient's factual knowledge with questions such as: What is the capital city of this state? How many inches are in a foot? What holiday do you celebrate on July 4? How many eggs make a dozen? What liquid comes from a cow?

Abstract Reasoning

Proverbs: Ask the patient to interpret a proverbial phrase
(e.g., "A stitch in time saves nine.").

Analogies: Ask the patient to describe how the following objects are alike:
a peach and an apple, a dog and a cat, a bathtub and a swimming pool.

Judgment

Ask the patient, "What would you do if your house was burning?" or "What would you do if you found a stamped, addressed envelope lying on the sidewalk next to a mailbox?"

Physical Examination

Physical examination was unremarkable except for poor eyesight and a mild hearing deficit. The patient had lost 8 lb in the last month, and his joints had arthritic changes. Rectal examination found a heme-negative fecal impaction and benign prostatic hypertrophy.

Laboratory

Serum chemistries, complete blood cell count (CBC), urine analysis (UA), and thyroid function tests were normal for R.L.'s age and health.

Diagnosis and Management

Clinically, R.L. had been diagnosed with major depression, chronic glaucoma, hearing loss, and chronic rheumatoid arthritis. Imipramine 25 mg BID was prescribed. Ophthalmic and audiology appointments were arranged.

Over the next several months, R.L. became more sociable, regained his weight, returned to his usual sleeping pattern, and began dressing and grooming himself. The imipramine dose was increased to 75 mg QD HS without severe side effects and his glaucoma was treated to slow its progression. He and his wife received counseling. A hearing aid improved his social interaction. Imipramine was continued for three months and then gradually tapered under close monitoring to see if the depressive episode had resolved.

Table 3.2

Common Abbreviations Used in Mental Status Examinations

A & O	Alert and oriented
A & O x 3	Alert and oriented to person, place, and time
ADL	Activities of daily living
LOC	Loss of consciousness
MSE	Mental status exam
O x 3	Oriented to person, place, and time
O x 4	Oriented to person, place, time, and situation

Discussion

Disease. R.L.'s depression was identified using mental status measurements. It is common for a third party, such as a family member or health professional, to notice a personality or behavioral change at variance with the patient's usual behavior. In this case, the nursing home nurses, who have considerable contact time with R.L., noticed subtle changes in his appearance and mood. Initially, he denied any problem and said he did not seek medical attention because he felt his life seemed meaningless. However, upon further questioning, he spoke more freely. His symptoms included aches and pains, withdrawal, self-neglect, difficulty in concentration, fatigue, slowness of thought and action, and sleep disturbance. The physical changes present in R.L. (e.g., poor appetite, weight loss, constipation) often accompany mental depression, but are nonspecific findings.

The patient's social history is an important source of information concerning mental disturbances. Inquire about the patient's interactions with family, friends, work associates, and, if institutionalized, with other patients. As treatment progresses, document changes in social interactions and determine whether supporting family and friends are available. Lifestyle habits, including a person's daily activities, outside interests, physical habits, and nutritional habits should be monitored throughout therapy. Of particular concern is the presence of worsening isolation, which increases suicidal risk. If the patient admits suicidal thoughts or articulates a suicidal plan, he should be hospitalized and treatment initiated immediately.

R.L. had symptoms suggestive of other concomitant diseases. Senile dementia and hypothyroidism have signs and symptoms similar to those of depression in the aged. Intellectual function and thyroid function tests were normal; therefore, dementia and hypothyroidism probably were not present.

Treatment. The four general methods of treating depression are counseling, socialization, drug therapy, and electroconvulsive therapy (ECT). R.L.'s depression did not require ECT. Upon counseling, he exposed his feelings about financial problems, concern for his sickly wife, and lack of contact with his children. The social worker, activities therapist, and nursing staff helped resolve these problems by encouraging social interactions.

As adjunctive therapy, antidepressant drug therapy helped treat his depression. Physical complaints such as constipation and sleep disturbance also support the decision for an antidepressant. The tricyclic antidepressant, imipramine, was selected because the patient exhibited psychomotor retardation symptoms without agitation. He had no known cardiac problems, but did have constipation and prostatic hypertrophy which are relative contraindications to imipramine. However, these potential problems are manageable. Another potential problem with antidepressant therapy was anticholinergic-induced glaucoma; however, R.L.'s glaucoma was treated. A low dose of imipramine was prescribed and the dose was adjusted by target symptoms.

Therapeutic Drug Monitoring Examples

SCHIZOPHRENIA

The approach to therapeutic drug monitoring by clinicians varies depending upon many factors. Some of these include preferences among clinicians in a given community or region; concurrent medical problems which dictate that certain drugs be used or avoided; the patient's response to selected medication. The following outlines of therapeutic drug monitoring offer examples which may serve to stimulate discussion and further understanding of initiating and monitoring drug use. The drugs and dosages presented should not be applied to any clinical situation without proper medical supervision.

Drug Therapy	Haloperidol 5 mg PO QID.
Monitoring	**Symptoms:** Interview for symptoms of delusion, illusion, and hallucination. Describe alertness and orientation. Note incoherent or loose-association speech patterns. Determine the patient's ability to perform activities of daily living (ADL), work, and socialization functions.
	Signs: *MSE:* Note the patient's hygiene, dress, and manner of speech. Observe motor functions for agitation or retardation. Pay particular attention to bizarre behavior, thought content, and form of thought dysfunction.
Laboratory Tests	The clinician may elect to order all, none, or some of these laboratory studies depending upon history and physical findings, as well as other specific clinical indications. Liver enzymes.
Adverse Drug Event Monitoring	Check blood pressure for orthostatic hypotension (see Chapter 10: Blood Vessels). Monitor for excessive sedation/cognitive impairment. Observe for signs/symptoms of: **Tardive dyskinesia:** oral/facial repetitive movements such as lip smacking, puffing of cheeks, and rapid, worm-like tongue movements. Document with the Abnormal Involuntary Movement Scale (AIMS).

Therapeutic Drug Monitoring Examples

SCHIZOPHRENIA
(continued)

Adverse Drug
Event Monitoring

Parkinson's features: shuffling gait, stiffness of arms and legs, loss of balance, fatigue, mask-like face, trembling and shaking of fingers and hands. **Dystonia:** muscle spasm of the neck and back (i.e., torticollis). **Akathisia:** anxiety-like state with restlessness or need to keep moving. Question/test for anticholinergic toxicities such as blurring vision, constipation, dry mouth, and weak urination or distended bladder.

Therapeutic Drug Monitoring Examples

BIPOLAR DISORDER: MANIC EPISODE

The approach to therapuetic drug monitoring by clinicians varies depending upon many factors. Some of these include preferences among clinicians in a given community or region; concurrent medical problems which dictate that certain drugs be used or avoided; the patient's response to selected medication. The following outlines of therapeutic drug monitoring offer examples which may serve to stimulate discussion and further understanding of initiating and monitoring drug use. The drugs and dosages presented should not be applied to any clinical situation without proper medical supervision.

Drug Therapy	Lithium carbonate 300 mg PO TID.
Monitoring	**Symptoms:** Question about mood swings, especially euphoria and exhilaration. Interview family and friends. Check for insomnia, reckless decisions without regard for personal safety or financial outcomes, over-confidence, delusions of grandeur.
	Signs: *Gen:* Question about recent weight change (e.g., excessive weight gain or loss). *MSE:* Observe appearance and behavior. Note rapid, compressed speech with flights of ideas. Observe for agitation and motor hyperactivity.
Laboratory tests	The clinician may elect to order all, none, or some of these laboratory studies depending upon history and physical findings, as well as other specific clinical indications. Serum creatinine, urinalysis, thyroid function studies (T_4, T_3, and TSH), electrocardiogram (ECG), complete blood count (CBC), serum lithium, and serum electrolytes (especially sodium).
Adverse Drug Event Monitoring	Ask about fainting, fast heart beat, nausea, vomiting, unusual thirst, and fatigue. Examine the hands for a fine tremor. Check for hypothyroid findings (e.g., dry skin, hair loss, cold intolerance, enlarged thyroid, and non-pitting lower leg edema). Record pulse rate and rhythm.

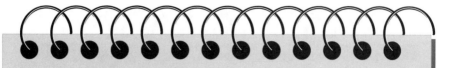

Therapeutic Drug Monitoring Examples

MAJOR DEPRESSION

The approach to therapuetic drug monitoring by clinicians varies depending upon many factors. Some of these include preferences among clinicians in a given community or region; concurrent medical problems which dictate that certain drugs be used or avoided; the patient's response to selected medication. The following outlines of therapeutic drug monitoring offer examples which may serve to stimulate discussion and further understanding of initiating and monitoring drug use. The drugs and dosages presented should not be applied to any clinical situation without proper medical supervision.

Drug Therapy	Desipramine tablet 25 mg PO TID.
Monitoring	**Symptoms:** Check for depressed mood (i.e., despondence), loss of interest in pleasurable activities, sleeping pattern (e.g., either hypersomnia or insomnia with early morning awakening and difficulty returning to sleep once awakened), lack of energy, and thoughts of death and/or suicide. Evaluate appetite as well as withdrawn or antisocial feelings. Observe emotional outbursts of crying. Ask about morning fatigue, not responsive to rest. Note any vague generalized physical complaints to multiple body systems. Check for loss of libido.
	Signs: *Gen:* Question about excessive weight gain or loss. *MSE:* View appearance, dress, and hygiene. Note facial expression for affect and mood. Listen to the manner of speech (e.g., slow, monotone). Watch for psychomotor agitation or retardation. Evaluate loss of thinking with judgment, abstraction, calculation, recent memory, and language testing. Test the patient's ability to decide between two options. *Neuro:* Observe slow body movements (gait).
Laboratory Tests	The clinician may elect to order all, none, or some of these laboratory studies depending upon history and physical

Therapeutic Drug Monitoring Examples

MAJOR DEPRESSION
(continued)

Laboratory Tests	findings, as well as other specific clinical indications. ECG.
Adverse Drug Event Monitoring	Check blood pressure for orthostatic changes and pulse for regularity and rate. Evaluate for signs and symptoms of anticholinergic effects (e.g., mental confusion, urinary hesitancy, blurred vision, dry mouth, or constipation). Evaluate for parkinson-like symptoms.

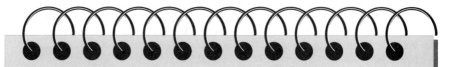

Therapeutic Drug Monitoring Examples

GENERALIZED ANXIETY DISORDER

The approach to therapeutic drug monitoring by clinicians varies depending upon many factors. Some of these include preferences among clinicians in a given community or region; concurrent medical problems which dictate that certain drugs be used or avoided; the patient's response to selected medication. The following outlines of therapeutic drug monitoring offer examples which may serve to stimulate discussion and further understanding of initiating and monitoring drug use. The drugs and dosages presented should not be applied to any clinical situation without proper medical supervision.

Drug Therapy	Alprazolam tablet 0.25 mg PO TID.
Monitoring	**Symptoms:** Ask about anxious feelings (e.g., feeling on edge), feeling shaky. Question about shortness of breath, palpitations, dizziness, hot flashes, dry mouth, frequent urination, and diarrhea. Question about inability to fall asleep and difficulty performing tasks requiring concentration (e.g., balancing a checkbook).
	Signs: *VS:* Record pulse, respiration, and blood pressure. *Skin:* Note excessive sweating or cold clammy skin. *MSE:* Observe behavior for signs of motor tension such as trembling, twitching, and restlessness. Test attention span and recent memory.
Laboratory Tests	None.
Adverse Drug Event Monitoring	Observe for ataxia, drowsiness, confusion, slurring of speech, and falls. Check performance of ADLs. Determine ability to recall information (i.e., recent memory) of current events. Monitor for delirium (e.g., abrupt combativeness, disorientation, cloudy sensorium, rambling speech, short attention span).

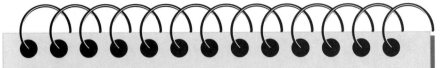

Therapeutic Drug Monitoring Examples

SLEEP DISORDER

The approach to therapuetic drug monitoring by clinicians varies depending upon many factors. Some of these include preferences among clinicians in a given community or region; concurrent medical problems which dictate that certain drugs be used or avoided; the patient's response to selected medication. The following outlines of therapeutic drug monitoring offer examples which may serve to stimulate discussion and further understanding of initiating and monitoring drug use. The drugs and dosages presented should not be applied to any clinical situation without proper medical supervision.

Drug Therapy	Triazolam 0.25 mg tablet PO Q HS.
Monitoring	**Symptoms:** Interview for sleep pattern (e.g., initiating and maintaining sleep, total length, restorative energy upon awakening).
	Signs: *MSE:* Observe for fatigue and alertness. Check ability to perform motor functions (e.g., walk, write). Record appearance, behavior, and orientation. Ask the patient to repeat and recall three words. Ask the patient to repeatedly subtract 7 from 100 until reaching 65.
Laboratory Tests	None.
Adverse Drug Event Monitoring	Check for performance of ADLs. Observe for confusion, drowsiness, slurred speech, and forgetfulness. Evaluate gait. Question about complaints of blurred vision and check for depressive symptoms.

Skin, Hair, and Nails

*T*he skin, hair, and nails are readily available for physical examination and can often be affected by various systemic and localized disorders (e.g., melanoma, systemic lupus erythematosus, scleroderma). Observable cutaneous lesions, therefore, can signal serious underlying systemic disorders. The pharmacist can advise patients on the use of nonprescription medications to self-manage common topical dermatologic conditions. However, patients who have cutaneous lesions that are symptomatic of more serious problems should be referred to a physician. To make this determination, the pharmacist should skillfully interview the patient, carefully examine the integument, and consider the possibility of an adverse drug reaction before suggesting a nonprescription medication or referring the patient to a physician.

ANATOMY AND PHYSIOLOGY

Skin is the most accessible, rugged, regenerative, and defensive organ of the body. It covers the entire body; protects underlying organs against microbial and traumatic injury; regulates body temperature by conduction, convection, and radiation of heat, as well as evaporation of sweat; recognizes sensory stimuli for reflex protection; regulates body fluids; and repairs wounds. The skin is composed of three distinct morphological layers: the epidermis, dermis, and hypodermis (subcutaneous layer). Sweat glands, sebaceous glands, sensory nerves, and blood vessels are distributed throughout its various skin layers (see Figure 4.1).

Epidermis

The epidermis is avascular and depends upon the dermis for nutrition and excretion of waste. Histologically, the epidermis is divided into several layers: the stratum corneum, the stratum lucidum, the stratum granulosum, the stratum spinosum, and the stratum basale. The stratum corneum consists of several layers of dead, keratinized cells that are continuously shed and regenerated. This layer protects the body against a hostile environment and limits the loss of fluids and electrolytes. These protective functions are partly due to the properties of keratin, a tough, impervious cellular material. Melanocytes, located in the basal layer, produce the brown skin pigment

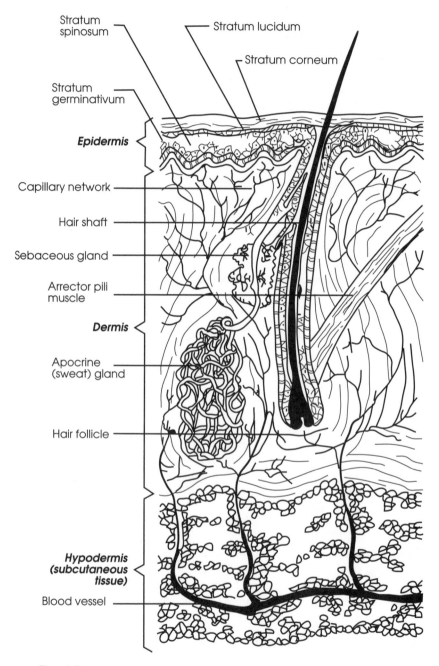

Fig. 4.1   Layers of skin and associated structures.

known as melanin. Melanin gives the skin its color and protects the dermis and hypodermis from the sun's harmful rays. Abnormal growth of melanocytes is associated with melanoma, a dangerous skin cancer which must be differentiated from normal pigmented nevi or birthmarks.

Dermis

The dermis separates the epidermis from the hypodermis. Blood vessels richly permeate the dermis and supply nutrients to the epidermis. Collagen and elastin are distributed throughout the dermis and provide strength, stability, and resilience to the skin. Autonomic nerves in the dermis regulate blood vessel diameter, sebaceous and sweat gland secretion, and arrector pili muscle contraction and relaxation. Sensory nerves in the dermis transmit the sensations of temperature, touch, vibration, and pain to the central nervous system (CNS). The dermis is especially thick over some structures (e.g., palms and soles) and especially thin over others (e.g., eyelids and scrotum).

Hypodermis

The hypodermis lies beneath the dermis and is composed of collagen and fat tissue. This subcutaneous layer gives the skin its soft, supple texture; provides insulation; and stores calories. As the skin ages, it loses its elastin and collagen support. This loss of support contributes to the skin's wrinkled appearance.

Glands

Eccrine (sweat), sebaceous, and apocrine glands are the major glands located in the dermal layers. **Eccrine glands** are controlled by cholinergic nerves and regulate body temperature by secreting an aqueous electrolyte solution, commonly known as sweat. When sweat evaporates, it cools the surface of the skin. Sweat glands are located throughout the dermal surface including that of the palms of the hands and the soles of the feet; however, they are not found in the glans penis, eyelids, lips, or ears. Thermal stress promotes perspiration over the entire body, especially on the forehead, upper lip, and neck. Normal insensible sweat loss is 300 to 600 mL/day; yet, considerably more can be lost with various clinical conditions (e.g., fever), and with extreme exercise a person can lose 6 to 8 L/day.

Sebaceous glands develop at puberty in response to androgenic stimulation and produce the lipid material, sebum. Sebum is transported via ducts to the follicular canal (see Figure 4.1) and out onto the surface of the skin. The water-repellent and mildly antibacterial sebum from sebaceous glands throughout the skin (except on the soles and palms) protects and lubricates the skin surface. The glyceride component of sebum is converted to free fatty acids and glycerol by *Propionibacterium acnes*. These free fatty acids presumably irritate the follicular wall, cause increased cell turnover and inflammation, and produce the inflammatory reaction known as acne, or, in its severe form, as acne vulgaris.

Apocrine glands are located in the axillae, breasts, eyelids, external ear canals, and anogenital area. These glands become active at puberty and secrete a white, odorless fluid in response to emotional stimuli. Decomposition of this fluid by skin bacteria results in the characteristic adult body odor.

Hair

Hair is histologically composed of a hair shaft with an associated follicle and arrector pili muscles (see Figure 4.1). The hair shaft, made of dead, keratinized, melanin-colored material, grows from a hollow bulb that fits over the hair papilla. Two types of hair are found in adults: vellus and terminal. **Vellus hair** is short, fine, soft, and lacks pigment. **Terminal hair** is longer, thicker, and pigmented. Hair length and diameter vary depending upon the location on the body. Scalp hair grows about one-half inch per month, but this varies with the season. Hereditary factors, gender, nationality, and endocrine function (e.g., pregnancy, thyroid function) influence hair growth, quantity, quality, and distribution.

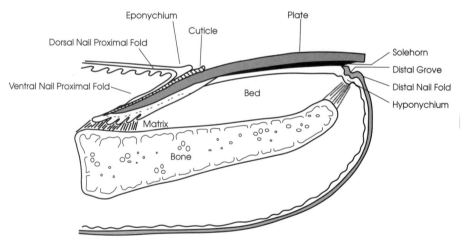

Fig. 4.2

Nails

The nail is a translucent keratin plate that rests upon, and adheres to, the highly vascular **nail bed**. Thus, the nail allows direct visualization of vascular content and activity in the hypodermis. In patients with a normal number of red blood cells (RBCs) and normal oxyhemoglobin, the nail bed is healthy pink. The cutis (i.e., eponychium) is the stratum corneum layer that covers the nail plate edge. The paronychium is the soft tissue surrounding the nail border (see Figure 4.2). The nail plate grows proximally from the deeply buried nail root. Fingernails grow faster than toenails, with replacement times of about 6 months and 12 to 18 months, respectively.

PHYSICAL ASSESSMENT

When examining the skin and its appendages, remember that normal findings will vary widely depending upon the genetic constitution, age, and gender of the patient. Although presented here as a separate procedure, the examination of the skin, hair, and nails is, for the most part, carried out while examining other body systems. Adequate lighting (e.g., natural light or fluorescent lights), a comfortable room temperature (i.e., neither too cold nor too hot), and appropriate exposure of the patient's skin are essential to the examination of skin conditions. The patient should be dressed in a gown to provide some dignity and modesty. However, serious mistakes can be made by an examiner too shy to fully evaluate the entire skin surface. Sometimes, the clinical situation may not demand total exposure of the skin surface and a limited assessment can be adequate when an identified problem is localized.

Skin Assessment

Inspect and palpate the integument in a careful, orderly manner. To assess normal skin function, note the color, temperature, and texture of the skin. Examine the hands, fingernails, arms, face, hair, scalp, and neck while the patient is in a sitting position. Then ask the patient to expose his or her upper body. Inspect the anterior and posterior chest, the lower back, and the abdomen. Next, examine the lower extremities. Do not forget to carefully inspect the axilla (i.e., arm pits), palms of the hands, areas between the toes, and the soles of the feet. Compare symmetrical regions to detect differences. Also note the anatomic distribution of lesions since some dermatological conditions have characteristic anatomic patterns (e.g., lupus erythematosus and acne; see Figure 4.4 on page 4–10).

Skin Color. Race, gender, nationality, occupation, and climate all affect normal skin colors, which range from pale pink to black. An individual's skin color also varies on different parts of the body and can be transiently altered by emotional stress, fever, or variations in environmental temperature. While many skin color changes represent such benign findings as freckles or birthmarks, others can indicate serious underlying conditions. The discovery of changes in skin color represents an important finding. When examining skin color, be sure to note whether color distribution is generalized or localized.

Diffuse cutaneous color changes result from the influences of blood, collagen, and pigment. Oxygenated hemoglobin in the skin capillaries brings a red color to the skin. Scarlet fever, lupus erythematosus, polycythemia, and first degree burns are characterized by an erythematous (red) appearance caused by the predominance of oxygenated blood in the skin. Yellow skin discoloration comes from the natural color of collagen and can be intensified by the abnormal presence of carotene or bile. Brown discoloration results from a predominance of melanin pigment and can be seen in patients with scleroderma or porphyria. (See Table 4.1 for a discussion of the causes and conditions associated with variations in skin color.)

Medications can also affect skin color. Quinacrine therapy can result in a brown discoloration of the skin. Birth control pills can cause melasma ("pregnancy mask"); gold injections and bismuth deposits can cause a gray or blue-gray discoloration; and some drugs (e.g., phenothiazines, isoniazid, and tetracycline) can cause yellowish-green jaundice. Photoallergic and phototoxic reactions can impart a reddish color to the skin and can be caused by demeclocycline, anticonvulsants, and phenothiazines. A yellow or orange stain is noticeable on the soles or palms of patients who ingest excessive amounts of carotene-rich foods (e.g., carrots) and in patients treated with isotretinoin or rifampin. Years of exposure to chlorpromazine causes dark hyperpigmentation. **Livedo reticularis** (a peripheral vascular condition characterized by a reddish-blue net-like pattern) has been associated with amantadine. Excessive exposure to glucocorticoids induces thinning, striae, and darkening of skin. Chronic iron intoxication imparts a bronze color to skin. Rapid infusion of vancomycin or codeine (histamine released) may lead to the so-called "red neck syndrome" (also termed "red man syndrome").

Vasodilation that is generalized (e.g., fever) or localized (e.g., inflammation) can cause an erythematous (red discoloration resulting from oxygenated hemoglobin) reaction in

Skin Color Variations

Table 4.1

Color	Cause	Condition
Pallor	Absence of melanin pigment Increased deoxyhemoglobin Reduced blood flow, tissue perfusion	Albinism, vitiligo Anemia Shock
Erythema	Increased skin blood flow, tissue perfusion	Fever, inflammation
Brown	Darkening melanin pigment	Pregnancy, nevi, Addison's disease
Blue	Increase in deoxygenated blood Abnormal hemoglobin	Heart or lung disease Methemoglobinemia
Yellow	Bile pigment deposited Predominance of collagen Increased carotene	Liver disease Anemia Carotene-rich diet

skin. Cyanosis (blue skin discoloration resulting from deoxyhemoglobin) is sometimes noticeable in patients with chronic bronchitis, anemia, or congestive heart failure. A white uremic frost can be found on the surface of the skin in severely ill, undialyzed, chronic renal failure patients. The congenital absence of pigment in the skin, hair, and eyes is known as albinism. Vitiligo is an idiopathic condition characterized by the skin's failure to form melanin resulting in patches of depigmentation. It is associated with a variety of systemic diseases (e.g., insulin dependent diabetes mellitus, Hashimoto's thyroiditis, pernicious anemia, local inflammatory disease, idiopathic adrenal insufficiency, Down's syndrome, mycosis fungoides, multiple myeloma, Hodgkin's disease, and melanoma).

Skin Temperature. While inspecting skin color, feel the skin surface with the backs of your fingers to detect unusual variations in *skin temperature*. Normal skin temperature varies with skin blood flow and feels warm to cool. At room temperature, a range of skin temperatures can be felt depending upon the body region (e.g., toes = 27° C; forehead = 32° C; oral = 37° C). Palpation of the skin surface provides a general estimate of heat loss especially when evaluating regional inflammation. When palpating the skin surface area, compare temperature differences bilaterally and be sure the areas have been exposed to the room temperature long enough to make a fair comparison.

Skin texture varies with age, gender, occupation, and body region. Skin texture is described in terms of softness, moisture, and lubrication and is classified on the basis of oiliness, dryness, coarseness, fineness, and moistness (see Table 4.2). Texture varies greatly with body region. The skin on the elbows, palms, and soles feels rough due to the frequent pressure placed upon these areas. In most other areas, the skin should be smooth and soft. You should feel minimal perspiration and oiliness except on the patient's face, scalp, palms, and axillae. Give particular attention to the anogenital and any obese areas where the skin folds. Evaluate **mobility** (i.e., the ease of lifting a fold of skin) and **turgor** (i.e., the rapidity with which skin returns to its original position). Mobility is affected by collagen content (e.g., the collagen, connective tissue disorder of scleroderma is associated with reduced mobility). Turgor primarily depends upon water content or changes in collagen structure with age. Measure skin turgor and mobility over a bony surface area (e.g., sternum, back of hand; see Fig. 2.2). Skin that does not quickly return to its original position is described as "tenting" or having poor turgor. Although skin turgor is sometimes used to evaluate dehydration, it is not a reliable sign in elderly patients because of the natural loss of elasticity associated with aging.

Skin Lesions. After noting skin color, temperature, and texture, carefully examine the patient for skin lesions. If lesions are present, measure them with a metric ruler and describe them in terms of: **type** (e.g., primary, secondary); **anatomic distribution** (e.g., localized, regional, generalized); **consistency** (e.g., firm, soft); and **color** (e.g., white, red). The description of these attributes serves as the foundation for evaluations of responses to treatment; serial comparisons of these attributes serve as guidepost markers. Even if you do not know the underlying cause of a lesion, providing an accurate description for a physician, especially a dermatologist, can help greatly in the patient's care.

Skin Texture Changes

Table 4.2

Texture	Possible Cause	Selected Disease
Oiliness	Excessive sebum	Parkinsonism
Dry	Decreased sebum	Normal aging
Coarse	Chronic edema	Stasis dermatitis
Fine	Loss of hypodermis	Hypothyroidism
Moist	Thermal, emotional, or disease	Fever

Several types of primary lesions are described in Table 4.3 on page 4–11 according to their elevation, size, shape, and consistency. The presence of these attributes determines the classification of lesions as: macules, papules, maculopapules, plaques, nodules, wheals, vesicles, bullae, pustules, cysts, or keratoses (see Figure 4.3). Secondary lesions are identified by changes in the primary lesion (see Table 4.4 on page 4–12), and are described as scales, lichenifications, crusts, atrophy, sclerosis, erosions, fissures, ulcers, and gangrene. Figure 4.4 lists the nomenclature for the various skin lesion distribution patterns. Although primary and secondary lesions usually appear together, secondary lesions may appear alone (see Figures 4.6 through 4.13 on page 4-14–4-16).

Hair Assessment

Assess distribution, color, texture, and quality of the patient's hair. The degree of fragility and the ease with which a hair can be removed from its follicle are measures of hair quality. Alopecia (i.e., excessive hair loss), changes in hair distribution, excessive hair growth, or changes in texture also are important findings. Drug therapy (e.g., alopecia induced by chemotherapy), diseases (e.g., fine, silky hair of hyperthyroidism), or normal physiology (e.g., pregnancy) can affect these attributes of hair. Scalp hair may feel coarse or fine, dry or oily. Check the color and note whether the patient uses a hair dye. Look for areas of abnormal hair growth and variations in the quantity of hair in relation to the gender of the patient. Normal male pattern baldness is associated with androgen excess. In men with prostate cancer, treatment with estrogens, antiandrogen, or bilateral orchiectomy can cause a female pattern of hair distribution. An excessive growth of hair is called hypertrichosis or hirsutism. In a female patient, hirsutism could indicate an endocrine disorder. Drugs, such as the vasodilator minoxidil, can cause hirsutism as well. Generalized and local alopecia can be caused by drugs (e.g., birth control pills), seborrheic dermatitis, alopecia areata, trichotillomania, tinea capitis, lupus erythematosus, or thyroid disease.

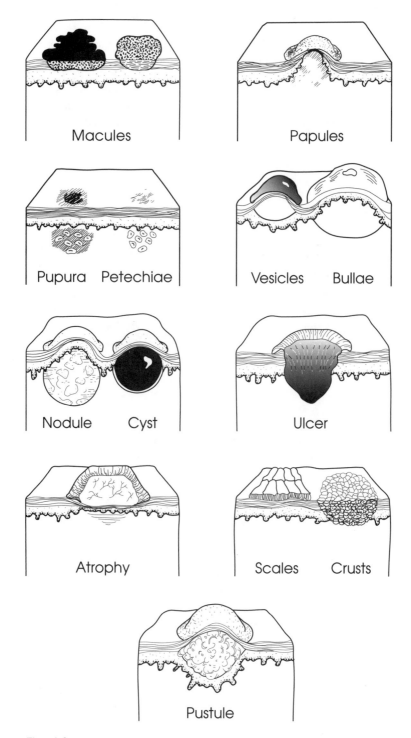

Fig. 4.3 Primary Skin Lesions.

Nail Assessment

Many physical signs of generalized disease can be identified through an examination of the fingernails. The nails also provide an opportunity for the examiner to directly view capillary changes that can be affected by systemic disease.

Inspect and palpate the patient's nails for secure attachment, color, and lesions. Note the angle between the nail plate and nail base. Normally, the nail base feels firm and forms an angle of less than 180° with the nail plate. The fingernails and nail beds

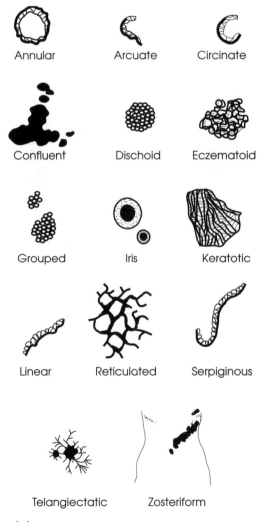

Fig. 4.4   Skin Lesion Distribution Patterns.

Table 4.3

Primary Skin Lesions

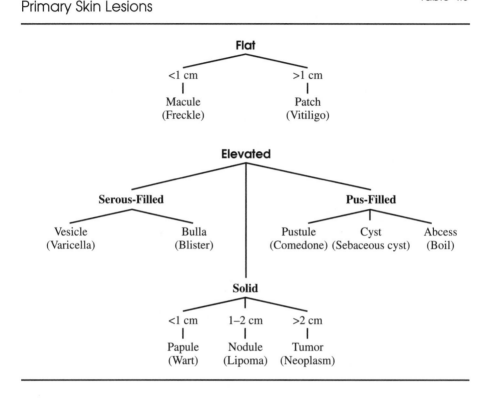

can be affected by a variety of respiratory and cardiovascular disorders. For example, a phenomenon known as **clubbing** occurs when the nail base softens and the angle between the nail plate and nail base increases beyond the 180° angle. This increased angle gives the tip of the finger a "club-like" appearance (see Figure 4.5). Clubbing has been associated with chronic hypoxia; however, it is also a normal variant, especially in black patients. To check for clubbing, place a ruler across the nail and distal finger joint, and look at the space between the nail plate and nail base. A **floating nail**, or a loose nail plate, also accompanies clubbing and can be demonstrated by holding the patient's finger by the tip of nail and pressing down at the distal nail plate.

Inspect the nail in bright light, preferably direct sunlight. Decreased hemoglobin oxygenation causes cyanosis (a bluish color) in the nail bed. Anxiety, a cold environment, heart or lung disease, or an abnormal hemoglobin (e.g., drug-induced methemoglobinemia) causes cyanosis. Pallor of the nail bed suggests decreased amounts of oxyhemoglobin (e.g., anemia) or decreased blood flow (e.g., syncope or normal variant). Nail bed color can be correlated to a serum hemoglobin or hematocrit concentration. After this correlation has been established for a specific patient, the hematocrit can be estimated merely on the basis of nail bed color.

Table 4.4

Secondary Skin Lesions

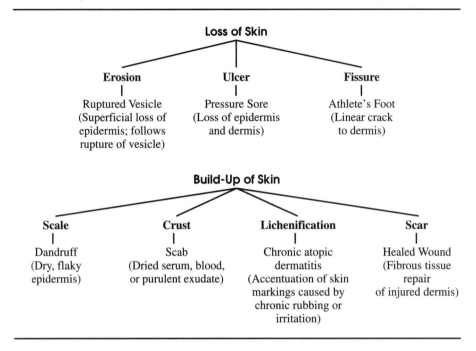

Loss of Skin

Erosion	Ulcer	Fissure
Ruptured Vesicle (Superficial loss of epidermis; follows rupture of vesicle)	Pressure Sore (Loss of epidermis and dermis)	Athlete's Foot (Linear crack to dermis)

Build-Up of Skin

Scale	Crust	Lichenification	Scar
Dandruff (Dry, flaky epidermis)	Scab (Dried serum, blood, or purulent exudate)	Chronic atopic dermatitis (Accentuation of skin markings caused by chronic rubbing or irritation)	Healed Wound (Fibrous tissue repair of injured dermis)

Yellowish discoloration of the nail bed and paronychial hypertrophy have been associated with psoriasis and fungal infections; greenish discharge under the nail with *Pseudomonas* species infections. Chronic, heavy cigarette smokers have yellowish-orange stained nails on the index and middle fingers. Splinter hemorrhages in the nail bed (red or brown parallel lines more than 1 mm wide) or Beau lines (transverse lines) indicate tiny emboli and interrupted nail growth; however, simple trauma is the most common cause of nail bed hemorrhages. Malignant melanoma can discolor the nail bed brown or black. Hypoalbuminemia may cause Muehrcke's lines (white, transverse, opaque bands) in the nail bed that disappear as the serum concentration of albumin returns to normal. These are unlike true nail plate lesions which disappear only with nail plate growth. White spots are usually a benign finding, showing cuticle damage. Thick, yellowish nail plates are normal findings with aging. Darkening of nail plate occurs with many cancer chemotherapies. Small pits in the nail plate are seen in psoriasis. Onycholysis (separation of the nail plate from the nail bed) can be caused by diseases (e.g., mycotic infections, psoriasis, hyperthyroidism) or drugs (e.g., chronic amphetamine use, doxorubicin, captopril, tetracycline). Patients with chronic iron deficiency anemia often display a classic condition known as koilonychia (spoon nail). The spoon nail has an indention in the center deep enough to comfortably hold a drop of water.

PHARMACOTHERAPEUTIC CASE ILLUSTRATION

History

R.J., a 67-year-old male, was admitted with the chief complaint (CC) of "itching everywhere." History of present illness (HPI) showed that the patient was in his usual state of health until three weeks prior to admission (PTA). Three days PTA, he noticed a generalized itching on his back which spread to his chest and axillae. He developed a fever and was lethargic.

Significant past medical history (PMH) included history of acute gouty arthritis, chronic glaucoma, benign prostatic hypertrophy (BPH), hypertension, and angina pectoris. A medication history (MH) noted prescriptions for allopurinol 300 mg PO QD, timolol 0.25% 1 drop each eye QD, diltiazem 30 mg PO TID, and nitroglycerin (NTG) 1/150 gr tablet sublingually (SL) PRN chest pain. The patient had no known drug allergies.

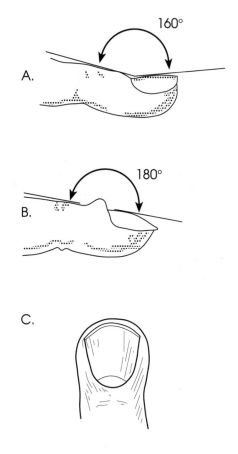

Fig. 4.5 Clubbing of the finger. A shows the normal angle of the nail. B shows an abnormal angle seen in late clubbing. C shows a top view of clubbing.

Physical Examination

R.J.'s vital signs (VS) were as follows: blood pressure (BP) 130/80 mm Hg (supine); pulse 75 beats/min and regular; respiratory rate (RR) 20/min, and temperature 39.2° C. Physical examination (PE) revealed a maculopapular rash with scales on erythematous bases on the chest, face, axillae, and back. The rest of the physical examination was unremarkable.

Laboratory

Laboratory data were within normal limits (WNL), except uric acid of 9.2 mg/dL (normal: 4.4–8.4) and eosinophil count of 700/mm^3 (normal: 150–300/mm^3).

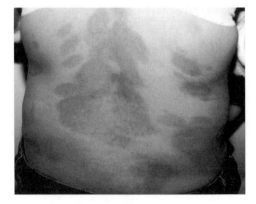

Fig. 4.6 Macules and papules.

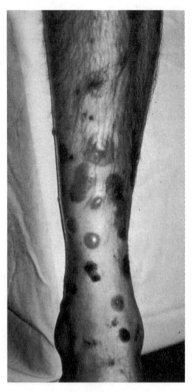

Fig. 4.8 Vesicles and bullae.

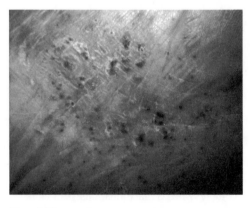

Fig. 4.7 Petechiae.

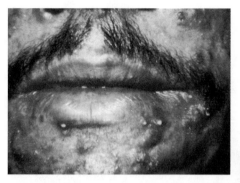

Fig. 4.9 Nodules and cysts.

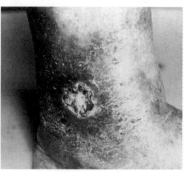

Fig. 4.10 Ulcer.

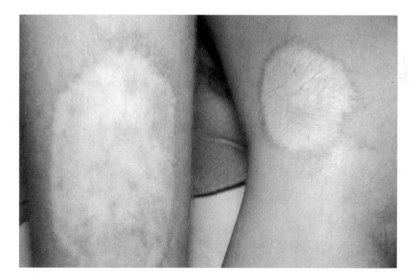

Fig. 4.11 Atrophy.

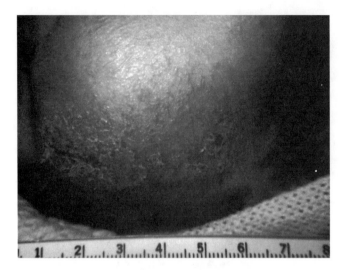

Fig. 4.12 Scales and crusts.

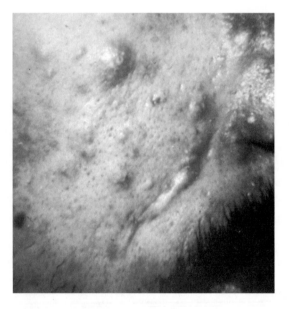

Fig. 4.13 Pustules.

Diagnosis and Management

R.J.'s admitting diagnosis was a drug reaction to allopurinol. He was treated with trimeprazine (Temaril) 2.5 mg PO QID, acetaminophen 325 mg PO Q 4 hr PRN fever >38.8° C oral, and prednisone 60 mg PO QD with a tapering schedule. His previous medications were continued with the exception of the allopurinol.

The itching resolved within 48 hours. However, R.J. complained that "I can't make my water." The trimeprazine was stopped, and terfenadine 60 mg PO Q 12 hr was ordered.

Discussion

Disease. The skin is a frequent target organ of adverse drug reactions (ADRs). The scope of the problem is unknown, but adverse drug reactions are especially common in hospitalized patients. The causes of adverse drug reactions are many and include overdoses, idiosyncrasies, exacerbations of other diseases, and allergies.

Dermatological allergic reactions are often pruritic, symmetrical, and most prominent on the trunk. They generally occur after seven to ten days of drug use following the first exposure, or within 48 hours following the second exposure. Allergic reactions are dose independent and subside upon discontinuation of the medication. Although eosinophilia is commonly noted with allergic reactions, it may be absent.

It is very difficult to precisely determine the type of dermatologic drug reaction based on a classical clinical presentation, or even by histological investigation. The most common drug-induced skin eruptions are urticarial, maculopapular, vesicular, bullous, photosensitive, vascular, exfoliative, pigmented, acneiform, and fixed reactions.

Many drugs, such as anticancer agents, hormones, and antibiotics, frequently cause adverse dermatological effects. Although one type of lesion is usually more common with a particular drug (e.g., maculopapular reactions with penicillin), drugs can cause a variety of skin eruptions. For instance, penicillin can cause urticarial, vesicular, or maculopapular eruptions.

Skin toxicities are a common problem with allopurinol. Although some deaths have been reported, the rash usually subsides with discontinuation of the drug. The primary lesions induced by allopurinol appear as pruritic maculopapules progressing to erythematous scales; however, they sometimes appear as exfoliative, urticarial, and purpuric lesions. Lethargy and fever may accompany the rash and linger after discontinuation of allopurinol therapy. These dermatological reactions are allergic in nature because they are dose independent, immediate in onset, pruritic, and accompanied by eosinophilia. Patients with hepatic or renal dysfunction may be particularly susceptible to allopurinol allergic reactions.

Management. The primary treatment for R.J. involved discontinuation of the suspected drug and symptomatic control. Although allopurinol was the most probable offending agent, the possibility that R.J.'s other medications could be involved should not be disregarded. Trimeprazine, a phenothiazine analog, was used to relieve the pruritus associated with the histamine mediated reactions, with the therapeutic goal of alleviating the itch and its associated anxiety. R.J.'s response to this treatment plan can be evaluated by monitoring complaints of itching, signs of excoriations, and the lack of new primary lesions. The strong sedative effect of trimeprazine (Temaril) alleviates itching; other antihistaminics such as hydroxyzine (Vistaril) or diphenhydramine (Benadryl) are equally effective. R.J.'s constitutional signs (fever and lethargy) were treated with prednisone. Corticosteroids can relieve allergic symptoms within a few days. Fever is an important sign of infections; therefore, acetaminophen was used only for an excessively high temperature.

The anticholinergic reaction R.J. experienced is a common side effect of antihistamines. Benign prostatic hypertrophy, a common problem of elderly males, predisposed R.J. to dysuria or urinary retention. The phenothiazine, trimeprazine, and commonly used antihistamines have strong anticholinergic properties and should be administered cautiously to patients with obstructive uropathies, primary angle closure glaucoma, or angina pectoris. Because R.J. was being effectively treated with diltiazem for angina pectoris and timolol for primary open angle glaucoma, these problems were not aggravated. His probable prostatic urinary difficulty was managed by simply changing to a less anticholinergic antihistamine such as terfenadine.

Therapeutic Drug Monitoring Examples

ACTINIC KERATOSIS (MULTIPLE LESIONS ON THE SAME AREA OF THE BODY)

The approach to therapuetic drug monitoring by clinicians varies depending upon many factors. Some of these include preferences among clinicians in a given community or region; concurrent medical problems which dictate that certain drugs be used or avoided; the patient's response to selected medication. The following outlines of therapeutic drug monitoring offer examples which may serve to stimulate discussion and further understanding of initiating and monitoring drug use. The drugs and dosages presented should not be applied to any clinical situation without proper medical supervision.

Drug Therapy:	Fluorouracil 2% solution applied with a cotton applicator to lesions BID for 4 weeks is one of several treatment modalities. If severely inflamed, reduce application to QD.
Monitoring	**Symptoms:** Ask when the person first noticed the lesions? Quiz about any bleeding or pruritus. Has rapid growth of a particular lesion happened recently?
	Signs: Describe the distribution and number of lesions. What do the borders look like (e.g., regular or irregular)? Is the pigment uniform? Is there more than one shade of color in the lesion? Are the lesions friable or oozing blood? Are the lesions nodular, cystic, sclerosing, or superficial?
Laboratory Tests	The clinician may elect to order all, none, or some of these laboratory studies depending upon history and physical findings, as well as other specific clinical indications. Biopsy for histology, CBC.
Adverse Drug Event Monitoring	Question about *excessive* burning sensation and pruritus with each application. Examine each lesion for normal treatment response: first erythema (week 1), then erosion (week 2), followed by necrosis (weeks 3–4), and healing (weeks 5–6).

Therapeutic Drug Monitoring Examples

PSORIASIS VULGARIS (SEVERE)

The approach to therapuetic drug monitoring by clinicians varies depending upon many factors. Some of these include preferences among clinicians in a given community or region; concurrent medical problems which dictate that certain drugs be used or avoided; the patient's response to selected medication. The following outlines of therapeutic drug monitoring offer examples which may serve to stimulate discussion and further understanding of initiating and monitoring drug use. The drugs and dosages presented should not be applied to any clinical situation without proper medical supervision.

Drug Therapy	Etretinate 25 mg capsule 1 PO TID with milk.
Monitoring	**Symptoms:** How long has the patient had psoriasis? Ask the patient to describe the distribution of the psoriatic lesions and how the problem has changed recently.
	Signs: *Skin:* Expose all affected areas. Inspect the color and distribution pattern. Are there lesions on the knees, elbows, buttocks, scalp, or intertriginous areas? Note the presence of scaly plaque formations. Are silvery scales present? Feel the texture (toughness) and temperature (inflammation). *Nail:* Assess the texture and attachment for psoriatic nails.
Laboratory Tests	The clinician may elect to order all, none, or some of these laboratory studies depending upon history and physical findings, as well as other specific clinical indications. Liver function tests, serum lipid profile because of the etretinate therapy.
Adverse Drug Event Monitoring	Determine any problem with *new onset* fatigue, visual disturbances, nausea, and vomiting. If the patient complains of excessive thirst, skin peeling (especially on fingers, palms, or soles), bruising, conjunctivitis, or nail dystrophies,

Therapeutic Drug Monitoring Examples

PSORIASIS VULGARIS (SEVERE)
(continued)

Adverse Drug
Event Monitoring

carefully examine the patient for supportive findings. Question about unusual nose bleeding (epistaxis), sore tongue (glossitis), and loss of hair (alopecia). Inspect the lips for excessive dryness with fissures (cheilitis); also look for dryness of the mouth and nose which are troublesome to the patient.

Therapeutic Drug Monitoring Examples

IMPETIGO CONTAGIOSA (NONBULLOUS)

The approach to therapuetic drug monitoring by clinicians varies depending upon many factors. Some of these include preferences among clinicians in a given community or region; concurrent medical problems which dictate that certain drugs be used or avoided; the patient's response to selected medication. The following outlines of therapeutic drug monitoring offer examples which may serve to stimulate discussion and further understanding of initiating and monitoring drug use. The drugs and dosages presented should not be applied to any clinical situation without proper medical supervision.

Drug Therapy	Mupirocin 2% ointment is often applied to lesions TID after washing with Phisohex.
Monitoring	**Symptoms:** Ask when the symptoms first appeared. Has the patient experienced any generalized symptoms such as fever or malaise?
	Signs: *VS:* Measure the oral temperature. *Skin:* Inspect for vesicles and pustules (primary lesions) and honey-colored crusted lesions (secondary lesions). Report their locations. Wearing gloves, palpate the areas.
Laboratory Tests	The clinician may elect to order all, none, or some of these laboratory studies depending upon history and physical findings, as well as other specific clinical indications. Skin culture/sensitive (rare).
Adverse Drug Event Monitoring	Question for local complaints of burning, stinging, or itching.

Eye

A n eye examination often reveals signs of systemic disease and intrinsic ocular disorders, as well as the effects of drugs that are administered either systemically or instilled onto the eye itself.

ANATOMY AND PHYSIOLOGY

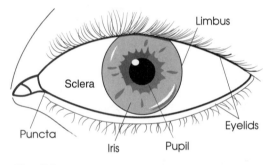

Fig. 5.1 External eye structures of the left eye. Note how the upper lid normally covers the upper rim of the iris and limbus.

The eye is composed of three anatomical divisions: the eyelids, the external eye structures, and the internal eye structures (see Figure 5.1). The **eyelids** are covered externally with skin and lined internally with conjunctiva. They protect the eyes from bright light and foreign objects, and distribute water and oil over the surface of the eye to prevent drying. The eyelid normally covers the upper border of the iris (the circular pigmented membrane behind the cornea) and contains hairs and their associated follicles (i.e., eyelashes), meibomian glands, palpebral conjunctiva, muscles, and tarsal plates (i.e., one of the plates of connective tissue forming the framework of the eyelid). **Meibomian glands** secrete sebaceous material to lubricate the inner lids. The oculomotor nerve (cranial nerve 3), the facial nerve (cranial nerve 7), and the sympathetic nervous system innervate the eyelids. The **conjunctiva** is a thin translucent membrane covering the anterior eye and folding onto the inner eyelids. The palpebral conjunctiva covers the inner aspect (i.e., internal side) of the eyelids and the bulbar conjunctiva coats the sclera. The normally transparent conjunctiva is richly supplied with blood vessels. It joins the corneal margin at the limbus.

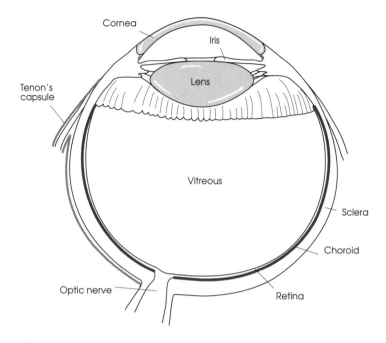

Fig. 5.2   The internal eye with its three layers: the retina, the choroid and the sclera; and the optic nerve, with its posterior chamber filled with vitreous fluid and anterior chamber containing the lens and retina.

The **external eye** consists of the lacrimal glands and lacrimal sac located in the temporal region of the bony eye orbit. The **lacrimal glands** secrete fluid to prevent drying and to ease removal of foreign matter with each blink of the eye. The lacrimal fluid bathes the anterior eye and drains into the lacrimal ducts and sac. The lacrimal sac, within the nasal bony orbit, drains into the nose via the nasolacrimal ducts. Normally, only the lacrimal sac openings (i.e., puncta) are visible on the medial lower eye lid.

The **internal eye** is the area immediately behind the **cornea**, the transparent avascular part of the sclera that refracts light. The eyeball divides into three concentric layers: the sclera, the choroid, and the retina (see Figure 5.2). The **sclera** is the whitish-creamy outer layer. The **choroid** is the middle layer of the eyeball. A dark-brown pigmented tissue, the choroid contains a rich network of veins and capillaries that supply nutrients to the inner concentric layer known as the **retina**. Within the retina, a sensory network of rods and cones transforms light into electrical impulses which are transferred over the optic nerve (cranial nerve 2) to the visual cortex of the brain. Veins and arteries supplying the retina are seen as they enter the posterior eye through the optic disc, the point of entry for the optic nerve. At the center of the disc is a cup-like physiologic depression which is normally less than one-half the optic disc diameter. Another important retinal landmark is the **macula**, in which rods and cones are highly concentrated. At the center of the macula is a depression known as the **fovea centralis**, or point of central vision.

Ciliary muscles control the lens to focus light on the retinal surface, particularly on the fovea centralis. The **iris** lies before the lens and its opening creates the pupil. Eye colors (blue, brown, green) depend upon the pigmentary cells in the iris.

The **eyeball** consists of an anterior and a posterior chamber. The jelly-like fluid of the vitreous body fills the posterior chamber of the eyeball, transmits light, and supports the lens and retina. Unlike the aqueous humor, the vitreous fluid (i.e., the vitreous humor) is not continuously replenished. The aqueous humor is a clear liquid that fills the anterior and posterior divisions of the anterior chamber of the eyeball. The ciliary body (muscular tissue controlling the shape of the lens) produces aqueous humor. Fluid secreted in the posterior chamber of the anterior eye flows through the pupil into the anterior chamber. It is then reabsorbed through a network of trabeculae into the canal of Schlemm, a venous channel at the junction between the iris and the cornea (see Figure 5.3). Any obstruction in this pattern of fluid flow causes acute or chronic increase in intraocular pressure (i.e., glaucoma).

Eye Movement

Autonomic and cranial nerves regulate eye movement and vision. The oculomotor nerve (cranial nerve 3) constricts pupillary muscles and directs eye movements in the

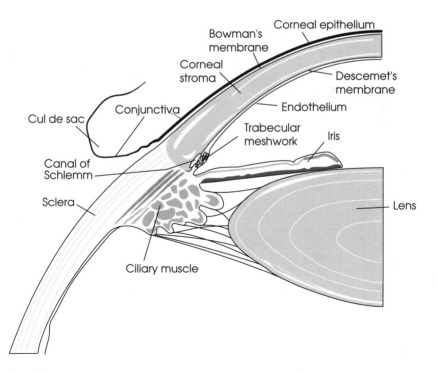

Fig 5.3   The anterior chamber of the eye. Aqueous humor forms in the area of the ciliary muscles, flows between the lens and iris to the anterior compartment to be absorbed into the canal of Schlemm through the trabecular meshwork.

fields of vision except the lateral and downward vision to the nose. Cranial nerve 4 controls downward, inward eye movement, and cranial nerve 6 controls lateral eye movement. Six extraocular muscles, 2 oblique and 4 recti, coordinate synchronous eye movements to facilitate depth of vision and prevent double vision. These extraocular muscles attach to the sclera and ocular orbit. Muscular imbalances cause various visual disturbances such as strabismus (i.e., wandering eye), diplopia (i.e., double vision), and ptosis (i.e., drooping of the upper eyelid; see Figure 5.9).

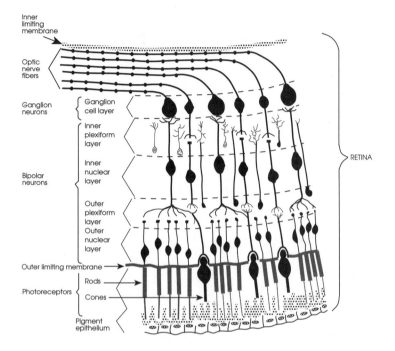

Fig 5.4   A cross-sectional view of the retina. Light passes through the lens to focus on the retina. Penetrating the inner limiting membrane, light is reflected off the pigmented epithelium and stimulates the rods and cones. The impulse is then transmitted through the optic nerve to the visual cortex of the brain.

Both sympathetic and parasympathetic nerves control autonomic functions. Stimulation of the adrenergic nerve endings contracts the radial iris muscle and relaxes the ciliary muscle for far vision. Cholinergic stimulation contracts the ciliary muscle and the sphincter iris muscle for near vision.

Vision

Each eye has a layer of receptors (i.e., rods and cones), a system for focusing light on these receptors (i.e., lens system), and a system of nerves (e.g., optic nerve) for conducting impulses from the receptors to the brain. For a patient to view an object, reflected light must pass through the cornea, pupil, lens, and vitreous body and focus on the retina. The light then stimulates the rods and cones on the retinal surface (see Figure 5.4). The rods (i.e., receptors for night vision) and cones (i.e., receptors for bright vision) transmit electrical impulses through the optic nerve (cranial nerve 2) and optic tract to the primary visual receiving area of the brain (i.e., the visual cortex).

The spatial arrangement of the optic nerve fibers in the optic nerve tract divides the eye into **visual fields**. The visual field of each eye is the portion of the external environment that is visible out of that eye. When a lesion disturbs the flow of impulses along the optic pathways, visual fields are lost. **Hemianopsia** is the term used to describe defective vision or blindness in half of the visual field. For example, a stroke patient may see only the right half of a visual field because of damage to the right optic tract. In this particular example, the visual pattern is termed left homonymous hemianopsia since the image projected by the eye reverses the side of the field. This patient only sees the right half of his body and environment because damage to the right optic tract has impaired his ability to see the left side of his visual field.

The eyes have protective reflexes. When a beam of light shines into one eye, the pupil automatically constricts (i.e., direct light reflex); simultaneously, the opposite pupil constricts (i.e., consensual light reflex). Consensual pupil constriction results when light-generated electrical impulses are transmitted over the optic nerve and optic tract. Upon reaching the midbrain, the electrical impulse diverges back through the oculomotor nerve to the opposite eye.

The process by which the curvature of the lens is increased to adjust the eye for viewing objects at various distances is called **accommodation**. Accommodation shifts the eye's focus from a distant object to a near object. For binocular accommodation (i.e., accommodation in both eyes), the eyes converge, the pupils constrict, and the lenses thicken, resulting in a bending of light rays onto the retina. Normal accommodation is the result of nerve impulse propagation from the occipital cortex, midbrain, parasympathetic control, and oculomotor nerve. Accommodation is also a function of compliance of the lens to refraction. After about 40 years of age, a person's lenses increasingly harden, resulting in a loss of accommodation that generally is sufficient to make reading and close eye work difficult. This loss of accommodation leads to the condition known as **presbyopia** which can be resolved by wearing glasses with convex lenses (i.e., reading eyeglasses).

PHYSICAL ASSESSMENT

Visual Testing

Visual acuity is a measure of a patient's central vision and the function of cranial nerve 2. It can be determined by comparing the clarity of the patient's vision at a

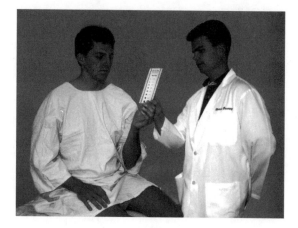

Fig 5.5 The hand-held Rosenbaum pocket vision screener is used to assess farsightedness (hyperopia).

specific distance to an expected norm using an eye chart. Visual acuity is expressed as a fraction (20/20). The numerator is the patient's vision and the denominator is normal acuity at 20 feet. Visual acuity can be tested at the bedside by evaluating the patient's ability to read lettering of various sizes in a magazine or newspaper; however, in the office or clinic, the Snellen Chart is used. Ask the patient to sit or stand 20 feet from the chart, to remove eye glasses (if worn), and to cover one eye. Point to the 20/20 line on the chart, and instruct the patient to read all letters. If the patient correctly identifies all letters, visual acuity need not be further evaluated. If the patient cannot read the 20/20 line, keep choosing a line with larger letters above the 20/20 line on the chart until the patient succeeds in correctly reading at least half the letters on one line. Record the number associated with that line (e.g., 20/30). Evaluate the visual acuity of the opposite eye in a similar manner. If the patient has **myopia** (i.e., nearsightedness), the denominator increases before the patient can read the letter (e.g., 20/200). **Hyperopia** (i.e., farsightedness) can be evaluated by asking the patient to read the letters of a handheld card (e.g., Rosenbaum pocket vision screener) at a distance of 14 inches (see Figure 5.5).

Tonometry is the measurement of **intraocular pressure** (IOP) and is determined by assessing the resistance of the eyeball to an applied force (e.g., a puff of air). Tonometry requires special equipment and is usually performed in the office of an ophthalmologist or optometrist. The volume of aqueous humor is the major determinant of intraocular pressure in the eye. Over-production of aqueous humor or obstruction of aqueous humor outflow increases intraocular pressure. One method of measuring IOP involves placing an applanometer upon the cornea of the anesthetized eye and using a table of conversion values to provide a result that is reported in mm Hg (normally less than 20 mm Hg). Another method of measuring IOP utilizes a sudden puff of air against the cornea (air-puff tonometer). Increased IOP characterizes a group of conditions known as glaucoma. In early stages of the disease, glaucoma may have no other accompanying symptoms or signs. With time, the increased intraocular pressure produces characteristic changes in the optic disc, visible upon inspection with an ophthalmoscope.

External Exam

Examine the **eyelids** for ptosis, edema, inflammation, and masses. Look for eyelid retraction, eyelid eversion (i.e., ectropion; see Figure 5.10), eyelid inversion (i.e., entropion; see Figure 5.11), and basal cell carcinoma. Inspect the eyelid margins for scaling, crusting, exudates, or pustules. Inflamed eyelids with associated scales and crusting at the base of the eyelashes, and with evidence of a secondary infection by *Staphylococci sp.* or *Streptococci sp.* can be encountered in patients with seborrheic dermatitis. Other eyelid diseases include: acute hordeolum or sty (an inflamed sebaceous gland resulting in a pustule on the eyelid margin; see Figure 5.12); chalazion (an infection of a meibomian gland; see Figure 5.13); xanthelasma (slowly growing, yellow plaques on the eyelids frequently associated with hypercholesterolemia; see Figure 5.14); and dacryocystitis (swelling anterior to the eyelid caused by obstruction of the nasolacrimal duct).

Systemic diseases can also cause physical changes in the appearance of the eyelids and surrounding tissues. Renal disorders, for example, can cause periorbital edema. Hypothyroidism is often accompanied by eyelids characterized by a dry, waxy type of swelling with abnormal deposits of mucin (i.e., myxedema). Hyperthyroidism can be accompanied by an abnormal protrusion of the eyeball (i.e., exophthalmos or proptosis; see Figures 5.15 and 8.12); tonic spasm of the orbicularis oculi muscle producing closure of the eyelids (i.e., blepharospasm); fasciculation or twitching of ocular muscles; failure of the upper eyelid to move downward with the eyeball when looking downward (i.e., lid lag or von Graefe's sign); or loss of the outer one-third of the eyebrows.

After completing the examination of the eyelids, continue the external eye evaluation by inspecting the **bulbar conjunctiva** and the blood vessels in the conjunctiva. A few conjunctival blood vessels may be dilated under normal conditions, or the vasodilation may reflect conjunctival irritation caused by allergens, viral or bacterial infections, or foreign bodies. When the conjunctivae are inflamed, patients complain that their eyes are itchy and feel as if they have sand in them. Conjunctival inflammation can also be accompanied by purulent discharge or a dry, crusted exudate on the lids. A physician should be consulted when moderate to severe eye pain, sensitivity to light, or blurred vision is experienced by a patient. The **pinguecula** is a small, raised, fatty tissue under the conjunctiva. When the pinguecula becomes inflamed, it can occasionally cause a vascular membrane called the **pterygium** to grow toward the cornea (see Figure 5.16).

To inspect the lower **palpebral conjunctiva** located at the anterior edge of the eyelid margins, gently pull the lower eyelid away from the eyeball. If indicated, inspect the conjunctiva of the upper eyelid by placing the handle-end of a cotton tip applicator about 1 cm above the upper eyelid margin, and gently evert the eyelid by turning up the upper lash and lid over the applicator. This procedure is uncomfortable for the patient and must be performed gently. Examine the conjunctiva for color. A pale-colored conjunctiva suggests possible anemia. A reddened conjunctiva is caused by multiple dilated blood vessels. When these dilated vessels radiate out from the iris and are accompanied by acute eye pain and mydriasis, acute glaucoma is a distinct possibility. Bright red blood under the conjunctiva could simply be caused by a benign subconjunctival hemorrhage.

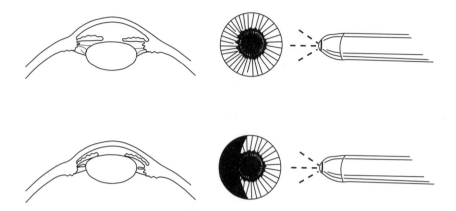

Fig. 5.6   With increased intraocular pressure in narrow angle glaucoma, the lens is pushed forward into the anterior chamber of the eye. This narrows the angle between the iris and the cornea. When light is directed across the cornea this change in angle results in the appearance of a shadow.

Continue the eye exam by inspecting the **cornea** which should be smooth and clear. Shining a beam of light at an oblique angle to the cornea helps to detect corneal scratches and opacities. When a crescent moon-like shadow is seen over the iris opposite the shining light, it could represent increased intraocular pressure. The size of the crescent generally increases as intraocular pressure increases (see Figure 5.6). The iris should appear flat. In closed angle glaucoma, however, the iris may bulge forward and cast the crescentic shadow described above. Next, examine the iris and lens for clarity and color by looking for opacities and growths.

Direct a beam of light tangentially onto the iris to inspect for possible lipid deposits in the periphery (**corneal arcus**; see Figure 5.17). Such lipid deposits are frequently seen in the aged (i.e., **arcus senilis**) or in the younger person with hyperlipidemia. When a penlight shines a beam of light at an angle through the pupil onto the lens, the appearance of a grayish area against a black background indicates an area of opacity in the lens (i.e., a cataract; see Figure 5.18). A cataract appears blackish against a reddish background when viewed through the ophthalmoscope. Although cataracts are commonly found in elderly patients, some drugs (e.g., allopurinol) can also cause cataracts.

After examining the eyelids, conjunctiva, cornea, iris, and lens, inspect the pupil and the iris. The **pupil** is the round "hole" in the center of the eye that is surrounded by the loosely pigmented iris. Normal pupils are round, of equal size, and react by constricting bilaterally, equally, and consensually to light. To examine the pupil, direct light from a flashlight at a 25° angle from the side into one of the patient's eyes in a darkened room. To minimize the patient's use of accommodation to fixate on the light, do not shine the light directly into the eye. Use a brief darting movement and avoid focusing the light continuously into the eye. When light shines into one eye, both pupils should constrict simultaneously, and to a nearly equal degree. Repeat the procedure with the other eye. The pupils normally should constrict equally, be round, and react promptly to light and accommodation (PERRLA). If bilateral, equal, and consensual constriction does not occur, the presence of a nerve lesion is suggested. **Anisocoria** is a normal variation in which pupils may be of unequal size but both react normally to light accommodation. The **tonic pupil** initially does not seem to be reacting, but with closer scrutiny, it is seen to be merely reacting slowly to light and accommodation. The tonic pupil, also known as Adie's pupil, is a benign condition. Bilateral, fixed, and dilated pupils that fail to constrict in response to light can be the result of anticholinergic drugs, severe brain damage, or sedative overdose. Bilateral, fixed, and constricted pupils can be the result of a pontine hemorrhage or narcotic overdose.

To test accommodation and convergence, ask the patient to focus on a distant object, then to focus on your finger. Your finger should be held stationary throughout the test about 12 inches from the patient's nose. Normally, the patient's eyes will converge and pupils constrict when focusing for near vision. A complaint of "seeing double" (diplopia) by the patient indicates an abnormal finding.

To test the **extraocular muscles** and **nerves**, instruct the patient to direct his eye movements in each of six cardinal directions. Holding the patient's chin to prevent head movement, direct the patient to follow your finger as you move it through the six cardinal fields of gaze. Move your finger to the right lateral position, to your right and up, then down, and return to the center position (see Figure 5.7.) Together these movements form the letter "H." Repeat these movements on the left side. Normally, both eyes move together and provide evidence that the extraocular muscles are intact (EOMI). Pause in the lateral and

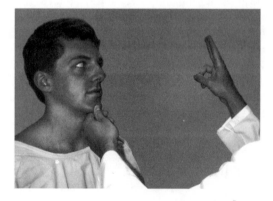

Fig. 5.7 The function of extraocular muscles and nerves is tested by having the patient focus on your finger as you move it through the six cardinal fields of gaze. Hold the patient's chin steady with your other hand.

upward positions to detect **nystagmus**. A few repetitive jerky movements of the eyes (i.e., nystagmus) are normal in the extreme lateral position. Nystagmus can be characterized according to the direction of the fastest eye movement. If the eyes move rapidly to the right and slowly return to the left, the nystagmus is termed horizontal or lateral nystagmus. Nystagmus also can be described as vertical or rotary in direction; fast or slow in speed; and fine or coarse in amplitude. Some drugs (e.g., phenytoin) disturb cerebellum function and induce nystagmus.

If hyperthyroidism is suspected as a cause of ocular muscle or nerve aberrations, instruct the patient to follow your finger as you move it rapidly downward. Normally, the eyes move downward with the upper eyelids covering the upper sclera and iris. If the patient's eyes move downward without movement of upper eyelid, and the upper sclera is exposed as a consequence, **lid lag** is present (Von Graefe's sign). The inability of either one or both eyes to move appropriately shows a potential muscle or nerve problem. To test **peripheral vision** when a neurologic problem or

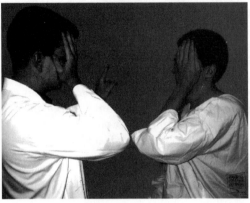

Fig. 5.8　The confrontation method is used to test a patient's peripheral vision when a neurologic problem or glaucoma is suspected.

glaucoma is suspected, use the confrontation method. When both you and the patient are at equal height, instruct the patient to cover one eye and to gaze directly into your opposite eye (i.e., the patient's right eye looking into your left eye). Positioned two feet in front of the patient, close your corresponding eye and wigwag two fingers moving in a clockwise direction in the periphery of the patient's field of vision. Hold your testing hand at an equal distance between the patient and yourself (see Figure 5.8). In the temporal field of vision, start slightly behind the patient. Assuming you have normal peripheral vision, compare your visual field with the patient's visual field. Repeat the procedure with the opposite eye.

Ophthalmoscopy

An important and informative part of eye assessment is the ophthalmoscopic evaluation of the eye. The ophthalmoscope enables the examiner to inspect the cornea, anterior chamber, lens, posterior chamber, and the retina along with its vasculature and anatomical landmarks.

A successful ophthalmoscopic examination requires cooperation from the patient and should be conducted in a darkened room. The pupils usually are not dilated during a routine examination; however, dilation of the pupil with a mydriatic agent allows inspection of a larger portion of the retina. The use of mydriatics are contraindicated if narrow angle glaucoma is suspected. Instruct the patient to remove contact lenses and ask whether either a cataract lens (aphakia) or artificial (e.g., "glass") eye have been implanted.

Several types of ophthalmoscopes are available with various apertures and colored filters. For most exams, use the large, round white beam and start the lens at "0" on the lens dial. Adjust the lens dial to lengthen the focus (red numbers) for the myopic (nearsighted) eye, or shorten the focus (black numbers) for the hyperopic (farsighted) eye. To get an approximation for a correct lens dial setting, hold your hand about three inches from the ophthalmoscope and adjust the lens dial to bring the skin lines of your hand into clear focus. An ophthalmoscopic exam requires a considerable amount of supervised practice; with experience, the wide range of normal variants can be differentiated from abnormal variants.

When corneal reflection interferes with good visualization of the retina, use the small spot aperture of the ophthalmoscope or direct the light beam to the edge of the pupil to correct this problem.

With the patient seated at your eye level in a dimly lighted room, ask the patient to focus on a distant object. With the ophthalmoscope held against your right eye, study the patient's right eye. Approach the patient's eye at a 25° angle lateral to the patient's line of vision. You should be about two inches away from the patient's right eye. While steadying the patient's head with your left hand, shine the light beam into the pupil and look for the "red reflex," which is light reflecting off the retina. Follow the red reflex and rotate the lens dial of the ophthalmoscope until you focus in on the retina. To examine the left eye, repeat these steps except hold the ophthalmoscope in your left hand, use your left eye, and stand at the patient's left side.

When conducting an ophthalmoscopic exam, remember there are wide variations in normal findings. The most conspicuous feature of the normal yellowish-pinkish **fundus** is the optic disc. Find a peripheral blood vessel and follow it until you find the optic disc. Look toward the patient's nose to find the disk. Examine the optic disc for size, shape, color, and margins. The optic disc has a sharp border demarcating its normally yellowish to creamy-pink color from the deeper color of the retina. The presence of dark pigment crescents along the disk's border is normal. The physiologic cup, a pale area on the side of the disc, does not contain nerve fibers and, as a result, forms a depression, or a cup. The normal cup size is less than one-half the total optic disc diameter. Major changes in the optic disc are associated with optic atrophy and glaucoma. With glaucoma, the physiological cup exceeds the normal diameter (see Figure 5.22). Changes characteristic of glaucoma within the disc result from increased intraocular pressure. The disc takes on an abnormal curvature and backward displacement and the color of an ischemic disc becomes pale. Prolonged, increased intraocular pressure leads to the death of the optic nerve and blindness.

Next, inspect the **retinal blood vessels**. When examining the vessels, view the principle vessel in each of the four eye quadrants (i.e., the right, left, upper, and lower quadrants). Then examine the periphery of the retina by looking through the ophthalmoscope while holding it steady and instructing the patient to look at a distant point. The size, color, and arteriovenous crossings of the retinal vessels should be noted. Arteries are easily distinguishable from veins because arteries are smaller in diameter, brighter red in color, and have a thin arteriolar light reflex (i.e., a white stripe) in the center of the artery. In the normal retina, arteries and veins cross in a random manner. These arteriovenous crossings are evaluated for the presence of abnormal venous indentations (i.e., A-V nicking) where the thickened artery "indents" the vein, narrowing it before and after it passes next to the artery (see Figure 5.19). A-V nicking is associated with atherosclerotic disease and is commonly seen in patients with chronic, untreated hypertension. Besides nicking, the retinal findings of hypertension include arteriolar narrowing ("copper wire-like"), hemorrhages, exudates, or papilledema. In addition to these abnormal findings, a diabetic patient with hypertension also may have neovascularization (see Figure 5.22).

Veins are slightly larger, darker, and do not have the prominent light reflex seen in arteries. A slight, visible pulsation appears at the proximal end of the vein where it overlies the optic disc margin. Retinal veins, in contrast to retinal arteries, normally pulsate.

The **macula,** an area on the retina lateral to the optic disc, deserves special study. If it is difficult to inspect, instruct the patient to look directly into the ophthalmoscope in order to place the macula in the center of your visual field. However, you only have a few brief moments to view the macula because the light creates considerable discomfort for the patient. The miniature spot of reflected light seen in the center of the macula is a small, fine depression called the **fovea centralis.** It is the point of central vision. Senile macula degeneration (SMD), or impairment of central vision, is a common problem in the elderly (see Figure 5.20).

PHARMACOTHERAPEUTIC CASE ILLUSTRATION

History

J.L., a 72-year-old male, was evaluated for a chief complaint (CC) of "blurred vision, especially in my left eye." History of present illness (HPI) noted occasional mild headaches. The headaches primarily seemed to originate from behind both eyes and he attributed them to the need for new eyeglasses. He also reported "my vision is worse."

Past medical history (PMH) was important for moderate essential hypertension, diabetes mellitus (diet controlled), and peptic ulcer disease. Social history (SH) was positive for cigarette smoking 1 pack per day for 35 years. He drank 1 to 2 glasses of wine at supper. Family history (FH) noted that his father died at age 72 of an acute myocardial infarction. His mother is living and in good health. Review of systems (ROS) was unremarkable except for the eye problems as described in the present illness. Drug history (DH) noted clonidine 0.1 mg tablet PO BID, potassium chloride slow-release tablet 10 mEq PO QD, and hydrochlorothiazide 25 mg tablet PO QD. The patient also self-prescribed magnesium/aluminum hydroxide gel 1 tablespoonful PO PRN indigestion, and ibuprofen 200 mg tablet 1 or 2 PO 4 to 6 times per day for headache.

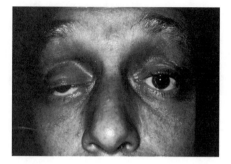

Fig. 5.9 Ptosis of the eyelid. Despite the patient's attempt to open the eyelid by also raising the eyebrows, the right eyelid remains almost closed. Weakness is present in the levators of both upper eyelids; however, the right is more marked than the left.

Fig. 5.10 Ectropion is an eversion of the eyelid resulting from aging or scar formation. It may lead to poor drainage of tears through the nasolacrimal system and thus prevent necessary moistening of the sclera and cornea.

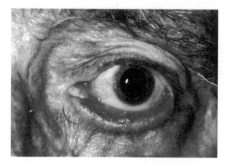

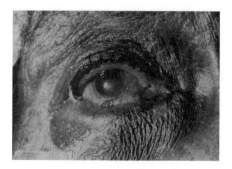

Fig. 5.11 Entropin results from aging and a loss of turgor of the eyelid or from scar formation. This inversion of the eyelid can cause irritation of the globe from eyelashes. If not managed properly, it may result in corneal ulceration and/or scarring.

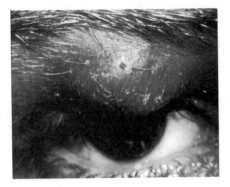

Fig. 5.12 Hordeolum (i.e., sty) is an acute localized pyogenic infection (usually staphylococcal) of the glands of the eyelid. Note the dark, swollen appearance.

Fig. 5.13 Chalazion is a chronic granulomatous enlargement of an eyelid meibomian gland. Often following inflammation, the gland duct becomes occluded. Eversion of the lower eyelid reveals a nodule of similar color and texture as the surrounding conjunctive.

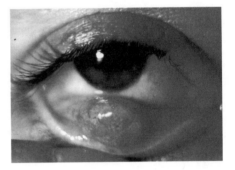

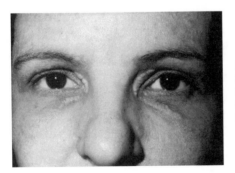

Fig. 5.14 Xanthelasma is a condition characterized by lipid-filled lesions of the skin commonly located in the periorbital arc. It is believed to be associated with marked hypercholesterolemia.

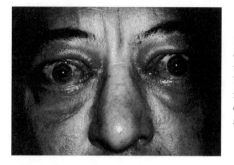

Fig. 5.15 Frontal view of exophthalmos (i.e., proptosis). Note how the sclera is easily seen both above and below the limbus of the cornea. The redness of the sclera suggests that the eyelids are not able to completely close and keep the cornea and sclera moist.

Fig. 5.16 Often found in dry, hot climates, a pterygium is a fleshy conjunctival growth onto the cornea that may distort the cornea, thus affecting visual acuity.

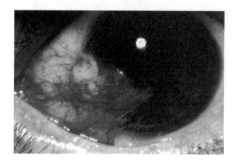

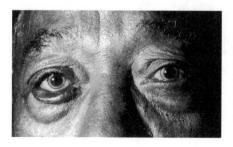

Fig. 5.17 Arcus senilis. In the area of the limbus where the cornea meets the sclera, there is a thickened white line representing deposits of fat. The outfolding of the lower lid of the right eye with exposure of the palperbral conjunctiva is called ectropion.

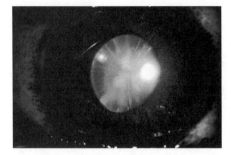

Fig. 5.18 Cataract. With aging, opacities form in the lens of the eye. As these opacities increase in number and size, less light passes through the lens, impairing vision.

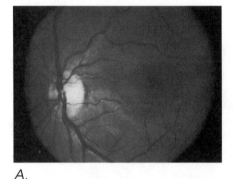

A.

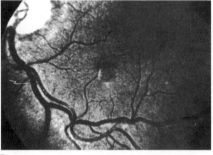

B.

Fig. 5.19 A. Normal retina with retinal blood vessels seen spreading from the site of the optic disk. B. Retina with signs of A-V nicking associated with atherosclerotic disease. Note the indentations in veins at points where they cross thickened arteries.

Fig. 5.20 Senile macular degeneration. In the center of the retina can be seen a blackened area with pale patches of retina immediately adjacent. This is where the fovea centralis is located. The changes represent early atrophy and degeneration of this macular area.

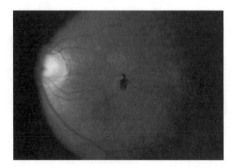

Physical Examination

The visual acuity of J.L.'s right eye was 20/40 and his left eye was 20/70. Applanation tonometry readings for the right eye were 30 mm Hg, and 50 mm Hg for the left eye. External structures of the eye were normal and extraocular muscles were intact (EOMI). Peripheral vision was determined to be decreased by confrontation testing; his pupils were equal, round, and reactive to light and accommodation (PERRLA). Funduscopic exam showed no cataracts. Retinal findings were normal, except for mild optic disc cupping.

Diagnosis and Management

A diagnosis of chronic open-angle glaucoma is consistent with J.L.'s symptoms and findings on physical examination. Pilocarpine 1% ophthalmic solution (1 drop in right eye and 2 drops in left eye QID) was prescribed. The patient was instructed to use only acetaminophen for pain and headaches. He was scheduled for follow-up tonometry in two weeks.

Discussion

Disease. Primary open-angle glaucoma (POAG) should be suspected when a patient is over age 40, has insidious worsening of vision, and mild headaches. The disorder is characterized by a slow, progressive loss of peripheral vision, a gradual rise in intraocular pressure, and, lastly, blindness. Unlike acute-angle-closure glaucoma, the pathogenesis of open-angle glaucoma is not due to blockage of aqueous humor drainage.

J.L. complained of blurred vision, which is a symptom of many common ocular disorders, including glaucoma. Glaucoma is fairly common in older people and some clinicians recommend that all people over the age of 40 should have a yearly evaluation of intraocular pressure (IOP), especially in diabetic patients and patients with a family history of glaucoma. Increases in IOP generally are not noticed by people until their vision is altered. J.L. was mildly diabetic and thus at an increased risk for POAG and cataracts. The IOP of 30 mm Hg in the right eye and 50 mm Hg in the left eye was elevated (normal: <20 mm Hg) and suggested chronic glaucoma. A repeated evaluation of IOP should confirm the persistence of the IOP elevation. J.L.'s peripheral vision was noted to be impaired and more detailed peripheral testing seems warranted. Seeing halos around electric lights and impaired adaptation to the dark are other visual symptoms associated with glaucoma.

Cupping of the optic disc is a characteristic finding in glaucoma; however, a normal cup to disc ratio (normal: 1:2) does not exclude chronic glaucoma. Chronic excessive intraocular pressure damages the optic nerve which leads to atrophy. The optic disc may appear pale.

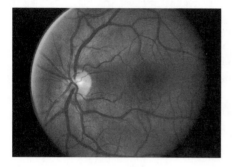

Fig. 5.21 Normal retina. The dark area to the left of the center is the fovea centralis with its concentration of rods and cones providing the point of greatest visual acuity. To the right of the fovea is the optic disc or head of the optic nerve. Note the retinal blood vessels spreading out over the retina from their point of entry at the optic disk.

Fig. 5.22 Glaucoma is the result of increased intraocular pressure. This is seen during retinal examination as increased pallor of the optic disk and a "curving under" of the vessels as they pass over the edge of the disk.

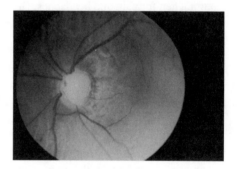

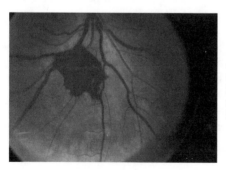

Fig. 5.22 Nonproliferative retinopathy of diabetes mellitus is characterized by increased capillary permeability, microaneurysms, hemorrhages (as seen here), exudates, and edema.

Management. Cholinergic drugs are administered topically to cause miosis and constrict the ciliary muscles in order to facilitate aqueous fluid drainage from the anterior chamber. Pilocarpine, a naturally occurring alkaloid, acts directly on the cholinergic receptor. Pilocarpine therapy should be initiated with a low dose of the weakest available preparation and the dose should be gradually increased in response to the results of sequential IOP measurements. No more than 2 drops of the cholinergic drug should be instilled into the conjunctiva sac. The most troublesome side effects of cholinergic drugs such as pilocarpine are blurred vision and poor night vision. The impairment of night vision by pilocarpine may limit its use in some patients. Systemic parasympathetic toxicities such as bradycardia, abdominal cramping, and wheezing may be a problem with concentrations of pilocarpine greater than 2%. J.L. should be instructed to occlude his lacrimal ducts by applying light pressure on the medial eyelids in order to decrease drainage into the gastrointestinal tract and thus reduce systemic absorption.

J.L. was initially prescribed pilocarpine 1%. Because IOP varied between eyes, a higher dose was prescribed for the left eye and this dose was adjusted based upon measurements of IOP. Epinephrine, or acetazolamide, could be added to J.L.'s cholinergic therapy if the IOP is reduced adequately. Timolol, a beta-blocker which purportedly reduces aqueous fluid formation, may not be a good choice in this diabetic patient because of its unpredictable ability to induce rare hypoglycemic reactions and cardiovascular side effects (e.g., bradycardia). In non-diabetic patients, a beta-blocking eye drop can be used safely and is the drug of choice in POAG.

Drugs may induce *de nova* or aggravate existing glaucoma. Primary-angle-closure glaucoma (PACG) is easily induced by many drugs with atropine-like properties. In this patient, ibuprofen, a nonsteroidal anti-inflammatory drug, may have contributed to increased IOP. Although J.L. was instructed to use acetaminophen rather than ibuprofen, adequate treatment of increased IOP by topical agents generally precludes the potential for increased IOP caused by systemic medications. Prolonged topical corticosteroid therapy, however, can increase IOP within the first two months. Any patient who experiences increasing intraocular pressure should have more frequent tonometry readings.

Therapeutic Drug Monitoring Examples

GLAUCOMA, PRIMARY OPEN ANGLE

The approach to theraputic drug monitoring by clinicians varies depending upon many factors. Some of these include preferences among clinicians in a given community or region; concurrent medical problems which dictate that certain drugs be used or avoided; the patient's response to selected medication. The following outlines of therapeutic drug monitoring offer examples which may serve to stimulate discussion and further understanding of initiating and monitoring drug use. The drugs and dosages presented should not be applied to any clinical situation without proper medical supervision.

Drug Therapy	Timolol ophthalmic solution 0.5% 1 drop each eye BID.
Monitoring	**Symptoms:** Quiz for visual field loss ("tunnel vision"), frequency of eyeglass changes, seeing halos around electric lights, or difficulty seeing at night.
	Signs: Check visual acuity with Snellen chart. Assess gross visual field loss with confrontation. Check pupil response to light and accommodation. Using tonometry, measure intraocular pressure. In funduscopic exam, inspect for enlarged cup-to-disc ratio, pale-appearing optic disc and retinal atrophy.
Laboratory Tests	The clinician may elect to order all, none, or some of these laboratory studies depending upon history and physical findings, as well as other clinical indications. Tonometry, serum blood glucose, ECG.
Adverse Drug Event Monitoring	Question about dizziness, headache, difficulty breathing, irregular heart beat, burning or stinging of eyes during eyedrop instillation. Measure blood pressure for hypotension. Palpate heart rate and rhythm for irregularity, slowness, or pounding. Listen to the chest for crackles or wheezes. Palpate lower extremities for signs of pitting edema (CHF).

Therapeutic Drug Monitoring Examples

ACUTE CONJUNCTIVITIS (BACTERIAL)

The approach to therapeutic drug monitoring by clinicians varies depending upon many factors. Some of these include preferences among clinicians in a given community or region; concurrent medical problems which dictate that certain drugs be used or avoided; the patient's response to selected medication. The following outlines of therapeutic drug monitoring offer examples which may serve to stimulate discussion and further understanding of initiating and monitoring drug use. The drugs and dosages presented should not be applied to any clinical situation without proper medical supervision.

Drug Therapy	Sulfacetamide 10% ophthalmic solution 1 drop both eyes QID. Wash affected eyelids with 50% baby shampoo BID.
Monitoring	**Symptoms:** Query for complaints of burning, itching, and purulent discharge, or complaints of "something in my eye" with mild visual blurring from eye discharge.
	Signs: Inspect for purulent discharge, moderate eyelid swelling, and diffuse peripheral conjunctival injection. Palpate preauricular nodes for enlargement. Check to see if conjunctival vessels are moveable.
Laboratory Tests	The clinician may elect to order all, none, or some of these laboratory studies depending upon history and physical findings, as well as other clinical indications. Gram's stain, culture, and sensitivity.
Adverse Drug Event Monitoring	Examine for symptoms and signs of eye irritation from sulfacetamide, such as stinging or burning sensation after instillation.

Therapeutic Drug Monitoring Examples

ACUTE CONJUNCTIVITIS (ALLERGIC)

The approach to therapuetic drug monitoring by clinicians varies depending upon many factors. Some of these include preferences among clinicians in a given community or region; concurrent medical problems which dictate that certain drugs be used or avoided; the patient's response to selected medication. The following outlines of therapeutic drug monitoring offer examples which may serve to stimulate discussion and further understanding of initiating and monitoring drug use. The drugs and dosages presented should not be applied to any clinical situation without proper medical supervision.

Drug Therapy	Fluorometholone ophthalmic solution 0.1% 1 drop in each eye QID.
Monitoring	**Symptoms:** Check for continuing complaints of watery, itching eyes without purulent discharge. Question about foreign body sensation and eye pain.
	Signs: Examine eyelids for redness and discharge. Palpate preauricular nodes for enlargement. Note if conjunctival vessels injected and blanch on pressure. Check to see if vessels are mobile over the sclera.
Laboratory Tests	None.
Adverse Drug Event Monitoring	Check for symptoms and signs of secondary infection with bacteria or virus. For long-term steroid use, periodic ophthalmologic examination by tonometry (glaucoma) and slip lamp (posterior subcapsular cataracts) is mandatory, especially in elderly and diabetic patients. Question about burning, stinging, or excessive watering of the eyes.

Therapeutic Drug Monitoring Examples

ACUTE HORDEOLUM (STY)

The approach to therapeutic drug monitoring by clinicians varies depending upon many factors. Some of these include preferences among clinicians in a given community or region; concurrent medical problems which dictate that certain drugs be used or avoided; the patient's response to selected medication. The following outlines of therapeutic drug monitoring offer examples which may serve to stimulate discussion and further understanding of initiating and monitoring drug use. The drugs and dosages presented should not be applied to any clinical situation without proper medical supervision.

Drug Therapy	Erythromycin 0.5% ophthalmic ointment applied in a small amount to affected eyelids at bedtime. Apply warm water compress TID. Wash affected external eyelid with 1:1 baby shampoo BID.
Monitoring	**Symptoms:** Check for eyelid pain and irritation.
	Signs: Examine the eyelids for redness and tenderness with a small, round, papule-like hair follicle. With suppuration, a small yellowish spot expresses a purulent discharge.
Laboratory Tests	The clinician may elect to order all, none, or some of these laboratory studies depending upon history and physical findings, as well as other clinical indications. Gram's stain, culture, and sensitivity.
Adverse Drug Event Monitoring	Question about clouding of vision by eye ointment. If symptoms and/or signs are not improved within 3–4 days, check for allergy to erythromycin or bacterial resistance.

Therapeutic Drug Monitoring Examples

BLEPHARITIS

The approach to therapuetic drug monitoring by clinicians varies depending upon many factors. Some of these include preferences among clinicians in a given community or region; concurrent medical problems which dictate that certain drugs be used or avoided; the patient's response to selected medication. The following outlines of therapeutic drug monitoring offer examples which may serve to stimulate discussion and further understanding of initiating and monitoring drug use. The drugs and dosages presented should not be applied to any clinical situation without proper medical supervision.

Drug Therapy	Apply a small amount of bacitracin ophthalmic ointment to eyelids HS. Wash both eyelids with 50% baby shampoo BID.
Monitoring	**Symptoms:** Inquire about foreign-body sensation, pain, itching, and photophobia. Determine if eyes are stuck together upon awakening.
	Signs: Inspect and palpate the eyelids for redness, swelling, loss of lashes, and scales. Note any crusting or discharge.
Laboratory Tests	The clinician may elect to order all, none, or some of these laboratory studies depending upon history and physical findings, as well as other clinical indications. Gram's stain, culture, and sensitivity.
Adverse Drug Event Monitoring	Question about blurred vision secondary to ointment. If symptoms and signs do not improve within 3 days, consider bacterial resistance or seborrheic component requiring topical corticosteroid.

Therapeutic Drug Monitoring Examples

ACUTE IRITIS (ANTERIOR UVEITIS)

The approach to therapuetic drug monitoring by clinicians varies depending upon many factors. Some of these include preferences among clinicians in a given community or region; concurrent medical problems which dictate that certain drugs be used or avoided; the patient's response to selected medication. The following outlines of therapeutic drug monitoring offer examples which may serve to stimulate discussion and further understanding of initiating and monitoring drug use. The drugs and dosages presented should not be applied to any clinical situation without proper medical supervision.

Drug Therapy	Atropine 1% eye drops, 1 drop TID. Dexamethasone 0.1% eye drops 1 drop QID.
Monitoring	**Symptoms:** Inquire about relief of eye pain, blurred vision, photophobia, and excessive lacrimation.
	Signs: Check change of visual acuity. Inspect the conjunctivae and irides for injected vessels (circumcorneal). Record excessive amount of lacrimal fluid. Note absence of small, fixed pupils (i.e., check light response). Palpate vessel for normal blanching. Look for posterior **synechiae** (adhesion of the iris to the cornea or to the lens) and **hypopyon** (an accumulation of pus in the anterior chamber of the eye).
Laboratory Tests	The clinician may elect to order all, none, or some of these laboratory studies depending upon history and physical findings, as well as other clinical indications. Tonometry, slit lamp.
Adverse Drug Event Monitoring	**Atropine:** Ask about troublesome night vision, blurring vision, and photophobia. Question about worsening eye pain and other findings suggesting acute glaucoma. Examine the eye for mydriasis. **Dexamethasone:** In long-term use, check intraocular tension (tonometry) and lens opacity (cataract–slit lamp examination). Ask if the patient sees halos around lights.

Therapeutic Drug Monitoring Examples

ACUTE IRITIS (ANTERIOR UVEITIS)
(continued)

Adverse Drug
Event Monitoring

Observe for signs associated with viral, bacterial, or fungal infection. Monitor frequently in diabetic patients.
Comment: Acute iritis can be a serious medical problem and should be managed by those experienced and trained to diagnose and manage the condition.

Ear

*T*he sensory receptors for hearing and equilibrium are found in the ear. The external ear, middle ear, and cochlea of the inner ear facilitate hearing by converting sound waves from the external environment into electrical impulses which are transmitted along the auditory nerves. The semicircular canals of the inner ear primarily control the sense of balance or equilibrium. Impaired sound transmission in the external or middle ear, or damage to neural pathways can cause clinical deafness. Diseases of the ear or ototoxic medications, therefore, can damage the ear and result in hearing or equilibrium dysfunction.

ANATOMY AND PHYSIOLOGY

External Ear

The external ear consists of the auricle and the external auditory canal. The most external part of the ear, the **auricle (pinna)** is composed of fibroelastic cartilage covered with skin. The prominent outermost fold of the ear is the **helix** and the inner concentric fold is the **antihelix**. Other landmarks of the external ear are depicted in Figure 6.1. The **auricle** is attached to the skull at the mastoid process. It usually forms a 30° angle with the side of the head and is innervated by cranial nerve 7 (facial). The adult auditory canal is about 2.5 cm long, and is surrounded by cartilage and bone. It is lined with sebaceous glands, hair follicles, and cerumen (wax) glands, and is served by sensory branches of the trigeminal and vagus cranial nerves. In the adult, the auditory canal points inwardly, then angles forward and down (see Figure 6.2). The inner bony part of the auditory canal is covered with very sensitive skin and flares to end at the tympanic membrane (eardrum) which is located in the middle ear.

Middle Ear

The middle ear is an air-filled, box-like structure that contains the tympanic membrane (the lateral wall), the three auditory ossicles, an opening to the eustachian tube (that, in turn, opens into the nasopharynx), and an opening to mastoid air cells. The **tympanic membrane** appears as a thin, semi-transparent, oval membrane that has the appearance of grayish-pink Saran™ wrap. The gray is the color of the membrane itself; the pink is the color of the normal mucous membrane lining the middle ear. The membrane is slightly concave because of its firm attachment to the handle of the malleus. When viewed through an otoscope, this concavity produces a

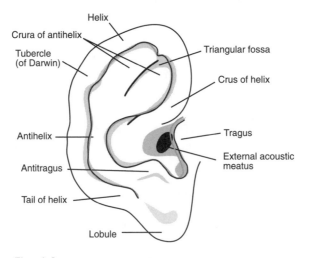

Fig. 6.1 External ear (auricle or pinna). The helix, lobule, tragus, and external acoustic meatus (opening into the external auditory canal) are frequently used during physical examination to evaluate deeper structures.

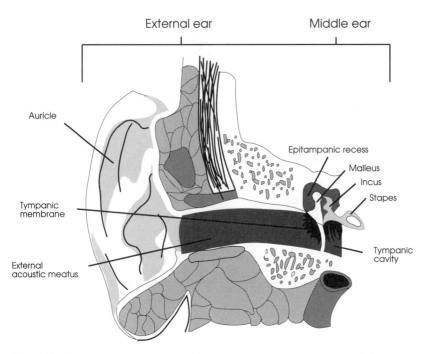

Fig. 6.2 The three compartments of the ear include the external ear (auricle to tympanic membrane), the middle ear (tympanic membrane to round window of inner ear) and the inner ear (see Figure 6.3).

landmark called the **cone of light** or **light reflex** located on the anterior inferior quadrant of the tympanic membrane; the apex, or center of the light reflex is called the **umbo** (see Figure 6.4).

The **ossicles** (**malleus, incus**, and **stapes**, which also are called the hammer, anvil, and stirrup, respectively) of the middle ear connect the eardrum to the cochlea of the inner ear behind the medial wall of the middle ear cavity. The mastoid air cells of the mastoid bone are connected posteriorly to the middle ear through an opening known as the ostium. The **eustachian tubes** open briefly during swallowing, yawning, or sneezing to allow air movement which equalizes pressure on both sides of the tympanic membrane. They also provide a passageway for the small amount of mucoid material continuously secreted by the middle ear mucosa to drain into the nasopharynx. In the adult, the eustachian tube is 3 to 4 cm long and forms an acute angle as it enters the nasal cavity. In infants and young children, the tube is shorter and has a less acute angle; this configuration hinders drainage and facilitates middle ear infections.

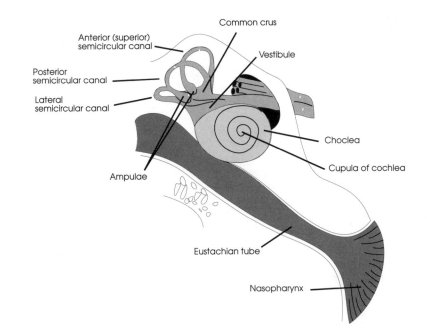

Fig.6.3 The primary structures of the inner ear, including the cochlea, which transmits sound, and the semicircular canals, which participate in maintaining equilibrium.

Inner ear

The inner ear contains the snail-shaped cochlea, the vestibule, and semicircular canals. The **cochlea** contains the organ of Corti, a structure housing small, hair-like auditory receptor cells suspended in fluid (see Figure 6.5). The cochlea receives sound and transmits it via the auditory branch of the eighth cranial nerve which passes through the bony internal auditory canal to the brain. The **semicircular canals** contain the sensing organs of balance. Sensing body position, these canals send messages along the vestibular branch of the eighth cranial nerve to the cerebellum.

Auditory and Vestibular Functions

The ear is functionally divided into two parts: the auditory and the vestibular systems.

Auditory Function. Sound waves travel along the ear canal and cause the tympanic membrane to vibrate (see Figure 6.4). As the tympanic membrane oscillates, the vibrations are then carried via the ossicles to the oval window of the cochlea. The vibrations are carried to the small hair-like sensors suspended in the organ of Corti. These sensors move and stimulate nerve endings which carry the impulses to the temporal lobe of the brain. Sound can also be conducted directly to the inner ear via bone, thereby bypassing the usual conductive sound pathway just described. This process is known as **bone conduction (BC)**. The detection of sound transmitted by way of the tympanic membrane and ossicles is termed **air conduction (AC)**. An audiogram is used to test for both air and bone conduction (see Figure 6.11).

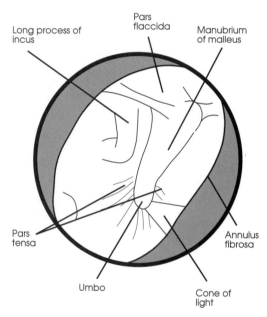

Long process of incus

Pars flaccida

Manubrium of malleus

Pars tensa

Annulus fibrosa

Umbo

Cone of light

Fig. 6.4 Landmarks of the tympanic membrane of the right ear.

Vestibular Function. Receptors located in the semicircular canals detect the body's orientation in relation to its environment (balance). These receptors sense changes in body (primarily head) position with respect to gravitational forces and then send impulses over the vestibular branch of the eighth cranial nerve to the cerebellum. Vision and proprioceptors (body position sensors) in the muscles and joints supplement the receptors in the semicircular canals in this process of maintaining the body in proper balance or equilibrium. A

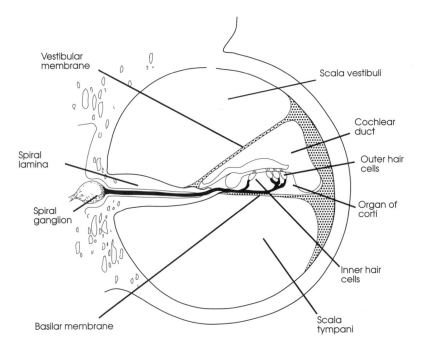

Fig. 6.5   Structure of the cochlea. This cross section of the cochlear canal demonstrates the vestibular membrane, the organ of corti, and auditory nerve fiber.

disturbance of the mechanisms that maintain balance (i.e., vision, proprioceptors, inner ear, cerebellum) results in **vertigo**.

Sound Pathways

Normal hearing depends upon two intact, functioning pathways: conductive and sensorineural. The conductive pathway requires normally functioning external and middle ear structures. The sensorineural pathway relies on a functioning inner ear and cochlea. Dysfunction in either pathway leads to reduced hearing or deafness.

When the ossicular conductive pathway is circumvented, the sensorineural pathway (acoustic branch of eighth cranial nerve) can be accessed by bone conduction. However, air conduction is normally more sensitive than bone conduction (i.e., AC>BC).

Hearing dysfunction can be the result of sensorineural loss, conductive loss, or sensori-conductive loss. Sensorineural hearing loss indicates a problem with the cochlea, the acoustic branch of the eighth cranial nerve, or the hearing center in the cerebral cortex. For example, as a person ages, demyelination of conductive pathways and degenerative changes in cortical centers result in diminished sensorineural function. These changes may result in the loss of a person's ability to discriminate sounds (e.g., pick out one person's spoken word in a noisy room). Patients affected by this disorder usually speak loudly and hear poorly in a crowded room or over the telephone. When sensorineural hearing is impaired, sounds are heard best in a quiet room. **Presbycusis** is another form of change in sensorineural hearing that occurs in the elderly and in middle-aged persons who have been exposed to high noise levels without proper ear protection. In this situation, the sensory hair cells of the cochlea lose their ability to sense certain frequencies of sound (usually higher frequencies first).

Conductive hearing loss results from a disturbance in sound transmission through the ear canal, tympanic membrane, middle ear, or ossicles. A person with conductive hearing loss generally speaks softly and is able to hear in a crowded room or over the telephone. Middle ear infections, a ruptured eardrum, and cerumen impaction in the ear canal can cause conductive loss. Sensori-conductive hearing loss is a combination of both conductive and sensorineural dysfunction.

PHYSICAL ASSESSMENT

External Ear

Routine assessment begins with inspection and palpation of the external ear. Examine the auricle for abnormal size, sebaceous cysts, skin cancers, and other skin lesions.

Fig. 6.6 Audiogram: Each ear is tested at pre-selected frequencies (H_2). For each frequency the chart is marked at the level (decibel) the sound is first heard. The circles indicate readings for the right ear; the Xs readings for the left. < represents bone conduction in the right ear; > represents bone conduction in the left. High frequency hearing loss encountered in elderly patients is termed presbycusis. This audiogram reflects this type of hearing loss.

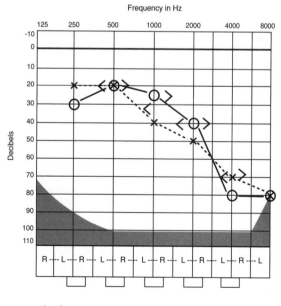

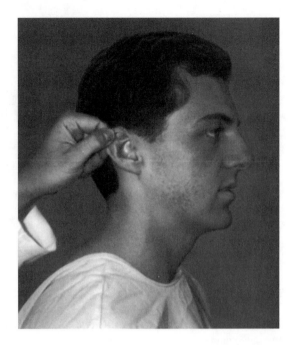

Fig. 6.7 Inspect and palpate the auricle for abnormal size, sebaceous cysts, skin cancers, and other lesions. As illustrated, grasp the helix and with a gentle tug, straighten the external auditory canal to facilitate visualization of the tympanic membrane with the otoscope.

Look for low-set auricles, congenitally large auricles (i.e., congenital renal disease or Down's syndrome), or disproportionately large auricles (i.e., acromegaly or normal aging). Sebaceous cysts in the lobule or behind the ear may become a problem for some patients. Wearing earrings may lead to swollen, tender, and infected earlobes (lobules). Although earlobe creases are believed to indicate a risk factor for coronary heart disease in young or middle-aged persons, this finding is confusing in the aged because of normal aging changes. The monosodium urate tophi of gout can appear as hard, pale, nontender nodules on the helix and antihelix of the auricle. Darwin's nodule, a thickening on the superior helix, is a benign finding. Venous lakes, actinic (solar) keratosis, and skin cancer (e.g., basal cell or squamous cell) may appear on the auricle, especially behind the ears. Seborrheic dermatitis also can be detected on and around the ears. When palpating the mastoid process for tenderness or swelling, look for a serous discharge coming from the auditory canal or for other signs suggestive of external or middle ear infection, such as swelling and erythema.

Otoscopic Exam

Use an otoscope to inspect the ear canal and tympanic membrane. Choose an aural speculum (the cone-shaped attachment for the otoscope) that comfortably fits into the patient's ear canal. To prevent nosocomial infection, use either a disinfected or disposable speculum. If in question about its sterility, wash the speculum with 70% alcohol or antiseptic soap, then rinse with sterile water.

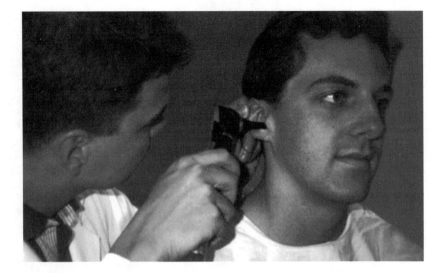

Fig. 6.8   Otoscopic examination of ear canal and tympanic membrane.

The larger the speculum opening you use, the easier it is to inspect the ear canal and tympanic membrane. Hold the otoscope comfortably in your hand (right or left). Most examiners hold the instrument as if they are holding a hammer. Another method is to hold the otoscope with its head pointing down so that the ulnar edge of your hand rests against the patient's head. This technique gives the examiner more stability and control which becomes especially important with an uncooperative patient.

Before inserting the speculum into the auditory canal, ask if the patient is experiencing any ear pain. Then press on the tragus and gently tug on the earlobe or auricle to detect a complaint of pain which could be a sign of ear canal infection. Pain can also be referred to the ear because of a dental abscess, oral cancer, or temporomandibular joint (TMJ) disease. If pain is elicited by this process, inspect the painful ear after examining the normal ear. Tilt the patient's head away and hold it at eye level. When examining an adult, grip the auricle at the superior helix and gently pull upward, back, and slightly out to straighten the normally curved auditory canal (see Figure 6.8). With young children, gently pull the auricle straight back. Hold the otoscope firmly at the entrance to the canal. Turn on the otoscope light and hold the speculum at the canal entrance. Look for abnormal findings, then lower your head to the otoscope and look into the orifice of the auditory canal. Next, with continuous viewing, gently insert and advance the otoscope speculum into the ear canal. Apply gentle pressure against the posterior canal wall to avoid stimulating the vagus nerve which may trigger coughing. Ask if the patient is experiencing any excessive pain or discomfort. If the patient cannot tolerate the procedure, discontinue this portion of the examination. The patient should be able to tolerate some degree of mild discomfort and novice examiners will overcome their hesitancy and nervousness with experience. Hair is usually seen at the entrance of the canal, especially in elderly men. Dark brown, black, or orange cerumen (earwax) sometimes occludes the auditory canal. Such an occlusion can be removed by gently instilling water at room temperature into the ear canal. Excessively hot or cold water instilled into the auditory canal can precipitate vertigo. Do not try to remove the wax with a cotton swab; this may cause the wax to become impacted against the eardrum. Sometimes, an ear wax removal drug (e.g., Cerumenex or Debrox) or warm mineral oil may be necessary to remove the wax. However, do not attempt this procedure if a perforated eardrum is suspected.

The normal auditory canal wall should look pale pink laterally and reddish medially. Continue inspecting the canal for fresh or dried blood; purulent or sanguineous discharge; serous fluid; polyps; bony, cartilage-capped projections (exostoses); or foreign bodies. If an infection is suspected (especially pseudomonas), carefully smell the speculum to check for an offensive odor. An external canal infection in

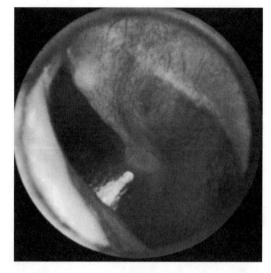

Fig. 6.9   An otoscopic view of a normal left tympanic membrane. The normal tympanic membrane has a see-through quality. Behind the membrane in the upper left corner is a faint horizontal line that represents the chorda tympani nerve as it transverses the middle ear cavity. The triangle shaped light reflex is normal and is lost or distorted with middle ear pathology. The umbo points posterior and the light reflex is directed anterior.

a diabetic patient is a serious finding because it may advance to fulminant external otitis. When viewed through an otoscope, the tympanic membrane appears as a transparent, gray-pink, glistening oval disc (see Fig. 6.9). Rotate the otoscope clockwise to view the periphery, and look for landmarks on the tympanic membrane such as the light reflex (cone of light), handle of malleus, and the umbo.

A few dilated blood vessels are normally seen on the membrane, especially radiating down the handle of malleus. The light reflex is found at the 5 o'clock position in the right ear and at 7 o'clock in the left ear. Behind the tympanic membrane, the middle ear bones and air-filled cavity should be visible. The presence of lesions or any aberration in the color of the tympanic membrane or in the position of the light reflex suggests abnormal physical findings.

Impaired movement of the tympanic membrane affects hearing and may slow development of a child's language skills. Immobility may result from a blocked eustachian tube, a middle ear effusion, a ruptured tympanic membrane, or acute otitis media. To check tympanic membrane mobility in both adults and children, attach a rubber bulb to the otoscope to create a pneumatoscope. Carefully place the speculum in the canal to create an airtight seal. Gently, but quickly, puff then suck with the bulb to create positive and negative air pressures in the canal. Observe for indications of tympanic membrane movement. This is best seen by watching the light reflex changing from its usual position or by observing the pars flaccida area of the ear drum for movement. The normal eardrum should move freely during this procedure.

Hearing Tests

Auditory Acuity Approximation. Obtain a global assessment of the patient's hearing acuity by engaging in normal conversation. If the patient speaks in a loud or monotone voice, or frequently asks you to repeat your questions, check for a hearing deficit. Ask if the patient has experienced a ringing sound in the ears (tinnitus) because this may be an early symptom of nerve damage. Several methods may be used to further assess hearing loss. For example, instruct the patient to occlude one ear. In a completely quiet room, stand behind or to the side of the patient to prevent lip reading. Exhale completely to reduce voice volume, then whisper some instruction such as "take your finger out of your ear." Increase the volume of your voice until the patient acknowledges the command. Alternate methods include holding a ticking watch (not digital) or gently snapping your fingers 5 cm from the patient's ear. Compare auditory response in one ear with the other. Then compare the patient's hearing to your own, assuming you have normal hearing. If the patient has reduced hearing, extend the examination to differentiate between conduction and sensorineural deafness using the Weber (lateralization) and Rinne tests described below.

Weber Test. In a quiet room, stand behind the patient and briskly tap a tuning fork of the 512 or 1024 Hertz frequency against your palm. Firmly place the vibrating tuning

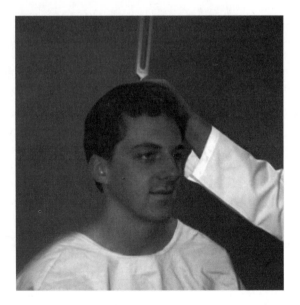

Fig. 6.10   The Weber Test is used to identify and differentiate defects in the conductive hearing pathways from defects in the sensorineural pathway.

fork in the center of the patient's forehead or on top of the patient's head in the midline (see Fig. 6.10). A sensitive alternative technique is to place the vibrating tuning fork base against the patient's top incisors. Ask the patient if she hears the tone equally in both ears or if it is louder in one ear than the other (lateralization). Normally, the tone is heard equally in both ears and sounds as if it is coming from the middle of the head. Be sure the patient reports a buzzing, humming, or tingling sound; simply reporting a vibrating sensation is not helpful. If the sound lateralizes, note the ear in which the sound is heard the loudest. If the conductive pathway is defective, sound lateralizes to the defective ear. If the sensorineural pathway (nerve) is dysfunctional, sound lateralizes to the normal ear. If the patient cannot hear the sound, ask the patient to close both eyes and repeat the test. Again ask the patient about the perception of sound. Also, check room noise. To report the result, describe normal findings as "midline" or "equal bilaterally." Abnormal findings are reported as "lateralizes to the left (or right)." To confirm if the problem is conductive or sensorineuronal, conduct the Rinne test (see Figure 6.11).

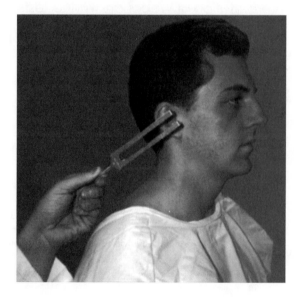

Fig. 6.11 The Rinne Test is used to confirm the conductive or sensorineural origin of abnormal findings identified by the Weber test.

Rinne Test. In a quiet room, stand behind the patient and tap a tuning fork as in the Weber test described above. Press the stem of the vibrating tuning fork against the mastoid bone and measure the time interval before the patient perceives the cessation of the sound (see Fig. 6.11). If the person cannot hear a buzzing or humming sound, then you can conclude there is sensorineural hearing loss and proceed to the other ear. If the patient can hear the sound, then have the patient indicate when the sound is no longer heard. At this point, quickly move the vibrating fork one inch from the same ear without allowing the tuning fork to touch the patient. Ask if the patient hears the sound. If the patient cannot hear the sound, the test is finished. If the sound is heard, have the patient signal when the sound is no longer heard. Then hold the tuning fork to your own ear to determine if there is any residual sound. Compare the time interval of air conduction with that of bone conduction. Normally, air conduction (AC) time lasts longer than that of bone conduction (BC). Patients with conduction defects cannot hear the tuning fork when it is held next to the ear and their hearing via bone conduction is longer than air conduction. Some patients may wait too long during the bone conduction phase, allowing the tuning fork to stop vibrating before it is moved next to the ear canal. This gives a false positive test. Any time you have a positive test, repeat it to confirm your results. Assuming you have normal conductive hearing, hold your ear near the tuning fork and listen to the vibration while testing to help minimize false positive results. Table 6.1 outlines the patterns of hearing loss. When reporting the results of this test, the abbreviation of "AU, AC>BC" indicates a normal finding of air conduction time greater than bone conduction time in each ear. For an abnormal right ear hearing loss, the abbreviation of "AD, AC<BC; AS, AC>BC" should be interpreted as "air conduction is less than bone conduction for the right ear" and "air conduction is greater than bone conduction for the left ear," respectively.

Table 6.1

Interpretation of Weber and Rinne Tests

	Weber Test	Rinne Test	
		Right Ear	Left Ear
Normal	Bilateral and equal	AC>BC (60 sec)	AC>BC (60 sec)
Left sensorineural partial loss	Lateralize AD	AC>BC (60 sec)	AC>BC (10 sec)
Total left sensorineural loss (totally deaf)	Lateralize AD	AC>BC (60 sec)	Cannot hear
Left conduction	Lateralize AS	AC>BC (60 sec)	BC>AC
Bilateral conduction loss[a]	Bilateral and equal	BC>AC	BC>AC
Bilateral sensorineural partial loss[b]	Bilateral and equal	BC>AC	BC>AC

[a] Conductive hearing loss results from decreased sound conduction through the external or middle ear. The most common causes are cerumen plug and otitis media.

[b] Sensorineural hearing loss results from a problem with the inner ear or eighth cranial nerve. It is most commonly caused by the changes of normal aging (presbycusis). Drugs such as aminoglycosides can induce sensorineural loss.

PHARMACOTHERAPEUTIC CASE ILLUSTRATION

History

R.L., a one-year-old male, was seen in clinic following several days of runny nose and nasal congestion. His parents said he had been more irritable than usual and had been crying and tugging at his ears. His appetite was normal. He has a past medical history of frequent episodes of otitis media.

Physical Examination

R.L. weighed 14 kg and his vital signs were as follows: rectal temperature of 37.8° C; a respiratory rate (RR) of 20/min regular; blood pressure (BP) 110/70; and a pulse of 105 beats/min. An examination of R.L.'s pharynx revealed no erythema, hypertrophy, or exudate. He had bilateral clear discharge from the nose with erythematous mucosa. Bilaterally, his ear canals were clear of cerumen without any discharge or tenderness. Tympanic membranes were inflamed with blurred light reflex. Serous fluid was bilaterally present in the middle ears. His lungs were clear and he had no enlarged lymph nodes.

Diagnosis and Management

R.L. was found to have bilateral acute otitis media, probably secondary to acute upper respiratory infection. He was treated with amoxicillin 125 mg/5 mL, 5 mL PO TID for 10 days; acetaminophen elixir 1 teaspoon PO Q 4 hr PRN fever; and oxymetazoline 0.025% 1 drop each nostril BID for 3 days.

Discussion

The Disease. Acute otitis media is an infection of the middle ear usually associated with an upper respiratory infection (URI). A disease primarily of infants and children less than three years of age, otitis tends to be recurrent and chronic and results in frequent physician office visits. It is an inflammatory disease of the middle ear which may affect the mastoid bone and eustachian tube and is classified into four types: chronic otitis media with or without effusion, acute otitis media with or without effusion.

The pathogenesis of the condition is based on two pathologic processes: infection or eustachian tube dysfunction. Infants and young children have frequent upper respiratory tract infections caused by bacteria and viruses and are at risk of disseminating the infection to the middle ear. In preschoolers (four years of age and younger), the eustachian tube is short and does not have a sharp drainage angle into the nasopharynx as it does in older children and adults. Normally, the tube is closed until the child chews, swallows, or yawns. The middle ear normally secretes a small amount of fluid that drains out the tube. When a child has an URI, however, the tube is obstructed and does not drain naturally. The condition can become chronic following repeated infections.

Otalgia (ear pain) is the most common symptom in the older child and adult. In the toddler, rather than pain, the parent first notices irritability, changes in appetite, and tugging or pulling at the ears. Other signs and symptoms are lethargy, hearing loss, vomiting, fever, diarrhea, and otorrhea. However, some children are asymptomatic.

The diagnosis usually is based upon otoscopic examination of the eardrum and middle ear. When viewed through the otoscope, the inflamed eardrum appears bright red, bulging like a doughnut, and immobile. Various effusions (e.g., purulent, serous, or bloody) are visible behind the eardrum. The eardrum may rupture spontaneously, discharging purulent fluid. If otitis media is untreated, the eardrum or middle ear ossicles may be permanently damaged. Otitis media may lead to complications such as mastoiditis, meningitis, and cerebral thrombophlebitis. Acute otitis media resolves with proper antibiotic therapy.

Management

Various antibiotics are available to manage bacterial otitis media. The most common bacteria, *Streptococcus pneumoniae*, account for about one-third of the acute otitis media infections. *Hemophilus influenzae* and *Moraxella catarrhalis* also are common causes of the disease and are clinically important because of their high incidence of beta-lactamase resistance. These three pathogens are the most common causes, but other bacteria such as *Staphylococcus aureus* or gram-negative enteric bacteria have been isolated depending upon the age group.

Amoxicillin is a good choice for empiric therapy of acute otitis media because it is active against most community-acquired *S. pneumoniae* and *H. influenzae*. Also, it may be given three times daily, is inexpensive, and has few side effects. If the child cannot tolerate its side effects (i.e., diarrhea) or is penicillin allergic, combinations of sulfamethoxazole/trimethoprim or erythromycin/sulfisoxazole are effective. Patients should be treated for 10 to 14 days.

In a hospital-acquired or suspected resistant infection, the antibiotic choices are a cephalosporin (cefixime, cefuroxime axetil, cefaclor), amoxicillin-clavulanate, or erythromycin-sulfisoxazole. Some children may need to be treated with parenteral antibiotics or a myringotomy.

Acetaminophen or ibuprofen reduces the child's fever and provides mild analgesia. Decongestants and antihistamines offer symptomatic relief. Topical decongestants open the eustachian tube to drain the inner ear and nasal passages; however, prolonged use causes rebound congestion and they should not be used for more than a few days.

Tell the parent to bring the child back if fever and pain persist for more than 48 hours. If the patient continues to be symptomatic, re-evaluate the problem and change the antibiotic if necessary. The continuation of fever and pain could signal the presence of a middle ear abscess which has to be drained by a myringotomy. Myringotomy should be performed by an experienced physician. Releasing the pressure on the eardrum by myringotomy often results in immediate pain relief. Often, a child screaming with pain suddenly stops after the fluid drains. The drainage from the ear should be cultured and tested for antibiotic sensitivity.

Therapeutic Drug Monitoring Examples

EXTERNAL OTITIS

The approach to therapuetic drug monitoring by clinicians varies depending upon many factors. Some of these include preferences among clinicians in a given community or region; concurrent medical problems which dictate that certain drugs be used or avoided; the patient's response to selected medication. The following outlines of therapeutic drug monitoring offer examples which may serve to stimulate discussion and further understanding of initiating and monitoring drug use. The drugs and dosages presented should not be applied to any clinical situation without proper medical supervision.

Drug Therapy	2% acetic acid otic solution; insert saturated wick; keep moist continuously. Instill separately 4–5 drops QID.
Monitoring	**Symptoms:** Otalgia, canal itching.
	Signs: *HEENT:* Inspect for canal swelling and erythema, purulent discharge. Ask the patient if the ear canal is pruritic. Check for ear pain by tugging on the auricle and pressing on tragus. Check for tympanic membrane (TM) hyperemia. Inspect for normal TM landmarks. Smell the otoscope speculum for foul pseudomonas odor.
Laboratory Tests	The clinician may elect to order all, none, or some of these laboratory studies depending upon history and physical findings as well as other specific clinical indications. Culture and sensitivity (C&S), if indicated.
Adverse Drug Event Monitoring	Check for signs of canal redness, itching, burning, swelling, and irritation not present before treatment. These findings indicate drug hypersensitivity.

Therapeutic Drug Monitoring Examples

ACUTE OTITIS MEDIA

The approach to therapuetic drug monitoring by clinicians varies depending upon many factors. Some of these include preferences among clinicians in a given community or region; concurrent medical problems which dictate that certain drugs be used or avoided; the patient's response to selected medication. The following outlines of therapeutic drug monitoring offer examples which may serve to stimulate discussion and further understanding of initiating and monitoring drug use. The drugs and dosages presented should not be applied to any clinical situation without proper medical supervision.

Drug Therapy:
Amoxicillin 250 mg PO Q 8 hr for 10 days, acetaminophen 325 mg PO Q 4 hr PRN ear pain/fever.

Monitoring
Symptoms: Question about otalgia (earache), "fullness in ear and popping sensation."

Signs: *GEN:* Fever, irritability. *HEENT:* Check for conductive hearing loss (check with whisper test, and/or Rinne and Weber tests). Note otorrhea and swelling. Check for pain by pressing on tragus or moving the auricle. Inspect the ear canal and tympanic membrane (TM). Note TM bulging, hyperemia, cone of light, and fluid behind TM. Inspect for TM perforation with purulent discharge. Check for improving TM movement upon insufflation.

Laboratory Tests
The clinician may elect to order all, none, or some of these laboratory studies depending upon history and physical findings as well as other specific clinical indications. Culture and sensitivity (C&S), if indicated.

Adverse Drug Event Monitoring
Question about diarrhea (especially antibiotic-associated pseudomembranous colitis), and check for skin rash, bacterial resistance, and anaphylactic reaction.

Therapeutic Drug Monitoring Examples

DRUG-INDUCED
SENSORINEURAL HEARING LOSS

The approach to therapuetic drug monitoring by clinicians varies depending upon many factors. Some of these include preferences among clinicians in a given community or region; concurrent medical problems which dictate that certain drugs be used or avoided; the patient's response to selected medication. The following outlines of therapeutic drug monitoring offer examples which may serve to stimulate discussion and further understanding of initiating and monitoring drug use. The drugs and dosages presented should not be applied to any clinical situation without proper medical supervision.

Drug Therapy — Avoid or carefully monitor drugs known to damage hearing.

Monitoring — **Symptoms:** Determine whether the patient speaks loudly; hears best in a quiet room; has difficulty hearing on telephone or in a noisy room; or has difficulty discriminating sounds (i.e., the patient hears garbled sounds). Identify high risk patients (i.e., patients with existing hearing loss; patients taking high doses of or multiple drugs known to damage hearing; patients with renal failure; and patients on prolonged treatment). Question for tinnitus (an early sign of impending hearing loss, however, this is not reliable in elderly due to presbycusis).

Signs: *HEENT:* Perform pre-treatment and post-treatment hearing tests. Screen with whisper test. Perform Weber and Rinne tests. *Note:* Conductive hearing loss indicates the presence of external canal obstruction (e.g., cerumen) or middle ear disease. Patients with conductive loss speak softly, hear best in a noisy room (compared to those with sensorineural hearing loss), and hear well on the telephone.

Laboratory Tests — The clinician may elect to order all, none, or some of these laboratory studies

Therapeutic Drug Monitoring Examples

DRUG-INDUCED SENSORINEURAL HEARING LOSS

(continued)

Laboratory Tests   depending upon history and physical findings, as well as other specific clinical indications. Audiometry.

Adverse Drug   Check for permanent hearing loss.
Event Monitoring

Therapeutic Drug Monitoring Examples

DRUG-INDUCED VERTIGO

The approach to therapeutic drug monitoring by clinicians varies depending upon many factors. Some of these include preferences among clinicians in a given community or region; concurrent medical problems which dictate that certain drugs be used or avoided; the patient's response to selected medication. The following outlines of therapeutic drug monitoring offer examples which may serve to stimulate discussion and further understanding of initiating and monitoring drug use. The drugs and dosages presented should not be applied to any clinical situation without proper medical supervision.

Drug Therapy	Avoid or monitor drugs causing vestibular dysfunction.
Monitoring	**Symptoms:** Question about nausea and vomiting, and hearing loss.
	Signs: *Neuro:* Check for positive Romberg sign (see Chapter 14: Nervous System); observe for nystagmus (see Chapter 5: Eye); ask patient to walk and check gait and ataxia. Check coordination (see Chapter 14: Nervous System) with finger-to-nose test.
Laboratory Tests	The clinician may elect to order all, none, or some of these laboratory studies depending upon history and physical findings, as well as other specific clinical indications. Electronystagmography.
Adverse Drug Event Monitoring	Check for acute vertigo.

Mouth, Nose, And Sinuses

D iseases involving the mouth, nose, and sinuses are common. In addition to illnesses such as upper respiratory infection, viral or bacterial pharyngitis, allergic rhinitis, and sinusitis, manifestations related to certain drug applications can affect these areas of the body (e.g., hypertrophy of the gums from hydantoin use, "hairy tongue" from certain antibiotic use, discoloration of the teeth from administration of tetracycline during childhood). An understanding of the anatomy and physiology of these areas, coupled with an orderly approach to clinical evaluation of the mouth, nose, and sinuses will aid in achieving an accurate clinical assessment and the formulation of an appropriate management plan.

ANATOMY AND PHYSIOLOGY

Mouth

The oral cavity, or mouth, includes the skin that externally covers the lips and the mucous membrane that lines the inside of the mouth. The mouth contains 32 teeth in the adult, including four incisors, two canines, four premolars, and six molars in each jaw (upper and lower). The parotid, submandibular, and sublingual salivary glands located in the mouth secrete large amounts of saliva to moisten the mouth, wet food for chewing and swallowing, and begin the digestion process.

The **parotid salivary glands** and their ducts (i.e., Stenson's ducts) can be seen in the mucosa on the inside of the cheek next to the upper second molars. The **submandibular salivary glands** and their ducts (i.e., Wharton's ducts) open on the floor of the mouth on either side of the lingual frenulum (i.e., the fold of mucous membrane connecting the tongue to the floor of the mouth at the midline anteriorly). Saliva squirts out from the submandibular salivary openings when we yawn. The **sublingual salivary glands** lie on either side underneath the tongue and have many duct openings on the floor of the mouth.

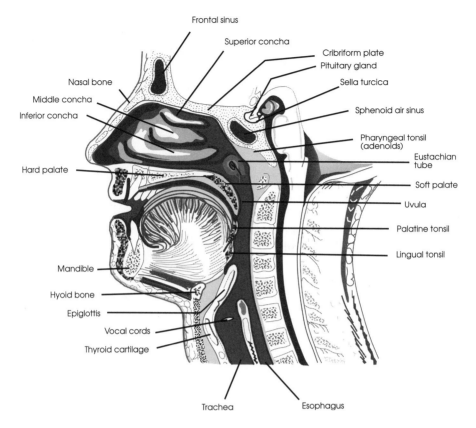

Fig. 7.1 A sagittal section through showing the primary structures of the face and neck. The nasal septum has been removed to expose the lateral wall of the nasal cavity.

Tongue

The primary functions of the tongue are to form words, taste substances, prepare food for digestion during the process of chewing, and propel food into the pharynx for swallowing. A narrow groove passes down the midline surface of the tongue. The anterior portion is attached to the floor of the oral cavity by the lingual frenulum. The anterior dorsal surface appears velvety, while the posterior surface looks more nodular. The anterior under surface appears moist and contains visible veins and small papules. The hypoglossal nerve (i.e., cranial nerve 12) controls muscle functions of the tongue, except those associated with the posterior part; this portion of the tongue is innervated by the vagus nerve (i.e., cranial nerve 10). Sensory nerves for tasting (i.e., the facial nerve) innervate the anterior two-thirds of the tongue.

Palate

The roof of the mouth, or palate, is composed of a **hard palate** and a **soft palate**. The hard palate is located in the anterior two-thirds of the mouth, while the soft palate is in the posterior third. Mucous membranes line the arching roof of the hard and soft palates. The soft palate tapers to form the conical, fleshy, free-hanging tissue known as the **uvula**, an important structure for assessing the function of the vagus nerve (i.e., cranial nerve 10). When a person swallows, the soft palate moves backward against the posterior pharynx to prevent regurgitation of material into the nasopharynx. The soft palate also plays a significant role in phonation (i.e., word formation).

Pharynx

The pharynx is the space lined by a thin, muscular tube connecting the nose, mouth, larynx/esophagus. It can be divided into three anatomical regions known as the nasopharynx, oropharynx, and laryngopharynx (see Figures 7.2 and 7.3). The **nasopharynx** is located above the soft palate and connects with the back of the nose

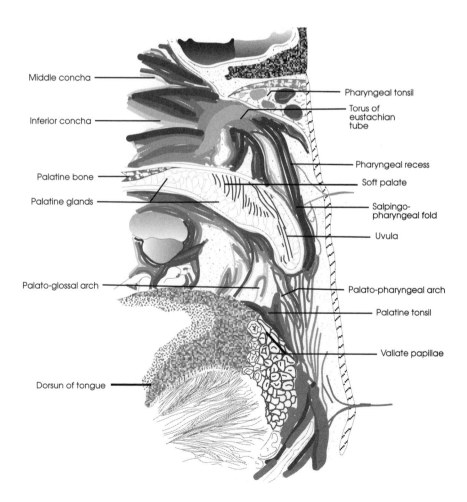

Fig. 7.2 A lateral view of the major structures of the interior of the pharynx, including the pharynx, oropharynx, and upper laryngopharynx.

and the auditory tube (superior-posterior aspect of the nasal cavity, superior to the oropharynx). The **laryngopharynx** lies below the upper edge of the epiglottis and opens into the larynx and esophagus (inferior between the oropharynx and the laryngeal folds). The laryngopharynx is innervated by the vagus nerve and controls swallowing and speech. The **oropharynx** is situated between the nasopharynx and laryngopharynx, lying between the soft palate and the upper edge of the epiglottis at the level of the base of the tongue.

Oropharynx

The oropharynx (throat) is a space defined by the following anatomical structures lying at its boundaries. Superiorly, it begins at the level of the soft palate, the pharyngeal tonsils, and the base of the nasopharynx. Anteriorly, the oropharynx is bounded by its opening into the mouth and the uvula. The muscles of the wall of the posterior pharynx mark the posterior boundary. The lateral boundary of the oropharynx is defined by its anterior and posterior arches and the palatine tonsils. The three pairs of tonsils (i.e., the palatine, lingual, and pharyngeal tonsils) act as a vanguard against bacterial and viral invaders in the head and neck, respiratory tract, and gastrointestinal tract. The palatine tonsils lie on the lateral wall of the oropharynx between the anterior and posterior arches. The lingual tonsils are located at the base of the tongue.

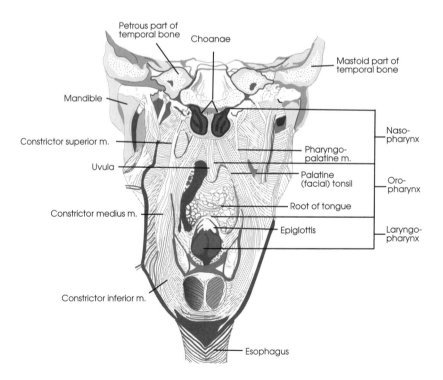

Fig. 7.3   Major divisions and structures of the pharynx viewed from behind.

Nose

The structures of the external nose include the columella (i.e., the tissue that separates the two naris or nostrils and continues internally as the nasal septum), the ala nasi (i.e., the fleshy, rounded eminence where the entrance of the nasal cavity meets the face), and the nostrils (naris) (See Figure 7.4). The **naris** open into the nasal cavity or vestibule. The nose is divided, usually equally, into right and

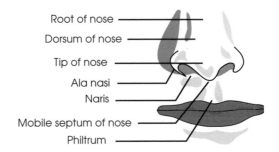

Root of nose
Dorsum of nose
Tip of nose
Ala nasi
Naris
Mobile septum of nose
Philtrum

Fig. 7.4 Nomenclature for structures of the nose and mouth.

left nasal passages by the **nasal septum**. The posterior nasal septum is composed of bone, while the anterior portion is cartilage. The floor of the nasal cavity is formed by the hard and soft palates of the oral cavity, and the roof of the nose is formed by the frontal and sphenoid bones. Mucous membranes cover the nasal septum. The paired openings where the right and left posterior nasal cavities join the nasopharynx are called the choana.

The mucous membranes covering the nasal cavity and the nasal hairs at the cavity's entrance remove particulate matter from inspired air as it travels through the nasal cavity, into and out of the sinuses, and across three vascular, mucous-covered turbinates (i.e., the inferior, middle and superior conchae) located on the lateral wall. The **turbinates** are bony protrusions with convolutions that curl downward. Each turbinate has a groove beneath it, giving it the appearance of a shelf-like structure. The inferior and middle turbinates are visible by inspection. The superior turbinate is located high in the nasal cavity and is not visible during routine examination. The turbinates increase the surface area of the nasal cavity, and thereby help warm, filter, and humidify inhaled air. The **nasolacrimal ducts** empty into the inferior turbinate. The superior, middle, and inferior **meatus** are recesses that lie under their respective turbinates. The nasolacriminal duct and the maxillary sinus orifice open into the inferior meatus. The middle meatus contains openings that drain the ethmoid, frontal, and maxillary sinuses. The superior meatus contains the posterior ethmoid sinus openings. The sphenoid sinus orifice is located above the superior turbinate. The eustachian tube opens into the nasopharynx near the posterior edge of the middle and inferior turbinates (see Figure 7.5).

The mucous membranes lining the nasal cavity swell and discharge secretions when irritated. These secretions can be clear and watery, or thick and sticky. The presence of excessive, thick, and sticky secretions may result in partial or complete obstruction of the nasal passages and/or the sinus openings. The nose is richly supplied by a network of blood vessels known as Kiesselbach's plexus that is located beneath a thin mucous membrane. This plexus of vessels can be easily traumatized, resulting in a nose bleed.

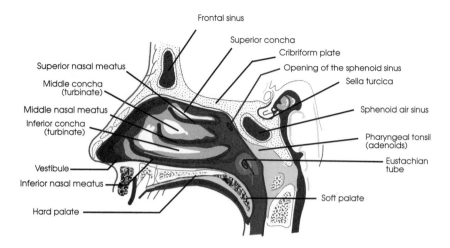

Fig. 7.5   Internal structures of the nose.

The nose is also the olfactory (i.e., smell) sensor. The sensory endings of the olfactory nerve lie anteriorly on the roof of the nose. The sense of smell is important because smells are often associated with pleasurable emotions and are used for defense to warn of the presence of malodorous or toxic substances. The loss of the sense of smell (i.e., anosmia) may be first noted by a patient as a disagreeable change in the taste of food. The olfactory receptors are extremely sensitive and transmit information over the first cranial nerve to the sensory cortex. The sense of smell commonly decreases with increasing age or chronic exposure to toxic substances in the air.

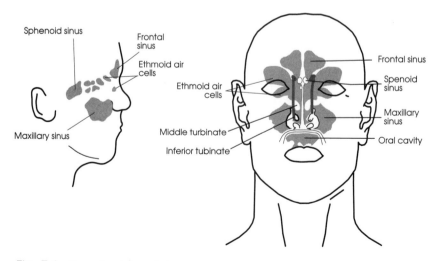

Fig. 7.6   Lateral and frontal views of the location of the paranasal sinuses.

Sinuses

The paranasal sinuses are air-filled, bony cavities that lighten the skull and give resonance to the voice. They drain into the nasopharynx and nasal cavity. The frontal sinuses are located above the eyes while the two maxillary sinuses lie below the eyes. The ethmoid sinuses located in the ethmoid bones and the sphenoid sinuses of the sphenoid bones are not accessible to routine inspection (see Figure 7.6). The mucosa of the sinuses is continuous with that of the nasal cavities and is composed of blood vessels and ciliated columnar epithelium.

PHYSICAL ASSESSMENT

Lips

With the patient's mouth loosely closed, inspect the lips for color, swelling, and lesions. The lips are normally pink, shiny, and symmetrical. Look for abnormalities such as **cheilitis** (inflammation of the lips), **angular stomatitis** or **cheilosis** (fissuring and dry scaling of the vermilion border of the lips at the corners of the mouth often associated with riboflavin deficiency). **Herpes simplex cold sores** or **fever blisters** (groups of small fluid-filled vesicles surrounded by areas of erythema) and several types of **skin cancers** (e.g., epidermoid carcinoma) are other potential abnormalities that most often affect the lower lip. Paralysis of the facial nerve (cranial nerve 7) causes muscle weakness of the affected side with loss of the nasolabial fold and drooping of the corner of the mouth.

Mouth

Sit opposite to and on the same level as the patient in an area with good lighting. Ask the patient to remove any dentures or partial dental plates and place them on a facial tissue. Use both inspection and palpation (wear latex gloves) to determine the presence of lesions such as cancer, cysts, or salivary calculi. Ask whether the patient has been smoking, chewing tobacco or snuff, or drinking excessively hot or cold beverages.

To check facial nerve functions and occlusion, ask the patient to clench his teeth and smile. Occlusion is probably normal when the patient's smile is symmetrical with the upper molars resting on the lower molars. Note the odor of the patient's breath. A sweet breath odor, similar to that of ripe bananas, is consistent with diabetic ketoacidosis. An ammoniacal or fishy odor of the breath is consistent with chronic renal failure. A sweet, musty odor of fetor hepaticus is present with liver failure. A foul odor (halitosis) can be caused by a dental or tonsillar infection. A putrid smelling breath might suggest an anaerobic lung infection. Be alert for the odor of alcohol, paraldehyde, chloral hydrate, or chloroform on the breath.

Use a tongue blade, latex gloves, and a flashlight to examine the patient's mouth. Retract the patient's lips and cheeks to inspect the buccal surfaces, gums, hard and soft palates, and teeth. The **buccal mucosa** should appear pink, moist, smooth, and shiny with yellowish spots (Fordyce's spots). A white line on the buccal surface next to the upper molars is a normal finding and commonly is caused by repeated biting or sucking on the cheek. Continue the examination of the buccal mucosa by looking for aphthous ulcers (i.e., small white spots), areas of chronic irritation, moniliasis (i.e., a yeast-like fungal infection), or leukoplakia (i.e., opalescent patches or leathery plaques resulting from keratinization of mucous membranes). To examine the **gums**, flip back the patient's upper and lower lips. The gums should be firm and pink in Caucasians or dark blue in blacks. Look for inflammation, swelling, bleeding, or infection of the gums. Enlargement (hyperplasia) of the gums can be associated with phenytoin therapy, leukemia, and pregnancy; and blue-black gum margins can be associated with bismuth and lead intoxication. Gums that bleed with minimal trauma (e.g., teeth brushing) suggest a possible hematologic disorder or anticoagulant therapy. Gingivitis and periodontal disease appear as bleeding, swollen gums that are retracted from the gingival margins of the teeth. Examine the teeth, noting dental caries, plaque, or missing teeth. Worn teeth with dentin exposure (i.e., attrition), and discoloration of the teeth by tetracycline, tobacco, coffee, or tea are common benign findings.

Look up at the **hard** and **soft palates**. The soft palate normally is pink with some fine blood vessels on the mucosa. Compared to the soft palate, the hard palate is whiter, and has a rougher surface (like a washboard anteriorly). Heavy smokers have tiny red spots scattered over the hard palate. A sometimes alarming, but benign, bony protuberance (exostosis) in the hard palate midline is torus palatines which commonly appears in adulthood. A similar growth, not in the midline, may be a cancer.

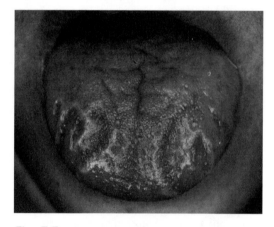

Fig. 7.7 Geographic tongue is characterized by irregular ridges on what is normally the smooth surface of the tongue. These denuded areas are usually not painful. This particular patient suffered from nutritional deficiencies secondary to marked anorexia and bulimia.

Next, examine the tongue by asking the patient to relax and let his or her tongue lie on the floor of the mouth. The tongue is normally pink, with a slight coating and small longitudinal furrows. Inspect the dorsal surface for the presence of **hairy tongue**. With this condition, hyperplasia of the papillae on the dorsal surface gives the tongue the appearance of being covered with patches of dark hair. This condition is caused by overgrowth of fungi that commonly results from antibiotic-inhibition of normal flora bacterial growth. Geographic tongue is a condition characterized by bright red denuded patches of epithelium surrounded by thickened epithelium. A tongue with this condition returns to normal within a few days when a "map" of newly involved patches appear (see Figure. 7.7). A smooth, bright red tongue that generates a burning sensation when in contact with hot or spicy foods is a sign of pellagrous tongue. This condition responds readily to 100 mg niacin within 48 hours. A grossly swollen, sore, inflamed tongue is an indication of glossitis.

The absence of saliva under the tongue is strongly associated with dehydration and is a more sensitive indicator of dehydration than dry buccal mucosa or tongue because these areas can appear dry from breathing through the mouth. To evaluate normal hypoglossal nerve (12th cranial nerve) function, ask the patient to stick out her tongue. Note any "contraction fasciculations" and whether the tongue remains in the midline without tremor or deviation. A fine tremor of the tongue is noticeable in patients with Parkinson's disease, and deviation of the tongue from the midline is consistent with tongue atrophy or stroke. Ask the patient to touch the tip of his tongue to the roof of his mouth, inspect the under surface and floor of the mouth. Look for swelling, leukoplakia, ulceration, and varicosities. Normally, the frenulum allows the tongue to touch the roof of the mouth (hard palate). The submaxillary salivary gland openings are on each side of the lingual frenulum. Some vein dilation on the underside of the tongue is normal.

Wearing a disposable glove, palpate any symptomatic or suspicious area in the mouth. Some oral lesions lie deep under the surface and may only be found with palpation. The tongue and its undersurface are common locations for oral cancer.

Oropharynx

Using a tongue depressor blade, latex gloves, and flashlight, inspect each half of the tonsillar region separately. With the patient's tongue relaxed on the mouth floor, firmly press the tongue depressor blade on the middle part of the tongue to see the oropharynx. Reassure the patient that you will not try to stimulate her gag reflex. Do not touch the pharynx with the tongue depressor blade to avoid initiating the gag reflex. Observe the tonsillar pillars and

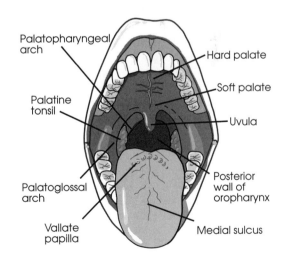

Fig. 7.8   Primary landmarks visible during inspection of the oral cavity.

tonsils for swelling, inflammation, ulceration, or exudate (i.e., pus). Normally, the palatine tonsils are moist, pink, and do not stick out beyond the edge of the pillars. A few white spots are normal on the palatine mucosa. Occasionally food particles may be seen in the tonsillar crypts and can sometimes be mistaken for infection.

The posterior pharyngeal wall is normally pink, moist, shiny, and smooth with small pink or red lymph nodules. A few red blood vessels are expected on the posterior wall. Pharyngeal erythema can be caused by viral infections or recent smoking. Bands are normally visible down the medial edge of the anterior and posterior pillar arches. An exudate on the tonsils and posterior wall is suggestive of a streptococcal infection, but can also be seen with certain viral infections. White, cotton-like patches on the

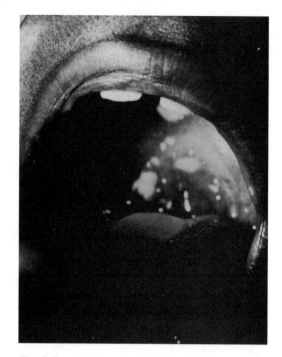

Fig.7.9 Monilia or oral thrush appears as white, cotton-like patches surrounded by irritated, erythmatous mucosa.

pharyngeal wall may be **Monilia** (i.e., oral thrush) or food particles (e.g., milk curds) and can be differentiated by scraping the patch off with a cotton swab. Monilia leaves a bleeding ulcer base, food does not (see Figure 7.9). Ask the patient to say, "ah" (phonate), place the tongue depressor blade on the tongue, and gently press downward and medial. Phonation raises the soft palate and elevates the uvula in the midline for better inspection of the oropharynx. Any deviation in the elevation of the uvula, or a lack of response by the uvula during phonation signifies loss of innervation of the 10th cranial nerve (i.e., the vagus nerve) which occurs with a stroke or injury to the nerve (e.g., a tumor). A congenitally long **uvula** may touch the tongue's base or posterior pharynx and cause gagging or coughing. Test the patient's gag reflexes (9th and 10th cranial nerves) by touching and pressing down on the roof of the tongue. Carefully observe the equal elevation of both sides of the tonsillar region. The first structure noted with the gag reflex is the **epiglottis** which lies between the larynx and base of the tongue. A swollen red epiglottis is seen in children with laryngotracheobronchitis. The epiglottis tends to be swollen and pale in patients with allergies.

External Nose

Inspect the external surface of the nose for deviation to one side or another, and for skin lesions that might represent squamous cell or basal cell cancer. A large, red, bulbous-shaped nose (i.e., rhinophyma) is a sign of rosacea and, sometimes, chronic alcoholism, while nasal flaring is a sign of respiratory distress. To check nasal patency, occlude one nostril and ask the patient to inhale through the other nostril. Repeat the procedure with the other nostril occluded. Normal nasal breathing is noiseless.

Internal Nose

Use either a penlight or otoscope to shine a beam of light into each nostril. Place your right hand on the forehead and your thumb on the tip of the patient's nose. Gently press against the tip of the nose to open the nostrils (anterior nares) for better inspection. Hold the nasal speculum in your left hand, tilt the patient's head backward about 10°, and gently insert the instrument about 1 cm into the nostril while constantly looking through the otoscope. Avoid pressing on the nasal septum. Remember, the floor of the nasal cavity is parallel with the roof of the mouth. Shine the light in one nostril and inspect the nasal septum for deviation to one side, perforation, or a mass. The nasal mucosa is normally pinkish in color. Check the mucosal surface for discoloration, swelling, or discharge (clear, colored, bloody, or purulent). Abuse of decongestants (i.e., rhinitis medicamentosus) causes a dry, red nasal mucosa. Also look for bleeding (i.e., epistaxis). Inspect the inferior and middle turbinates for swelling, exudate, or polyps. A pale to blue, boggy mucosa on the turbinates is suggestive of allergic rhinitis. Polyps are associated with chronic allergic rhinitis. Look carefully at the middle turbinate for purulent discharge from the frontal, maxillary, and ethmoid sinuses.

The sense of **smell** is tested by presenting familiar odors to the patient (e.g., an alcohol pad). When the patient's eyes are closed, occlude one nostril and ask the patient to inhale and identify various odors. Test each nostril separately. Although the sense of smell is usually tested as part of the neurological examination, it can be evaluated during a routine nasal examination. As with other neurological function tests, be alert for possible false positive responses due to fatigue or the patient's strong desire to please the examiner. Bilateral olfactory (cranial nerve 1) deficits can be attributable to various causes including infection, excessive smoking, drugs, or cocaine sniffing. Unilateral olfactory loss without nasal disease raises the possibility of an intracranial, frontal lobe lesion.

Sinuses

To check the frontal sinuses, press with both of your thumbs just above the patient's eye orbit ridge on either side of the midline (see Figure 7.10). Be careful not to press the supraorbital nerve in its supraorbital notch since this will elicit pain. Use the same technique to palpate the maxillary sinuses located just below the zygomatic bones. Do not press the infraorbital nerve, since this would also be painful for the patient. Percuss each maxillary and frontal sinus for tenderness. Normal sinuses are neither tender nor swollen. Facial pain, especially upon awakening, tenderness to pressure, and nasal purulent drainage are signs of acute sinusitis. Sinus infections are extremely dangerous because of their potential for spreading to the eyes, ears, or brain.

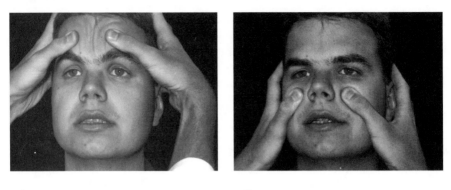

A.   B.

Fig. 7.10   A. Palpate the patient's frontal sinuses with both your thumbs pressing just above the patient's eye orbit ridge on either side of the midline. B. Palpate the maxillary sinuses just below and medial to the patient's zygomatic bones.

The frontal and maxillary sinuses are also examined using transillumination. In a dark room, shine a beam of light on the zygomatic bone over the maxillary sinuses. Look inside the patient's mouth for an equally distributed red glow on the palate. Diseased sinuses give an unequal glow between the two sinus areas. To examine the frontal sinuses, shine the light through the orbital bone above each eye. If normal, the frontal sinuses also glow equally (see Figure 7.11).

PHARMACOTHERAPEUTIC CASE ILLUSTRATION

History

M.L., a 16-year-old white male, was examined following several days of sneezing, nasal congestion, rhinorrhea, and pruritic eyes and nose. These symptoms occurred often, especially during the spring and summer months.

His social (SH), past medical (PMH), and family (FH) histories were not significant to this problem. The review of systems (ROS) was pertinent only as described in the history of present illness (HPI). Drug history revealed the use of over the counter antihistamines and decongestants. The patient admitted to the frequent use of oxymetazoline hydrochloride (Afrin) nasal spray.

Physical Examination

This white male (WM) patient was well-developed, well-nourished (WDWN), in no acute distress (NAD), and afebrile. His vital signs were stable (AFVSS). Eyes showed excessive lacrimation, dilated conjunctivae vessels, and swollen eyelids. Nose had clear, watery discharge. Nasal mucosa was swollen, boggy, and bluish-pink. Pharynx exhibited moderate inflammation without ulceration or cobblestone appearance. Exam of neck was negative for enlarged or tender lymph nodes. Lungs were clear to auscultation without inspiratory or expiratory wheezes.

Laboratory Tests

Microscopic examination of stained nasal secretions revealed sheets of eosinophils.

Diagnosis and Management

M.L. was diagnosed as having allergic rhinitis. The physician prescribed astemizole (Hismanal) one 10 mg tablet per day and flunisolide (Nasalide) nasal solution 2 sprays in each nostril BID. M.L. saw an allergist to identify the possible allergens.

Discussion

Disease. Allergic rhinitis is an IgE-mediated reaction of the nasal mucous membranes to an allergen. Nasal congestion; a profuse, watery nasal discharge; lacrimation;

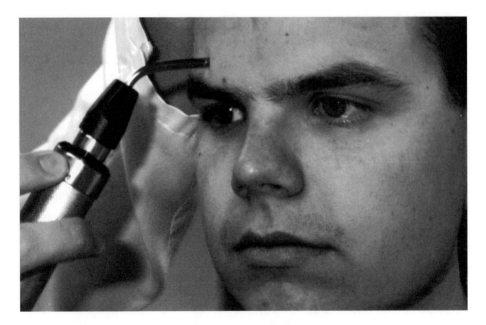

Fig. 7.11   Transillumination can be used to examine the sinuses. Here, the frontal sinuses are examined by shining a light through the orbital eye bone of each eye. Normally, the frontal sinuses will glow equally.

sneezing; and itching, burning nose and eyes are characteristic symptoms of mild allergic rhinitis. In severe stages of the disease, nasal passages can be completely occluded resulting in frequent, forceful sneezing episodes. Airborne pollen, dust, mites, animal epithelium, mold spores, and insect body parts are some of the most common allergens that cause allergic rhinitis. This disorder is usually, but not always, a seasonal problem.

Antigen and immunoglobulin E interact on mast cells, mononuclear phagocytes, and T-lymphocytes to release mediators of immediate allergic reaction. These antigen-antibody-mediator interactions lead to increased capillary permeability and interstitial swelling. Histamine is an important chemical mediator in this reaction that results in the characteristic symptoms described above.

The history is the most important diagnostic tool to identify allergic rhinitis, although some physical changes can be found upon examination. The copious flood of lacrimal and nasal secretions results in considerable rubbing of the eyes and nose. The so-called "allergic salute," a common hand gesture made by pushing the palm of the hand up and out against the tip of the nose, may result in a skin crease across the lower part of nose. In children it is common to see darkened areas under the eyes (i.e., "allergic shiners"). Nasal congestion may be unilateral or bilateral, or may alternate from one nostril to the other. The continuous drainage of nasal secretions into the throat (i.e., postnasal drip) often produces a dry, nonproductive cough which can disturb sleep. Other problems such as paranasal sinusitis, otitis media, and conjunctivitis can also complicate the management of allergic rhinitis.

The nasal mucosa of a patient with allergic rhinitis generally appears pale blue while edematous turbinates are coated with a clear nasal secretion. The presence of purulent drainage accompanied by facial headache and halitosis may represent a complicating bacterial infection of the sinuses. Scleral and conjunctival redness accompanied by excessive tearing are also common features of allergic rhinitis. Enlarged tonsils or cervical adenopathy are signs of complicating infections.

Laboratory studies may reveal an elevated eosinophilia count in nasal discharge. Other suggested studies include: a set of sinus x-rays (only if sinusitis is suspected), allergy skin testing, and radioallergosorbent test (RAST). The use of sinus x-rays is controversial because they do not always reveal sinusitis (false negatives). A computerized tomography (CT) scan is an expensive, but more accurate tool for examining sinusitis.

The most precise, least expensive, and quickest method of determining whether a person has allergies is skin testing. Allergens are applied to the patient's skin by an allergist or person well-trained and experienced with the test. The number of eosinophils may be normal or increased in the peripheral and nasal secretions of patients with either allergic or nonallergic rhinitis; therefore, the presence of eosinophilia is of limited value. Nasal cytology is primarily used to differentiate infectious rhinitis (many neutrophils) from allergic rhinitis (many eosinophils). The RAST measures serum IgE levels and is useful in a limited number of cases.

In summary, the diagnosis of allergic rhinitis depends upon a careful history and physical examination, and may or may not be supported by additional testing procedures.

Management. Allergic rhinitis can be managed by the avoidance of antigens, the administration of allergen-specific immunotherapy, and/or the administration of antihistamines and other drugs to relieve symptoms. First and foremost, environmental measures should be taken to avoid allergens. Exposure to dust can be limited by using dust-proof covers, avoiding outdoor activities during peak pollen season, and wearing protective clothing. Air filter devices also are helpful in reducing the numbers of some airborne allergens.

M.L.'s case of allergic rhinitis was managed by an antihistamine and nasal corticosteroid spray. Antihistamines competitively inhibit the binding of histamine to mast cells when given continuously; therefore, antihistamines are most effective in controlling the acute symptoms of nasal itching and sneezing when taken before exposure to the allergen. Astemizole was chosen for M.L. because it has minimal sedative effects and is given once daily.

Sympathomimetics can also be given topically to constrict nasal passages, but overuse can cause rebound congestion. Orally administered sympathomimetics have the added disadvantage of cardiovascular and central nervous system stimulation.

When the symptoms of allergic rhinitis are not sufficiently controlled by antihistamines an intranasal corticosteroid spray is especially effective in alleviating nasal symptoms in about two weeks. Patients with nasal eosinophilia are especially responsive to topical nasal steroids. After symptoms improve, the lowest effective dose of corticosteroid that maintains control should be used; generally two sprays in each nostril twice a day are adequate. The use of short-term (1 week) oral steroid therapy is limited to severe cases.

Cromolyn sodium is effective in preventing allergic rhinorrhea when administered two weeks before the known allergy season. The intranasal solution of cromolyn provides symptomatic relief of nasal congestion, sneezing, and rhinorrhea by preventing the release of mast cell mediators. Nasal irritation and sneezing are common adverse effects to cromolyn.

If the symptoms of allergic rhinitis are not adequately controlled by drug therapy and avoidance therapy, allergen-specific immunotherapy should be considered. Extracts of identified allergens are given intradermally at weekly intervals in increasing doses: desensitization takes approximately 6 to 12 months.

Therapeutic Drug Monitoring Examples

BACTERIAL PHARYNGITIS

The approach to therapuetic drug monitoring by clinicians varies depending upon many factors. Some of these include preferences among clinicians in a given community or region; concurrent medical problems which dictate that certain drugs be used or avoided; the patient's response to selected medication. The following outlines of therapeutic drug monitoring offer examples which may serve to stimulate discussion and further understanding of initiating and monitoring drug use. The drugs and dosages presented should not be applied to any clinical situation without proper medical supervision.

Drug Therapy	Cephalexin (Keflex) 250 mg PO Q 6 hr × 14 days is most commonly prescribed because Group A *beta hemolytic streptococcus* is the pathogen associated with rheumatic fever and its associated heart damage. Other causative organisms, of course, would require other antibiotics to which these organisms are sensitive.
Monitoring	**Symptoms:** Dysphagia, odynophagia (pain with swallowing).
	Signs: *Gen:* Fever. *HEENT:* Examine throat for signs of swelling, redness of tonsils, pillars, and uvula. Inspect for white or yellow patches (exudate) on anterior and posterior pharyngeal areas. Exudative material easily wiped off. Palpate for enlarged, tender cervical adenopathy (especially tonsillar nodes).
Laboratory Tests	The clinician may elect to order all, none, or some of these laboratory studies depending upon history and physical findings, as well as other specific clinical indications. Throat culture, white blood cell count (WBC), antistreptolysin O titer, rapid strep screen.
Adverse Drug Event Monitoring	Anaphylactic reaction, diarrhea, bacterial resistance, thrush and other candida overgrowth, hairy tongue.

Therapeutic Drug Monitoring Examples

CANDIDIASIS, OROPHARYNGEAL

The approach to theraupetic drug monitoring by clinicians varies depending upon many factors. Some of these include preferences among clinicians in a given community or region; concurrent medical problems which dictate that certain drugs be used or avoided; the patient's response to selected medication. The following outlines of therapeutic drug monitoring offer examples which may serve to stimulate discussion and further understanding of initiating and monitoring drug use. The drugs and dosages presented should not be applied to any clinical situation without proper medical supervision.

Drug Therapy	Ketoconazole (Nizoral) 200 mg PO QD or other imidazole fungal agents such as fluconazole (Diflucan).
Monitoring	**Symptoms:** Question about odynophagia, appetite, and dysphagia.
	Signs: *HEENT:* Inspect the oral structures for pathognomonic patches of white curd-like exudate. Using a cotton applicator, scrape off some of the exudate, revealing a hyperemic area with slight bleeding.
Laboratory Tests	The clinician may elect to order all, none, or some of these laboratory studies depending upon history and physical findings, as well as other specific clinical indications. Serum liver enzymes, potassium hydroxide smear for hyphae and spores.
Adverse Drug Event Monitoring	Hepatitis signs/symptoms: dark urine, pale stools, right upper quadrant abdominal pain, hepatomegaly, yellow sclera or skin (jaundice), tiredness, poor appetite. Ketoconazole also inhibits the hepatic metabolism of drugs such as terfenadine (Seldane), rifampin, and cyclosporine.

Therapeutic Drug Monitoring Examples

SINUSITIS

The approach to therapuetic drug monitoring by clinicians varies depending upon many factors. Some of these include preferences among clinicians in a given community or region; concurrent medical problems which dictate that certain drugs be used or avoided; the patient's response to selected medication. The following outlines of therapeutic drug monitoring offer examples which may serve to stimulate discussion and further understanding of initiating and monitoring drug use. The drugs and dosages presented should not be applied to any clinical situation without proper medical supervision.

Drug Therapy	Amoxicillin/clavulanate (Augmentin) 500 mg tablet PO Q 8 hr; normal saline spray 2 puffs each nostril 5 times daily and PRN nasal congestion; acetaminophen two 325 mg tablets PO Q 4 hr PRN fever/headache.
Monitoring	**Symptoms:** Face/paranasal headache, fever, facial pressure when bending forward, pain over sinus upon coughing or straining, anorexia, photophobia, or malaise.
	Signs: *HEENT:* Inspect for nasal discharge. Palpate paranasal sinuses for tenderness. Check for sinus fluid by transillumination.
Laboratory Tests	The clinician may elect to order all, none, or some of these laboratory studies depending upon history and physical findings, as well as other specific clinical indications. WBC with differential, sinus x-ray, CT scan.
Adverse Drug Event Monitoring	Diarrhea, skin rash, bacterial resistance, anaphylactic reaction.

Therapeutic Drug Monitoring Examples

RHINITIS, ALLERGIC

The approach to therapuetic drug monitoring by clinicians varies depending upon many factors. Some of these include preferences among clinicians in a given community or region; concurrent medical problems which dictate that certain drugs be used or avoided; the patient's response to selected medication. The following outlines of therapeutic drug monitoring offer examples which may serve to stimulate discussion and further understanding of initiating and monitoring drug use. The drugs and dosages presented should not be applied to any clinical situation without proper medical supervision.

Drug Therapy	Flunisolide (Nasalide) nasal solution 2 sprays each nostril BID.
Monitoring	**Symptoms:** Ask about sneezing episodes, fever, and cough.
	Signs: *HEENT:* Check for watery rhinorrhea, nasal patency, postnasal drip, pharyngeal redness, and watery eyes. Inspect nasal mucosa for pale blue, swollen, boggy appearance. Inspect for nasal polyps.
Laboratory Tests	The clinician may elect to order all, none, or some of these laboratory studies depending upon history and physical findings, as well as other specific clinical indications. Nasal discharge stain for eosinophil count. Allergen skin testing.
Adverse Drug Event Monitoring	Nasal burning, candida overgrowth.

Head, Face, and Neck

8

Since diseases of the head and neck are common, it follows that health complaints related to these areas are also common. Examples of diseases that generate these complaints include various headache syndromes, thyroid diseases, a variety of head and neck cancers, acute injuries, meningitis, torticollis, subarachnoid hemorrhage, referred pain of acute myocardial infarction, and cervical spine disorders (e.g., arthritis). These problems can be medically managed in many ways including the use of a myriad of drugs. Like all drugs, they must be carefully chosen, evaluated, and monitored for their efficacy and safety.

ANATOMY AND PHYSIOLOGY

Head and Face

The skull protects the brain and helps to protect other structures such as the eye, which is set deep in its bony socket. At birth the sutures of the skull are not fixed, allowing the bones of the skull to overlap and be molded during the vaginal birth process. As a child grows, the bony skull thickens, the fontanels close, and the bones fuse at their suture lines. In the adult, the skull is composed of seven bones (i.e., one occipital, two temporal, two parietal, and two frontal bones). The bones of the face are the nasal, ethmoid, sphenoid, maxillary, zygomatic, frontal bones, and mandible (lower jaw). A variety of facial muscles control speaking and facial expression. Two cranial nerves supply the motor and sensory innervation to the face. The **facial nerve** (cranial nerve 7) divides into five major branches (i.e., temporal, zygomatic, buccal, mandibular, and cervical) and primarily serves as a motor nerve to innervate the muscles of the face and neck. The **trigeminal nerve** (cranial nerve 5) has three branches (i.e., ophthalmic, maxillary, and mandibular) and carries skin sensory perception to the brain. The head and face are abundantly fed by blood vessels. The temporal arteries of the head are especially noticeable and can be felt pulsating about one finger breadth in front of each ear canal opening. (See Figures 8.1 and 8.2.)

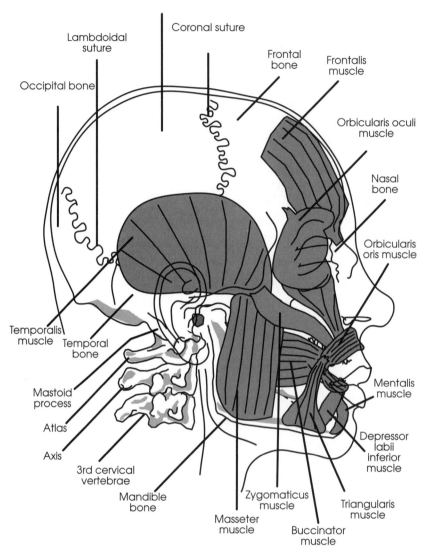

Fig. 8.1 Muscles of the face. Lateral view including bones of head and upper cervical spine.

Neck

The sternocleidomastoid, trapezius, and anterior neck muscles are the major muscles of the neck. On each side of the neck, the sternocleidomastoid muscles course from the base of the skull just behind the ear (i.e., the mastoid process) down and anterior to the area of the sternal notch (see Figure 8.3). To easily identify the sternocleidomastoid muscle, place your hand on the right side of the patient's chin. Ask the patient to turn her head to the right against the resistance of your hand. This maneuver causes the left sternocleidomastoid muscle to contract. The trapezius muscles form the posterior lateral border of the neck and are easily identified by having the patient shrug her shoulders against the resistance of your hands. The larynx, thyroid gland, spinal cord, cervical vertebrae, esophagus, trachea, carotid arteries, jugular veins, and vagus and phrenic nerves are located in the neck. The spinous processes of the seven cervical vertebrae are located on the posterior neck at the midline. The anterior midline structures of the neck from top to bottom are: the hyoid bone, thyroid cartilage, cricoid cartilage, trachea, and sternal notch. The thyroid cartilage, or "Adam's apple," protects the larynx. It is the most prominent structure of the neck's anterior midline and is especially noticeable in thin-necked persons and in males. The hyoid bone is located 1 to 2 cm above the thyroid cartilage and can be felt moving up and down when the patient swallows. The cricoid cartilage is the uppermost cartilaginous ring of the trachea and is positioned immediately below the thyroid cartilage.

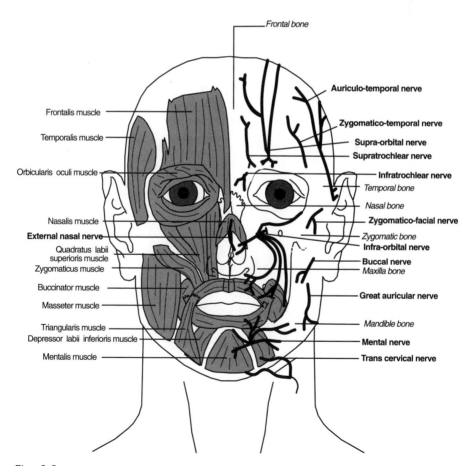

Fig. 8.2 Bones, muscles, and nerves of the face.

The esophagus lies behind the trachea and extends from the back of the mouth, through the neck, the mediastinum, and the diaphragm, to the stomach. The two recurrent laryngeal nerves lie between the trachea and esophagus, one on either side. The close proximity of these recurrent laryngeal nerves to the thyroid gland makes them vulnerable to injury during thyroid surgery or neck trauma, resulting in possible speech and breathing impairment.

Trachea

The trachea is about 11 cm long and 2.5 cm in diameter. It continues into the thorax to about the sternal notch, and then divides into the two main bronchi. Several tracheal cartilaginous rings can be felt while palpating down the trachea (see Figure 8.4).

Endocrine Glands

The highly vascular thyroid gland is composed of two lobes connected by a narrow isthmus. The right and left lobes lie against the sides of the trachea and are mostly

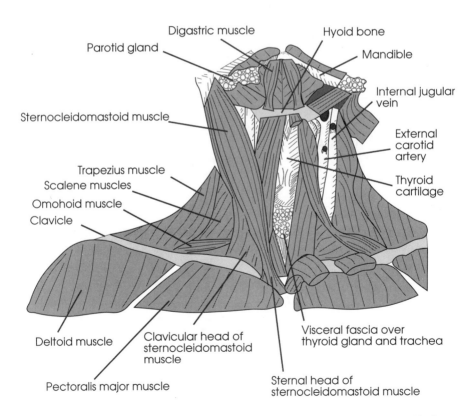

Fig. 8.3 Muscles of the anterior neck, as viewed when looking upward under the chin from the chest. Note digastric muscle going to point of chin (mandible).

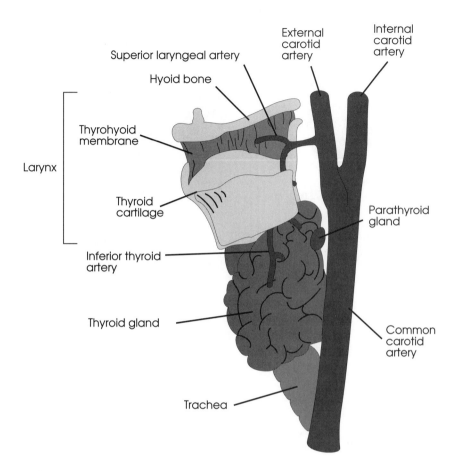

Fig. 8.4   Major structures of neck.

buried beneath the sternocleidomastoid muscles. The isthmus joining the two lobes is located about 2 to 2.5 cm below the thyroid cartilage. The adult gland weighs about 25 gm and is soft and consistently smooth. Unless a person has an extremely thin neck, the normal gland is not seen, and is only sometimes palpable.

The thyroid responds to the thyroxine stimulating hormone (TSH) or thyrotropin released from the anterior pituitary by secreting thyroxine (T_4) and triiodothyronine (T_3). These thyroid hormones increase the oxygen consumption of almost all metabolically active tissues (i.e., increase metabolic rate), affect growth and maturation, regulate lipid metabolism, increase absorption of carbohydrates, and increase oxygen disassociation from hemoglobin.

Behind the thyroid gland, and embedded in it, are four parathyroid glands (two on each lobe; see Figure 8.5). These pea-sized glands regulate calcium metabolism by secreting parathyroid hormone. The parathyroid glands are not detectable by physical examination.

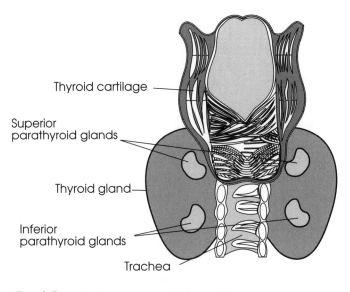

Fig. 8.5   Relationship of thyroid gland to larynx and trachea.
Posterior view (looking from back to front).

Blood Vessels

The right and left **common carotid arteries** branch off from the brachiocephalic artery which originates from the arch of the aorta. The common carotid arteries enter the neck just beneath the sternoclavicular joint and bifurcate into the internal and external carotid arteries at the upper level of the thyroid cartilage.

The **external carotid arteries** give rise to multiple arterial branches that flow to the pharynx, the occipital area, and the thyroid gland (e.g., superior thyroid artery). These arteries each send one branch (i.e., right and left **middle meningeal arteries**) to the dura (i.e., the lining of the brain). The **internal carotid arteries** supply blood to the brain, pituitary gland, orbit of the eye, middle ear, and other structures (see Figure 10.4 in Chapter 10: Blood Vessels).

Two **vertebral arteries** enter the cranial vault where the spinal cord exits and also supply blood to the brain. These arteries pass on each side of the vertebral column, through a hole in the transverse processes of the cervical vertebrae. The carotid and vertebral arteries join inside the cranium near the base of the brain to form the "Circle of Willis." Because of these anastomoses, the brain has a redundant blood supply that is crucial when one of the four arteries becomes partially or completely obstructed (see Figure 10.5 in Chapter 10: Blood Vessels).

Blood returns from the head and neck to the heart though the external and internal jugular veins. The **external jugular veins** receive blood from the superficial structures of the head and neck and the deep parts of the face, then empty into the subclavian veins. Blood from the brain and the deeper structures of the neck and face empty into the **internal jugular veins** which then join with the subclavian veins to form the **brachiocephalic veins.**

On either side of the neck, the **vagus nerves** lie behind the common carotid artery and on top of the internal jugular vein as it courses from the brain stem through the neck to the chest. In the upper chest, the vagus nerve gives off a branch that provides sensory and motor innervation to the larynx. Another branch continues on to supply parasympathetic innervation to the abdominal and thoracic viscera including the heart. The **phrenic nerves,** located deep in the neck, originate from the third, fourth, and fifth cervical nerves. They provide motor innervation to the diaphragm and affect the process of breathing.

Lymph Nodes

The lymphatic system supplements the circulatory system of the blood vessels, and, in conjunction with lymph nodes, plays an important role in defending the body against infection. Lymph, a fluid derived from blood and tissue fluid, drains from peripheral areas of the body through the lymphatic vessels into the cardiovascular system (see Figure 8.6). For example, these lymphatic channels transport proteins, certain enzymes (e.g., lipase), long fatty acids, and cholesterol from interstitial spaces to the blood stream. The lymphatic system in the head and neck consists of collecting ducts, tonsils, adenoids, and lymph nodes.

Lymph fluid from the right upper body drains into the right subclavian vein; lymph fluid from the rest of the body empties into the left subclavian vein. The total lymphatic system is a closed circuit of lymph channels that ultimately drains into the cardiovascular system. Most **lymph nodes** are found in groups or clusters in specific areas of the body. These clusters of nodes are generally found in the deeper aspects of the subcutaneous tissue adjacent to deep fascia of muscles. The lymph nodes are usually grouped in chains and drain specific regions of the body. As a result, they are often referred to as regional lymph nodes. Some lymph nodes are deeply embedded near fascia of muscle and other deeper body tissues. The head and neck are two areas of the body where several chains of lymph nodes are accessible to examination. [There are other areas besides head and neck where lymph nodes are accessible (e.g., axilla, inguinal area, epitrochlear, and popliteal).] Enlargement of lymph nodes may be a presenting sign of various conditions such as a local infection or neoplasm. However, since the lymph nodes drain extensive areas of the body, it may be difficult to localize a specific area or cause to explain an enlarged lymph node.

Most lymph nodes are about the size of an okra seed (1 to 5 mm) or garden pea (5 to 10 mm). **Submental** and **submandibular lymph nodes** are located along the edge of the mandible. **Preauricular** and **parotid lymph nodes** are found in front of the ear overlying the ramus of the mandible. **Postauricular** lymph nodes that serve the scalp and ear are located behind the ear in the area of the mastoid process. These lymph nodes drain the deep and superficial structures of the head and face. **Superficial** and

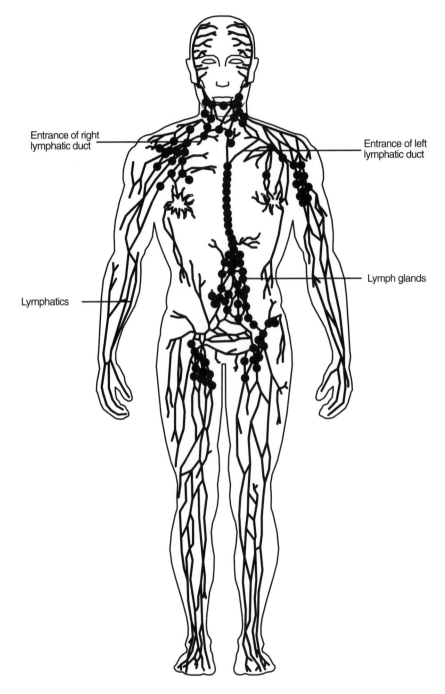

Entrance of right
lymphatic duct

Entrance of left
lymphatic duct

Lymph glands

Lymphatics

Fig. 8.6   Lymphatic system with major lymph node areas shown.

deep **anterior cervical nodal** groups are located in the anterior triangle along the anterior edge of the sternocleidomastoid muscles. A **deep cervical lymph node** chain lies alongside each carotid artery, and a posterior superficial cervical lymph node chain lies on the posterior edge of the sternocleidomastoid muscle. The **supraclavicular lymph nodes** are located along the superior edge of the clavicle in the fossae and drain the breasts, head, and neck. The **occipital lymph nodes** are located at the base of the skull posteriorly and drain the scalp area.

PHYSICAL ASSESSMENT

Head and Face

Examine the face for symmetry, expression, skin lesions, color, abnormal movement, paralysis, edema, and hirsutism. Normal head and facial features can be described as "normocephalic" (i.e., normal head shape) and "atraumatic" (i.e., without visible injury).

Abnormal head movements are associated with dyskinetic and dystonic disorders such as tardive dyskinesia (a late-appearing, potentially irreversible neurological syndrome associated with antipsychotic drug use and characterized by abnormal movements of the face, mouth, and extremities) and torticollis (the contracted state of cervical muscles that produces a twisting of the neck and an unnatural position of the head). Unique facial appearances are consistent with some diseases such as Cushing's syndrome, myxedema (primary hypothyroidism), scleroderma, and systemic lupus erythematosus. Facial features (e.g., affect) also can provide clues in the assessment of psychiatric illnesses (see Chapter 3: Mental Status Examination).

Conduct the examination of the head with the patient sitting in a well-lighted room. Inspect the patient's scalp for skin lesions and dandruff. Also, note the pattern, texture, and color of hair. Using your fingertips, palpate the scalp for scars, lumps, and areas of tenderness. If the patient describes any tender spots on the scalp, pay particular attention to those areas during the exam.

Neck

Anatomically, the neck can be divided into four triangles lying on either side of the midline. These two anterior and two posterior triangles are used as imaginary anatomic markers for describing the location of physical findings. Each **anterior triangle** is defined by the mandible (superiorly), the sternocleidomastoid muscle (posteriorly), and the imaginary midline (anteriorly) (See Figure 8.7.). A carotid artery and an internal jugular vein are located in each anterior triangle. The external jugular veins cross the surface of the sternocleidomastoid muscles as they course downward

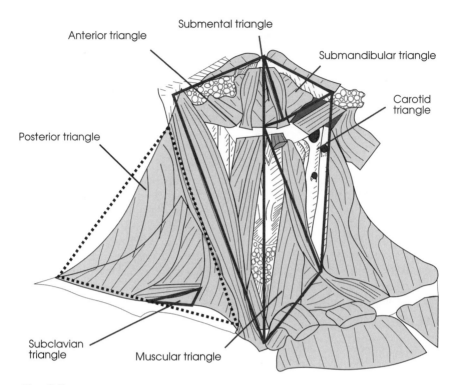

Anterior triangle

Submental triangle

Submandibular triangle

Carotid triangle

Posterior triangle

Subclavian triangle

Muscular triangle

Fig. 8.7 Anatomical divisions of the anterior neck: anterior triangle (with its subdivisions) and posterior triangle.

from just behind the angle of the mandible to the level of the clavicle where they empty into the internal jugular vein. These arteries and veins are the major blood vessels that carry blood to and from the head, neck, and brain. An anterior cervical chain of lymph nodes is also located in each of the anterior triangles.

The borders of each **posterior triangle** are determined by the sternocleidomastoid muscle (anteriorly), the trapezius muscle (posteriorly), and the clavicle (inferiorly). (See Figure 8.7.) Nerves, arteries, veins, and the posterior cervical chain of lymph nodes are located in each of the posterior triangles.

To examine the neck, stand in front of the reclining patient. Evaluate the neck for symmetry, abnormal pulsations, masses, scars, goiter, neck vein distension, lymph node enlargement, deviation of the trachea, and range of motion (see Chapter 13: Musculoskeletal System). With the patient's head slightly rotated to the left, look at the right side to identify the sternocleidomastoid muscle, the external jugular vein, and the visible pulsation of the common carotid artery. Repeat these steps with the patient's head rotated to the right. With the patient looking straight ahead, observe the position of the thyroid cartilage and the trachea at the midline. The trachea may be displaced to the right or the left with lung atelectasis, thyroid enlargement, neck or mediastinal tumor, or pleural effusion. A thoracic aortic aneurysm can pull the trachea downward with each heartbeat, creating the so-called "tracheal tug." (*Note:* An aortic aneurysm of the abdominal aorta will *not* demonstrate a "tracheal tug"). Although the thyroid gland is usually not visible; if seen, note the position, shape, and size of the gland. The normal neck should be soft and supple without thyromegaly or masses.

Cervicofacial Lymph Nodes

With the patient still reclining, palpate the lymph nodes of the head and neck in the following lymphatic areas: 1) the occipital area at the base of the skull for the occipital nodes; 2) behind the ears near the mastoid bone for the postauricular nodes; 3) in front of the ears at the level of, and above, the temporomandibular joint for the preauricular nodes; 4) beneath the angle of the mandible for the tonsillar nodes (superior aspect of the anterior cervical lymph node chains); 5) along the inferior edge of the mandible for the submandibular nodes; and 6) behind the tip of the mandible (chin) for the submental nodes (see Figure 8.8).

Progressing down the neck with the exam, palpate: 1) the anterior superficial nodes along the anterior edge of the sternocleidomastoid muscle; 2) the posterior superficial nodes along the posterior edge of the sternocleidomastoid; 3) the posterior cervical nodes along the anterior edge of the trapezius; and 4) the supraclavicular fossae between the sternocleidomastoid and trapezius for the supraclavicular node chain. Although normal lymph nodes may not be visible, they still may be palpable. To bring

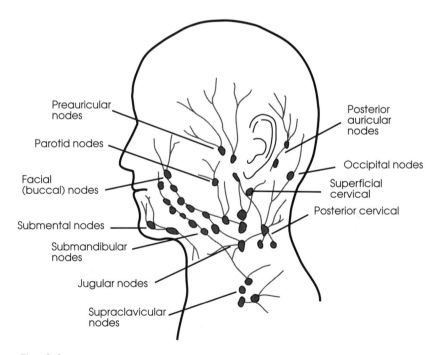

Fig. 8.8 Location of the primary lymph nodes of the neck and face.

the lymph nodes to the surface for easier examination, have the patient take a deep breath and increase intrathoracic pressure by forcibly exhaling against a closed glottis and using the tightened abdominal muscles to increase intra-abdominal pressure to push up on the diaphragm (i.e., the Valsalva maneuver). Do this with caution in cardiac disease patients.

Using the index and second fingers, palpate the superficial lymph nodes with a gentle, slow, rotating movement around each lymph node group. Note the mobility, size, shape (e.g., round, oblong, smooth, or irregular), consistency [e.g., hard, rubbery, or fluctuant (i.e., undulate as a wave)], and presence or absence of tenderness. The cervical lymph nodes, submandibular nodes, and supraclavicular nodes should be examined; the other lymph nodes are seldom clinically important and need only be examined when medical history dictates. Upon finding enlarged lymph nodes (i.e., lymphadenopathy), examine the area that the lymph nodal group drains. Localized cervical lymphadenopathy has been associated with infections of scalp, teeth, ear, or pharynx, as well as with Hodgkin's disease, tuberculosis, syphilis, actinomycosis, cysts, and carcinomas. Generalized cervical lymphadenopathy also has been associated with a variety of diseases (e.g., rubella, catscratch fever, drug allergy). Soft, red, movable, tender lymph nodes suggest inflammation or antigenic response. Hard, nontender, irregular, fixed lymph nodes suggest malignancy. Nontender node enlargement greater than 3 cm is a common sign of lymphatic metastasis from a distant cancer or lymphoma. Therapeutically, measuring the size and number of lymph nodes helps to evaluate a patient's response to chemotherapy. Carefully check the lymph nodes in a patient with a fever of unknown origin. The term "shotty" nodes is used to describe lymph nodes that feel like buckshot (i.e., firm but not connected). "Matted" nodes feel as if they are stuck together and move as a single mass under the skin. They are associated with metastatic cancer and primary lymphatic malignancy; however, they also occur in certain chronic inflammatory states (e.g., erythema nodosum).

Blood Vessels

Next, with the patient reclining at a 30° angle, examine the blood vessels of the head and neck by returning the patient's head to the midline. Place your index and middle fingers on the common carotid artery in the inferior part along the medial edge of the sternocleidomastoid muscle. Do not palpate both carotid arteries simultaneously. Bilateral or unilateral stimulation of the carotid sinus can cause dangerous vagal slowing of the heart and syncope.

While palpating the carotid artery, evaluate the rate and rhythm of the carotid pulse wave for possible partial obstruction (bruit) and note any tenderness that might be experienced by the patient (e.g., possible carotid arteritis). Then inspect each jugular vein for a normal venous pulse wave. The jugular veins are not easily palpable, if at all, because normal venous pressure is considerably less than arterial pressure. Jugular venous pulses, however, can be seen and reflect heart actions of systole and diastole. (See Chapter 11: Blood for a detailed discussion of neck blood vessels.)

Auscultate the carotid arteries with the diaphragm of the stethoscope placed at the carotid bifurcation. This area can be located by following a horizontal line from the top of the thyroid cartilage to a point just below the jaw angle. Ask the patient to hold his or her breath to eliminate breathing noises. Listen over both carotid arteries for bruits that signify turbulent blood flow past a partial obstruction. (See Chapter 11: Blood for details on assessing vascular sounds.)

Auscultation of the larynx with the diaphragm is important in patients with suspected laryngeal edema or obstruction (e.g., epiglottis). Turbulent air flow across the larynx can be heard as an inspiratory or expiratory wheeze. A wheeze heard in the chest, however, may be from either the chest or larynx. If auscultation over the larynx does not uncover a wheeze, then it can be concluded that the wheeze probably originates in the bronchial airways of the lung.

Thyroid

Seat the patient in a comfortable position. Palpate down the midline using your thumb, index, and middle fingers to feel the hyoid bone, thyroid cartilage, cricoid cartilage, and trachea. Check tracheal deviation from the midline position by drawing a perpendicular line with the index finger. Diseases within the mediastinum and lung or within the neck may cause the trachea to deviate from the midline.

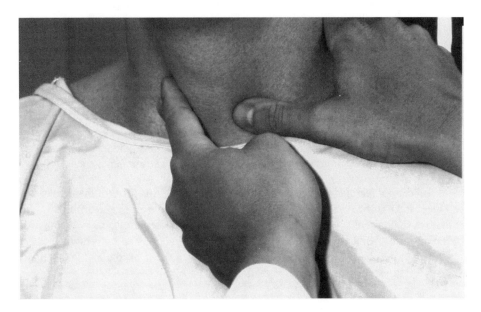

Fig. 8.9   To palpate the right lobe of the thyroid gland from the front of the patient, displace the trachea slightly to the patient's right side with your right hand. Hold the trachea steady and examine the right lobe with your left index and second fingers. Reverse the procedure to examine the left lobe.

The thyroid gland can be palpated from either the front or the back of the patient. Since either approach is workable, find the one that is most comfortable for you.

Standing behind the patient, move the chin down toward the sternum until the anterior neck muscles relax. Then slightly rotate the patient's head to the right side. Relax both hands on the patient's neck. Curve your fingers around the neck until they both touch the thyroid cartilage. Using the tips of the index and middle fingers, feel down the midline structures until about 1 cm below the cricoid cartilage. Follow the trachea laterally to examine the right and left lobes of the thyroid gland. Using the fingers of your left hand, displace the trachea slightly to the right. Hold the trachea steady with your left hand and examine the right lobe with your right index and second fingers. To examine the left lobe, reverse the method (i.e., push with your right fingers and feel with your left).

To identify the glandular thyroidal tissue, ask the patient to swallow; the gland, which is attached to the tracheal fascia, should move up and then down under your fingers. If you detect that the patient has difficulty swallowing, have him or her sip from a glass of water while you feel the gland. The swallowing action moves the thyroid upward beneath your fingers and allows examination of the paratracheal structures that lie beneath the manubrium. With this technique you may discover a substernal thyroid gland.

The frontal approach to examine the thyroid gland is similar to the rear method just described; however, use your thumbs instead of your index and middle fingers of one hand. Standing in front of the patient, flex the patient's head anteriorly, moving the chin toward the sternal notch. Then slightly rotate the chin toward the side of the neck to be examined, relaxing the neck muscles. Place both thumbs in the midline on the gland. Displace the gland to the examining side and feel with the examining fingers medial and deep to the sternocleidomastoid muscle for the thyroid gland. If the right lobe is being examined, stabilize the trachea with the right thumb and palpate with the left thumb (see Figure 8.9). To check the other lobe, reverse these steps. An alternate technique is to use the index and second fingers instead of the thumb to feel the gland. A third technique is to use the thumb, index and middle fingers of the same hand palpating the gland between the thumb on one side and the index and middle finger on the other side. Some examiners use a combination of these three methods.

If you still cannot feel the gland, repeat the above steps, but this time tilt the patient's head back and ask the patient to stare at the ceiling. When you are first learning to examine it, the normal thyroid gland is difficult to palpate. However, you will gain proficiency after many examinations. Also, the thyroid gland generally is more easily palpated in patients who have thin necks. Examination of the thyroid gland in a patient with a short, thick neck is particularly challenging.

Assess the glands for size, consistency (e.g., cystic, rubbery, or hard), shape (e.g., nodular or irregular), tenderness, temperature, and mobility. The gland is normally smooth, soft, nontender, and of normal body temperature. If an enlarged gland is tender and hot, auscultate the gland with the diaphragm of the stethoscope and listen for a bruit. The presence of a bruit is associated with increased blood flow through the large thyroid arteries in the hyperplastic thyroid. A true thyroid bruit will be heard as an intermittent sound. The presence of a continuous venous hum is a false positive finding that can be easily stopped by light compression of the ipsilateral jugular vein.

PHARMACOTHERAPEUTIC CASE ILLUSTRATION

History

L.B., a 38-year-old female, complained of insomnia, fatigue, and nervousness that had progressively worsened during the last several months. She stated that she had lost weight, but had not experienced any change in her appetite or bowel habits. She also complained of blurred vision. Past medical history (PMH), social history (SH), and family history (FH) are not clinically contributory.

Physical Examination

Physical examination revealed an anxious woman with the following vital signs: blood pressure (BP) 135/75 mm Hg; pulse 140 beats/min and regular; a respiratory rate (RR) of 18/min; and a temperature of 37.5° C. Eyes were prominent, with generalized weakness of extraocular muscles; no lid lag. Diplopia was present. Skin was warm and moist from excessive perspiration. Hair was thin and silky. Neck/thyroid: diffuse enlargement of thyroid gland, with the left lobe larger than the right. Gland palpated as firm but not tender; no bruits were heard over either lateral lobe. Neck vessels: no distension, carotid pulse strong and regular, no bruits. Nodes: submandibular, supraclavicular, anterior, and posterior cervical lymph nodes not enlarged, not tender. Heart: normal heart sounds, tachycardia with no arrhythmias, no murmurs, no extra heart sounds. Neurologic: hyperactive deep tendon reflexes, proximal muscle weakness in lower extremities, and hand tremor.

Laboratory

Thyroid function studies showed a high total thyroxine (T_4), large free thyroxine index, and low thyroid-stimulating hormone (TSH).

Diagnosis and Management

L.B. was found to have primary hyperthyroidism (Graves' disease). Methimazole (Tapazole) 20 mg PO QD and propranolol (Inderal) 40 mg PO BID were prescribed. A complete blood cell count (CBC) was ordered.

Discussion

Disease. Primary hyperthyroidism is a disease of hypermetabolic or sympathomimetic activity associated with abnormally high levels of T_4, T_3, or both. Specific causes of hyperthyroidism include diffuse toxic goiter (Graves' disease), toxic nodular goiter, toxic adenoma (Plummer's nodule), drug-induced hyperthyroidism, thyroiditis, pituitary adenoma, TSH-induced pituitary tumor, and choriocarcinoma.

Graves' disease is the most common cause of thyroid hormone overproduction, and occurs most often in women between 20 and 40 years of age. The signs and symptoms of hyperthyroidism can be attributed to increased catecholamine activity and hypermetabolism. The symptoms and signs of catecholamine excess include increased pulse, systolic hypertension, hand tremor, prominent cardiac apical impulse, excessive sweating, palpitations, and systolic heart murmur. Some hyperthyroid patients complain of generalized muscle weakness (especially in proximal muscle groups), insomnia, weight loss with a good appetite, anxiety, heat intolerance, and diarrhea. The thyroid gland is diffusely enlarged, but not tender, with a smooth lobular contour and easily palpable lobes. A bruit may be audible over the thyroid gland. Other physical findings include palmar erythema, onycholysis, staring gaze, and lid lag (see Chapter 5: Eye).

Proximal muscle weakness in the legs is often indicated by complaints of weakness when walking up stairs or when arising from a seated position. Deep tendon reflexes (DTRs) are usually hyperactive without myoclonus and can be demonstrated with Achilles tendon jerk (DTR) testing (see Chapter 14: Nervous System). With experience, a clinical assessment at the bedside can be reliable without the use of expensive equipment.

Ophthalmopathic complications are unique to Graves' disease. The extraocular muscles often become inflamed and weak, and, thereby, limit the movements of the eye. When orbital fat and retro-ocular pressure increase, the eye protrudes forward in the classic stare known as

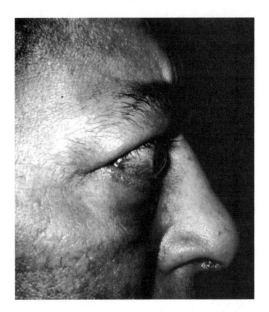

Fig. 8.10 Exophthalmos, a protrusion of the eye resulting from increased orbital fat and retro-ocular pressure, is a classic symptom of Graves' disease (also see Chapter 5: Eye, Fig. 5.15).

exophthalmos or proptosis (see Figure 8.10 and Figure 5.15 in Chapter 5: Eye). Exophthalmos may be unilateral or bilateral, and symmetrical or asymmetrical. Conjunctivae and cornea are also usually inflamed and the patient's optic nerve (cranial nerve 2) may be damaged with associated loss of vision.

Pretibial myxedema, a nonpitting edema of the lower leg caused by subcutaneous accumulation of mucopolysaccharide, gives a hyperthyroid patient's overlying skin an orange peel appearance on the anterior lower leg.

The extent to which a patient's bodily function and metabolic rate increase depends, in part, upon the rapidity of onset of the hyperthyroid state. Slowly progressive hyperthyroidism may go unnoticed for many years. In most cases, florid Graves' disease is easily recognizable; however, in some patients the clinical presentation is more subtle. For example, the clinical features of Graves' disease in the elderly are often limited to a single organ system and lack the clues commonly associated with sympathomimetic excess. The elderly person may only have atrial fibrillation, unexplained congestive heart failure, an unexplained weight loss, personality changes (e.g., depression), or chronic diarrhea.

Management. The correct diagnosis directs the selection of treatment: drug therapy, radioactive iodine (RAI), and subtotal thyroidectomy. The therapy of choice varies among clinicians and is affected by the age and gender of the patient. Radioactive iodine with or without anti-thyroid drugs generally is the treatment of choice in persons over 40 years of age. Radioactive iodine is absolutely contraindicated in pregnancy and must be used very cautiously in any female who might become pregnant. If the patient is less than 40 years of age, drug therapy is the treatment of choice. Subtotal thyroidectomy provides quick relief from symptoms and is often preferred by patients who are concerned about radioactive therapy, and by persons with contraindications to antithyroid drugs.

When choosing a treatment, the risks and benefits of each treatment approach must be carefully explained to the patient, and the patient needs to take part in the treatment selection process. When hyperthyroid symptoms must be quickly brought into control, treatment with an antithyroid drug in combination with a beta-adrenergic blocking agent can be started. After the acute hyperthyroid symptoms are under control, the patient feels better and can rationally talk about choosing among the three treatment choices.

Hyperthyroidism has a variable course once treatment is started. About one-third of patients remain euthyroid after treatment; however, some relapse after an initial remission. Therefore, once hyperthyroidism is diagnosed the patient must be monitored regularly for recurrence of hyperthyroidism and for iatrogenic hypothyroidism. Over-treatment is the most frequent cause of hypothyroidism, especially with ablative therapies (e.g., radioactive iodine or subtotal thyroidectomy). Hypothyroidism can also be caused by antithyroid drugs. The onset of hypothyroidism can be very subtle and insidious, and is best detected by periodic TSH testing and clinical evaluation. Hypothyroidism must be treated with thyroid hormones (e.g., levothyroxine) on an ongoing basis.

To achieve symptomatic control, methimazole was prescribed for L.B. Two antithyroid compounds (thioamides) are available: propylthiouracil (PTU) and methimazole. The dosage of these drugs varies with the severity of the disease. The usual initial dose of propylthiouracil is 100 mg Q 8 hr; methimazole is 10 mg Q 8 or 12 hr. Methimazole can be administered once daily (i.e., 10 to 30 mg as a single daily dose), is less costly, and does not have a bitter taste like PTU. Usually, doses less than 30 mg/day of methimazole are sufficient to convert the patient to a euthyroid state. PTU is preferable to methimazole during pregnancy and thyroid storm. Unlike methimazole, PTU also inhibits the peripheral conversion of T_4 to T_3. The important side effects of thioamides are skin reactions and agranulocytosis. Some patients may have an itching rash, particularly early in the course of therapy. A more serious, but rare, complication of the thioamides is agranulocytosis. Drug-induced agranulocytosis most commonly affects patients older than 40 years of age who are being treated with more than 30 mg/day of methimazole or 250 mg/day of PTU. The patient must be alerted to report the abrupt onset of rash, fever, sore throat, or flu-like symptoms. A complete blood cell count (CBC) with differential is recommended before initiation of thioamides, a few weeks after initiation of therapy, and at the first sign of agranulocytosis.

About two to three weeks of thioamide therapy is needed before clinical symptoms resolve. Therefore, the beta-adrenergic blocker propranolol was ordered for L.B. Propranolol (Inderal), nadolol (Corgard), atenolol (Tenormin), or other beta blockers improve some of the hyperthyroid symptoms such as excessive sweating, nervousness, tremor, and palpitations. L.B. can feel better quickly while waiting for the full onset of benefits from the thioamide. The beta blockers, however, must be used cautiously in patients with asthma, AV conduction block, or congestive heart failure. Propranolol may have an advantage over other beta blockers because it inhibits the peripheral conversion of T_4 to T_3. The daily dose of propranolol is 160 mg, atenolol about 200 mg, and nadolol 80 mg. The dose, however, is determined by therapeutic response and the presence of side effects.

Although not used in L.B., Lugol's solution and a saturated solution of potassium iodide (SSKI) are often used to gain rapid control of symptoms or to rapidly prepare the gland for surgery. Large doses of iodide administered for two weeks before surgery, increase the firmness of the thyroid gland by decreasing its size, vascularity, and friability. Iodides are simple to administer, inexpensive, have few side effects, and do not ablate the gland; however, an early release of thyroid hormone, unpleasant taste, relapse after 7 to 14 days of treatment, and interference with radioactive iodine therapy are disadvantages. In the hyperthyroid patient, monitor the reversal of hypermetabolic signs and symptoms such as a slowing pulse, increasing muscle strength, temperature tolerance, improved ophthalmopathy, decreased nervousness, and normalizing DTRs. After several months, the myxedema will be less noticeable, regular menses will resume, and sleeping patterns will normalize.

After one year of continuous thioamide therapy, the methimazole dose will be gradually reduced to see if L.B. remains euthyroid. She has about a 30% chance of remaining euthyroid after one year of thioamide therapy; however, after two years of continuous thioamide suppressive therapy, the remission rate is about twice that of one year of continuous suppressive therapy. The goal of thioamide therapy is to achieve symptomatic relief and spontaneous remission. Because the onset of remission is by chance, the most appropriate time to withdraw treatment is not known. Thioamide therapy must be gradually withdrawn, and be analogous to the gradual opening of the corral gate to see if a penned-up bull comes out raging or meandering.

Therapeutic Drug Monitoring Examples

HYPERTHYROIDISM (GRAVES' DISEASE)

The approach to therapuetic drug monitoring by clinicians varies depending upon many factors. Some of these include preferences among clinicians in a given community or region; concurrent medical problems which dictate that certain drugs be used or avoided; the patient's response to selected medication. The following outlines of therapeutic drug monitoring offer examples which may serve to stimulate discussion and further understanding of initiating and monitoring drug use. The drugs and dosages presented should not be applied to any clinical situation without proper medical supervision.

Drug Therapy

Propylthiouracil 100–200 mg PO Q 6 hr, then maintenance dose of 100–300 mg/day; or methimazole 5–20 mg PO Q 8 hr × 2 months, then maintenance dose of 5–15 mg/day.

Monitoring

Symptoms: Question about heat intolerance, weight loss, excessive appetite, and excessive sweating.

Signs: *MSE:* Rapid speech and nervousness. *Skin:* Palpate scalp hair for fine texture. *HEENT:* Inspect eyes for lid retraction, proptosis; test for lid lag and ophthalmoplegia by EOM and accommodation testing (see Chapter 5: Eye). Inspect and palpate thyroid gland for size, consistency, and temperature. Auscultate thyroid gland for bruit. *CVS:* Count pulse rate and rhythm for sinus tachycardia or irregular rhythm of atrial fibrillation (see Chapter 10: Heart). Auscultate the heart for systolic murmur. Palpate for pretibial non-pitting edema (see Chapter 11: Blood). *Neuro:* Check for knee or Achilles DTR hyperactivity (see Chapter 14: Nervous System).

Therapeutic Drug Monitoring Examples

HYPERTHYROIDISM (GRAVES' DISEASE)
(continued)

Laboratory Tests: The clinician may elect to order all, none, or some of these laboratory studies depending upon history and physical findings, as well as other specific clinical indications. T_4, RT_3U, FT_4I, and WBC with differential.

Adverse Drug
Event Monitoring Check for pruritic maculopapular rash, arthralgia, fever, sore throat, transient leukopenia, agranulocytosis, hepatitis signs and symptoms.

Therapeutic Drug Monitoring Examples

HYPOTHYROIDISM

The approach to therapeutic drug monitoring by clinicians varies depending upon many factors. Some of these include preferences among clinicians in a given community or region; concurrent medical problems which dictate that certain drugs be used or avoided; the patient's response to selected medication. The following outlines of therapeutic drug monitoring offer examples which may serve to stimulate discussion and further understanding of initiating and monitoring drug use. The drugs and dosages presented should not be applied to any clinical situation without proper medical supervision.

Drug Therapy	Levothyroxine 50–100 µg PO QD.
Monitoring	**Symptoms:** Ask about weight gain with reduced food intake, cold intolerance, constipation, and decreased libido.

Signs: *MSE:* Assess mental status for signs of apathetic affect or depression (see Chapter 3: Mental Status Exam). *Skin:* Palpate for cold, dry, scaly, or thick skin and hair loss. *HEENT:* Note any vocal hoarseness or low pitch/rough quality. Palpate for puffy non-pitting facial edema. Inspect for an enlarged tongue and lateral eyebrow loss; note ptosis. *CVS:* Auscultate the heart S_3, S_4, or gallop rhythm; count the apical pulse (bradycardia). Palpate heart for left lateral shift of point of maximal cardiac impulse (PMI) (cardiomegaly). Hypokinetic, weak pulse (see Chapter 11: Blood). *Abd:* Check for ascites by shifting dullness and fluid wave tests (see Chapter 12: Abdomen). *Mus:* Grade muscle strength for weakness (see Chapter 13: Musculoskeletal System). *Neuro:* Evaluate knee and Achilles hyporeflexia and sign of median nerve compression (hand paresthesia) by lightly percussing median nerve at the wrist and hand (Tinel's sign) (see Chapter 14: Nervous System).

Therapeutic Drug Monitoring Examples

HYPOTHYROIDISM
(continued)

Laboratory Tests	The clinician may elect to order all, none, or some of these laboratory studies depending upon history and physical findings, as well as other specific clinical indications. Thyroid stimulating hormone (TSH), T_4, complete blood count (CBC), electrocardiogram (ECG).
Adverse Drug Event Monitoring	Watch for atrial fibrillation (irregular rate and rhythm), palpitations, MI, chest pain of angina pectoris, symptoms and signs of iatrogenic hyperthyroidism.

Chest
and Lungs

The ribs and attached muscles of the chest work together with the lungs to support the respiratory metabolic needs of the body. This respiratory system is structurally divided into three major components: the trachea, the lungs, and the thoracic cage with its associated muscular diaphragm. Drugs can significantly affect the respiratory system.

ANATOMY AND PHYSIOLOGY

Thorax

The skeletal components of the thoracic wall consist of bones and cartilage that join together to form the sternum, thoracic vertebrae, and ribs (see Figures 9.1 and 9.2). The **sternum** (i.e., breast bone) can be differentiated into three distinct anatomic segments: the **manubrium**, the **body** (i.e., corpus), and the cartilaginous **xiphoid process**. Measuring about 17 cm in length in an adult, the sternum supports the heads of the clavicles at their junction with the manubrium. The point at which the manubrium joins the body of the sternum is known as the **"angle of Louis."** The second ribs attach anteriorly to the sternum at the angle of Louis, making it an important anatomic landmark for counting and locating ribs.

Twelve pairs of ribs form the superstructure of the thoracic cage. The first seven pairs of ribs, known as the **vertebrosternal** (i.e., "true ribs") start from thoracic vertebrae one through seven and are joined anteriorly to the sternum by costal cartilage. The remaining five pairs of ribs are known as "false ribs." The first three pairs of false ribs join the cartilage of the rib immediately above. (i.e., the eighth rib joins the cartilage of the seventh rib, the ninth rib that of the eighth, and the tenth that of the ninth). These ribs are also known as **vertebrochondral** ribs. The last two pairs of false ribs (i.e., the eleventh and twelfth ribs) originate at the eleventh and twelfth vertebrae. Rather than attaching to the sternum, these last two ribs are free at their anterior ends and are called **vertebral** ribs (i.e., "floating ribs"). The intercostal space (ICS) between each rib is described in terms of the rib immediately above the space (e.g., the space between the first and second ribs is the first intercostal space.)

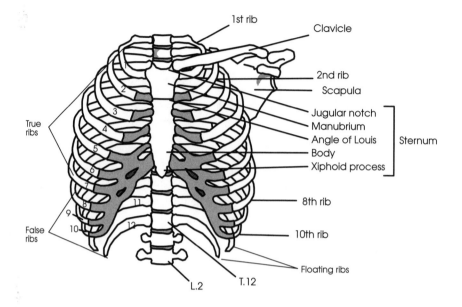

Fig. 9.1 Anterior view of the bony thorax.

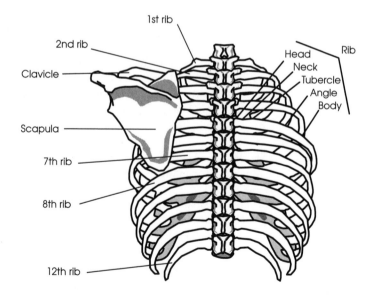

Fig. 9.2 Posterior view of the bony thorax.

Respiratory Muscles

Inspiration is an active process requiring the work of many muscles. The **diaphragm**, a musculomembranous partition between the abdominal and thoracic cavities, contracts to increase the vertical dimension of the chest cavity during normal inspiration. Innervated by the phrenic nerves, the diaphragm moves about 1.5 cm downward during normal tidal respiration and can move as much as 7 cm with deep inspiration. The other important inspiratory muscles are the **external intercostal muscles**, which are innervated by intercostal nerves (see Figure 9.3).

Contraction of the external intercostal muscles raises the lower ribs upward and forward, pushes the sternum outward and increases the expansion capacity of the lungs by increasing the anteroposterior and lateral (i.e., transverse) diameters of the chest. The diaphragm and the external intercostal muscles can maintain adequate ventilation while a person is at rest. During vigorous inspiration, the **sternocleidomastoid muscles** of the neck, along with the **anterior serrati** and **scaleni muscles**, serve as accessory inspiratory muscles that lift the ribs from an oblique position to one more perpendicular with the spine.

After inspiration, the **internal intercostal muscles** contract to pull the ribs downward, thereby decreasing the intrathoracic volume and facilitating expiration. Lung and chest wall elasticity and compliance; pliability of ligamentous rib articulations; shifts in the position of abdominal contents, actions of abdominal muscles; and the force of gravity are other factors that work together with respiratory muscles to facilitate expiration.

Tracheobronchial Tree

Inspired air passes through the nasal passages and pharynx, down the trachea, through the right and left bronchi to secondary bronchi, and into progressively smaller bronchioles and alveolar ducts to the air sacs known as alveoli.

The **trachea** is the top of the respiratory tree. Measuring about 2.5 cm in diameter and 11 cm in length in adults, the trachea is kept open by C-shaped cartilaginous rings. It originates at the thyroid cartilage (i.e., Adam's apple) and extends to about the fifth thoracic vertebra before it bifurcates to become the **right** and **left bronchi**. At the point of bifurcation, the right bronchus diverges less acutely than the left. Because of this configuration, aspiration pneumonia is more likely to result in right lobe consolidation. Similarly, inhaled foreign objects are more likely to lodge in the right bronchus. The right bronchus is approximately 2.5 cm in length compared to the left, which measures 5 cm. These two bronchi further subdivide into secondary bronchi which correspond to the lobes of the lungs. The bronchi continue to divide into smaller and smaller airways until they reach the alveoli.

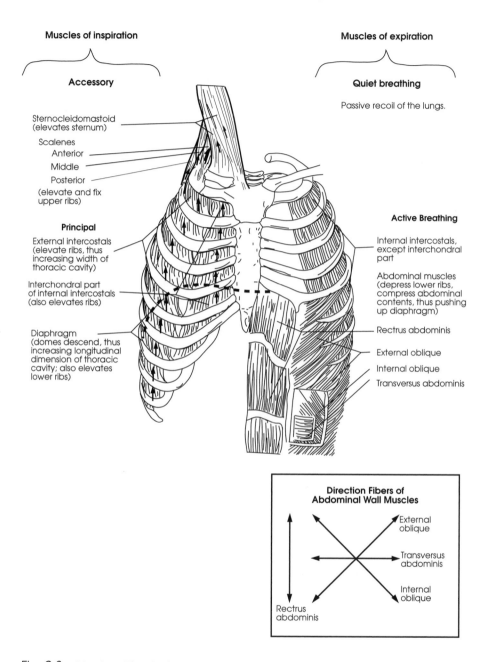

Muscles of inspiration

Accessory

Sternocleidomastoid
(elevates sternum)

Scalenes
Anterior
Middle
Posterior
(elevate and fix
upper ribs)

Principal

External intercostals
(elevate ribs, thus
increasing width of
thoracic cavity)

Interchondral part
of internal intercostals
(also elevates ribs)

Diaphragm
(domes descend, thus
increasing longitudinal
dimension of thoracic
cavity; also elevates
lower ribs)

Muscles of expiration

Quiet breathing

Passive recoil of the lungs.

Active Breathing

Internal intercostals,
except interchondral
part

Abdominal muscles
(depress lower ribs,
compress abdominal
contents, thus pushing
up diaphragm)

Rectrus abdominis

External oblique

Internal oblique

Transversus abdominis

**Direction Fibers of
Abdominal Wall Muscles**

External
oblique

Transversus
abdominis

Internal
oblique

Rectrus
abdominis

Fig. 9.3   Muscles of Respiration.

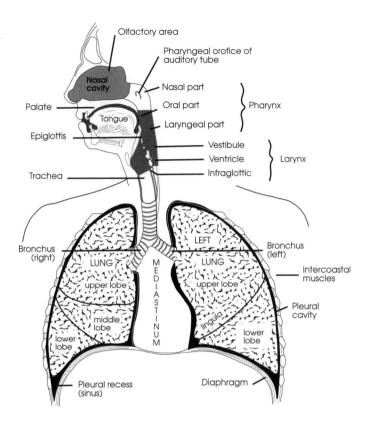

Fig. 9.4 Components of the respiratory system from the nose to the alveolus.

Lungs

The lungs are separated by a mass of tissues and organs known as the **mediastinum**. The right lung is divided into three lobes: **the right upper lobe, the right middle lobe**, and **the right lower lobe**. The left lung is divided into only two lobes: **the left upper lobe** and **the left lower lobe**. (See Figure 9.4.)

Each lobe is further divided into subunits known as **bronchopulmonary segments**. A serous membrane or **visceral pleura** covers the surface of each lung. The **parietal pleura** lines the chest wall, mediastinum, and diaphragm, and joins the visceral pleura as it reflects off the lung at the hilum (i.e., the point at which the veins and arteries enter and exit the lung). The fluid-filled space between the visceral and parietal pleura is called the **pleural cavity** and functions to ease lung expansion and contraction (see Figures 9.5 and 9.6). The pleural cavity normally is not visible on chest x-rays; however, it can be seen when disease or injury causes it to fill with air (i.e., pneumothorax) or excessive fluid (i.e., hydrothorax). Sometimes, when the parietal and visceral pleurae become inflamed, a friction rub may be heard over the involved area during auscultation. However, increased fluid (i.e., pleural effusion) can diminish this sound by reducing the friction between two inflamed pleural surfaces.

Respiration

Each breath, or respiratory cycle, is composed of an **inspiratory phase** and an **expiratory phase**. Under normal conditions, the lung and chest wall are elastic and recoil during expiration to their initial positions. However, with airway diseases (e.g., asthma), accessory neck muscles are needed to assist in expiration. During forceful expiration (e.g., coughing), the abdominal muscles, including the **transversus abdominous, internal** and **external oblique muscles**, and **rectus abdominis**, contract (see Figure 9.3). Contraction of the abdominal recti muscles forces the abdominal contents upward against the diaphragm. This action pushes the diaphragm upward and pulls the thoracic cage downward, decreasing the space in the thorax and forcing more air out of the lungs.

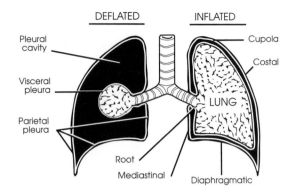

Fig. 9.5 Lungs. Lining of the pleural space (parietal and visceral plura) and relation to other thoracic structures. The deflate lung represents what might be seen if the lung was collapsed and the deflated lung surrounded by fluid (hydrothorax) or air (pneumothorax).

Respiratory centers in the brain stem (i.e., the pons and medulla oblongata) regulate respiration (i.e., gas exchange) by responding to impulses originating from peripheral and central chemoreceptors, as well as changes in arterial pH and the concentration of oxygen and carbon dioxide in the blood. The lungs also have receptors that react to stretching, irritants, and hemodynamic changes. These sensors control respiration by sending information to the respiratory centers, which stimulate or inhibit the respiratory muscles.

PHYSICAL ASSESSMENT

Landmarks

The horizontal lines of the ribs and vertical lines of various thoracic structures form an imaginary grid that is used as a foundation for physical assessment of the chest. Thus, you must be familiar with chest wall landmarks to accurately describe the locations of your physical findings (see Figure 9.7 on page 9–8).

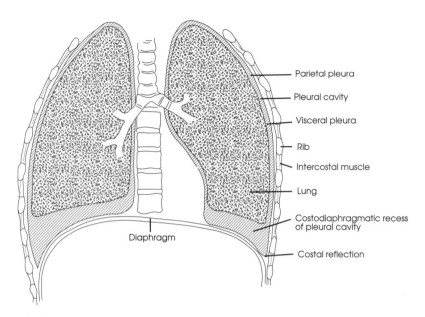

Parietal pleura

Pleural cavity

Visceral pleura

Rib

Intercostal muscle

Lung

Costodiaphragmatic recess
of pleural cavity

Diaphragm

Costal reflection

Fig. 9.6 Pleural space in relation to diaphragm, ribs, and mediastinum. The volume of the pleural space does not change with breathing. The volume of the lung changes with inspiration and expiration.

Anteriorly, the second rib connects to the sternum at the angle of Louis. The space beneath this rib is the second intercostal space. Starting at this point, the ribs and interspaces are numbered to denote the horizontal lines of the grid. The imaginary vertical lines are called the midsternal, midclavicular, anterior axillary, midaxillary, and posterior axillary lines.

The **midsternal line** extends vertically from the middle of the sternal notch through the tip of the xiphoid process. The **midclavicular line** extends vertically from the midpoint of the clavicle down through the nipple. Moving laterally to the armpit (i.e., axilla), imagine three equidistant vertical lines starting anteriorly and moving posteriorly (i.e., the anterior, mid, and posterior axillary lines). The **anterior axillary line** extends inferiorly from the anterior fold of the axilla (i.e., the point at which the pectoralis muscles attach to the proximal humorus). The **posterior axillary line** extends inferiorly from the posterior axillary fold (i.e., the point at which the latissimus dorsi muscle attaches to the proximal humorus). The **mid axillary line** begins at a midpoint between these two folds and extends vertically in an inferior direction.

On the back, think of a line passing straight down the spine touching each of the spinous processes; this is the **vertebral line**. Next, envision a line coming off the mid-shoulder and passing vertically through the middle of the scapula; this is the **scapular line**. When describing a physical finding on the chest, use the imaginary lines and ribs with intercostal spaces to pinpoint its location (e.g., "A friction rub is heard maximally on the anterior chest wall at the level of the fourth intercostal space, right midclavicular line.")

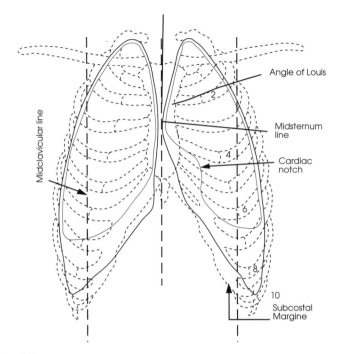

Fig. 9.7 The location of physical findings in the chest exam are described in terms of an imaginary grid formed by the horizontal lines of the ribs and vertical lines corresponding to key anatomical landmarks.

Posterior Chest: Inspection

The examination should be conducted in a warm, comfortable, quiet, and well-lighted room. Ask the patient to disrobe from the waist up and to sit with his arms relaxed at his sides. A posterior chest inspection is more difficult with some bedridden patients who are unable to sit up. These patients must be rolled from side to side with someone's help to complete the exam. Wheelchair patients can be asked to lean forward to facilitate access to the posterior chest.

Examine the patient in an orderly manner, beginning with the upper posterior chest and proceeding downward. Note the skin color, temperature, and texture. Is it cyanotic, red or inflamed, hot and dry, or excessively sweaty? Observe the chest through a complete respiratory cycle. Throughout the assessment, try to visualize the underlying structures and compare one side of the chest with the other to detect any differences. Standing at the patient's right side, note the ratio of the anteroposterior (AP) diameter to lateral diameter. This ratio normally ranges from 1:2 to about 5:7. The anteroposterior to lateral ratio can be affected by normal aging, kyphosis (a deformity of the spine characterized by extensive flexion), or chronic pulmonary disease (i.e., emphysema and its associated barrel chest). In patients with emphysema, the AP diameter may approach a 1:1 ratio.

The normal respiratory rate is 12 to 20 breaths per minute. Normal rhythm is regular and the depth should be neither excessively deep nor shallow. Tachypnea (i.e., a rate greater than 20 breaths per minute) occurs with many diseases (e.g., pleurisy) or injuries (e.g., rib fractures). As a result of volume changes with aging, pseudo-tachypnea may be normal in a resting elderly patient. Bradypnea (i.e., a rate of less than 12 breaths per minute) is associated with conditions such as central nervous system (CNS) drug overdose, psychiatric illnesses, and coma. Figure 9.8 depicts various breathing patterns which should be carefully studied so that they are recognizable. Once seen in a patient, these patterns are easily remembered.

Observe and note the **contour** of the chest and the patient's **posture** and **motions** associated with breathing. Some variations in contour (e.g., kyphosis or scoliosis) limit the free movement of the ribs and cause abnormal breathing patterns (see Figure 9.9). Follow the downward slope of the ribs (e.g., elevated in emphysema), and look at the intercostal spaces throughout the respiratory cycle (e.g., retraction). Normally, the space between each rib bulges outward during expiration and retracts inward with inspiration. This process is generally difficult to notice during periods of quiet breathing. However, with airway dysfunction (e.g., an acute asthma episode) generalized intercostal space retraction is exaggerated during inspiration. Focal inhalation space retraction can occur with pleural effusion or lobar pneumonia. Inspect for abnormal bulging of the intercostal spaces during expiration (e.g., emphysema) and for the use of accessory muscles.

While seated, patients with advanced chronic obstructive airways disease (COAD) tend to lean forward and prop themselves up with their hands on their knees. This position elevates the patient's clavicles and provides leverage for the accessory breathing muscles to expand the chest. Excessive abdominal muscle contraction and nasal flaring are other signs of breathing difficulty. Some patients may purse their lips as if they are trying to blow out a candle. This movement increases pressure within the bronchioles, keeps them from collapsing (a result of the disease process), and allows more air to be exhaled.

Clubbing of the fingers is often present with chronic lung and heart disease; however, it is also a normal variant finding (see Figure 4.5 in Chapter 4: Skin, Hair and Nails). **Splinting** is a protective reaction to chest pain associated with rib fractures, pleurisy, pneumothorax, and pleural fibrosis. Patients with these disorders tend to hold their painful chest area to limit its expansion, especially during deep breaths. Along with splinting to one side, these patients breathe with a shallow, rapid pattern.

Posterior Chest: Palpation

After completing the inspection of the posterior chest, palpate the area with the palm of your hand and fingertips. Be sure to warm your hands (e.g., by vigorously rubbing them together) before touching the patient. Begin at the apex and move down the posterior chest, comparing one side with the other. Feel for areas of tenderness, masses, and crepitation on the chest. **Crepitus** (or subcutaneous emphysema) is

Breathing Patterns

Normal Breathing

The rate is between 12 to 20 breaths per minute. The depth (i.e., volume) is neither excessive nor brief; it is active during inspiration and passive on expiration. The patient uses chest muscles. The rhythm is regular.

Rapid, Deep Breathing (Hyperpnea, Hyperventilation)

The rate is more than 20 breaths per minute. The depth is deep and the rhythm is regular. This pattern is seen with exercise, anxiety, and metabolic acidosis.

Slow, Regular Breathing (Bradypnea)

The rate is less than 12 beats per minute and the rhythm is regular. The depth is normal. This pattern is seen with coma, CNS depressant drug overdose, and increased intracranial pressure (e.g., brain tumor).

Rapid, Shallow Breathing (Tachypnea)

The rate is more than 20 breaths per minute, the volume is shallow, and the rhythm is regular. This pattern happens with restrictive lung diseases, pleuritis, and emphysema.

Cheyne-Stokes Breathing

A cyclic pattern with periods of apnea followed by crescendo-decrescendo breathing. Cheyne-Stokes breathing happens in drug-induced respiratory depression, heart failure, uremia, and brain trauma.

Kussmaul Breathing

A pattern of fast and deep breathing seen in patients with metabolic acidosis as they attempt to "breathe off" the acid accumulating in their blood.

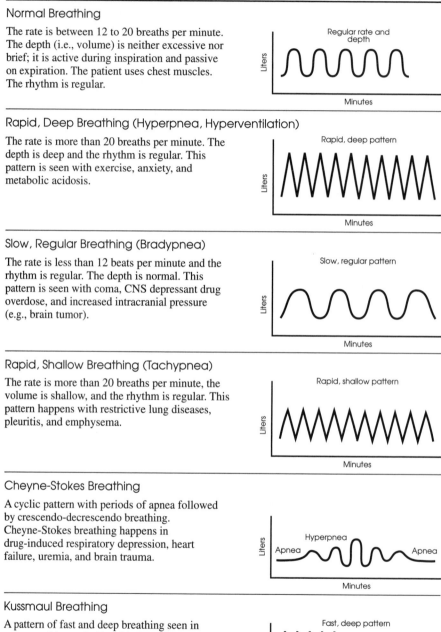

Fig. 9.8 Breathing patterns.

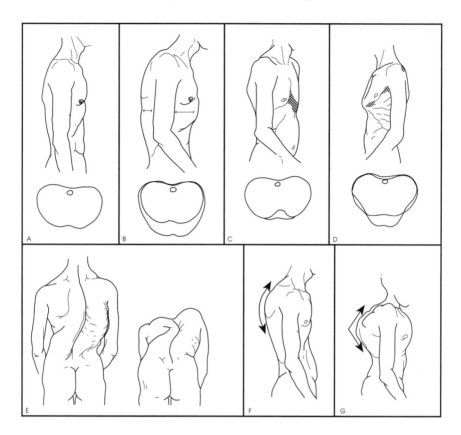

Fig. 9.9 Chest wall contours: A. Normal. B. Barrel chest associated with emphysema. C. Pectus excavatum (i.e., funnel chest). D. Pectus carinatum (i.e., pigeon breast). E. Scoliosis. F. Kyphosis. G. Gibbus (i.e., extreme kyphosis).

caused by subcutaneous air bubbles and is felt as a coarse, crackling sensation similar to the feeling of plastic, air-filled packing material. When palpated, the air bubbles move around freely under the skin.

To check for **tactile fremitus** (i.e., palpable vibration) place both palms on the chest and ask the patient to repeat the phrase "bad boy." Compare the intensity and symmetry of the palpable vibrations. Tactile fremitus is easiest to sense if the patient places her hands on her hips. Looking at the patient's back, press your palms and fingertips firmly over the apices of the right and left lung. Work your way down the back, feeling the following areas: the apices; the space between the abducted (i.e., spread apart) scapulae; and down the paravertebral area to the twelfth rib. Then ask the patient to raise both arms to the ceiling and feel the lateral chest wall. Normally, you should feel a cat-like purring sensation that is symmetrical and almost equal in intensity on each side of the chest.

Because the trachea lies in contact with the right lung apex tactile fremitus is normally felt to vibrate more over the right upper lobe of the lung than over the left upper lobe. Although tactile fremitus is more intense in the second right intercostal space in the front and between the scapulae on the back, the ability to discern this differentiation usually comes only after considerable practice and experience.

Identifying an area of decreased tactile fremitus suggests either the presence of an obstruction in the bronchial tree or that the lung has moved away from the chest wall. Displacement of the lung from the chest wall may be caused by fluid (e.g., blood or pus), air, or solid matter (e.g., tumor). Atelectasis, pneumothorax, pulmonary effusion, and bronchial obstruction are pathophysiologic conditions that decrease tactile fremitus.

Accentuated or increased **vocal fremitus** can be palpated when there is a direct or solid communication from the bronchus through the lung directly to the chest wall. Vocal fremitus is classically associated with lobar pneumonia in which the alveoli fill with a fluid (i.e., pus) which transmits bronchial tree vibrations of breathing better than the air normally present.

Respiratory excursion is a measure of lung expansion, and is measured by placing both your thumbs at the tenth rib with your hands grasping around the lower lateral back. With gentle pressure, slide your thumbs to the patient's spine to create a skin fold between the thumbs. Then ask the patient to inhale deeply. Normally, the thumbs move laterally an equal distance from the spine. If one thumb does not move or lags behind, check for asymmetric expansion, a sign of unilateral disease (e.g., pleurisy). Again, stand behind the patient with your hands resting laterally at the mid-scapular line and ask the patient to take a deep breath. Then watch to see if both your hands move equally outward. If one side moves more than the other, additional testing for unilateral disease is indicated.

Respiratory excursion can also be evaluated by placing a soft, cloth tape measure around the chest at nipple level and asking the patient to inhale as deeply as possible. Measure the circumference of the chest before and after the patient deeply exhales. Note whether the external intercostal muscles contract on inspiration, being careful not to confuse these muscles with the pectoralis major or the latissimus dorsi. Most adults can expand their chest about two inches on inspiration; however, the normal aging process can limit chest expansion. Severe chronic lung diseases generally limit the expansion to about one inch.

Posterior Chest: Percussion

After inspection and palpation, proceed with percussion of the posterior chest. This procedure causes the underlying tissues to vibrate and produces various sounds that help distinguish whether fluid, air, or a solid mass is in the chest or lungs. The vibrations penetrate to depths of 3 to 6 cm.

Percussional Sounds

Table 9.1

Sound	Description	Example
Resonant	Loud, low pitch of long duration	Normal lung
Flat	Soft, high pitch of short duration	Thigh
Dull	Moderately loud, moderate pitch and duration	Liver
Tympanitic	Loud, high pitch of moderate duration	Air-filled stomach
Hyperresonant[a]	Very loud, very low pitch, long duration	Hyperinflated lung

[a] An abnormal percussional sound. Other sounds may or may not be abnormal depending upon the site of percussion and underlying tissue density.

Percussion is usually difficult to master and feels very awkward at first. (See Chapter 2 : Physical Examination and Techniques for a description of percussion techniques.) As shown in Table 9.1, five percussional sounds (i.e., **tympanitic, hyperresonant, resonant, dull**, and **flat**) can be both heard and felt. Test your ability to discern these sounds by percussing surfaces of varying density such as a table top (i.e., flat), a book (i.e., dull), and the upper part of a half-empty, 2-liter plastic soda bottle (i.e., hyperresonant). Practice listening to the percussive sounds that can be elicited from your own body. For example, percuss your deflated cheek for a **flat** note; press your tongue against the cheek to elicit the sound and feel of **dullness** upon percussion; distend your air-filled cheek to elicit **hyperresonance**; and lastly, percuss the water-filled cheek for **resonance.**

There are many variations in percussion methods. One method begins with placement of the distal interphalangeal joint (DIP) of the third finger (i.e., the pleximeter finger) firmly in the intercostal space and utilizes a quick, brisk blow from the third, second or both fingers (i.e., plexor fingers) as described in Chapter 2: Physical Examination and Techniques. Be sure to keep your fingernails trimmed. Deliver the blow briskly and directly on the DIP joint. (Many inexperienced examiners strike the plexor blow too gently.) No other part of your hand should touch the surface in order to minimize the retardation of the vibrations.

Ask the patient to sit down and hold onto his right kneecap with left hand, and his left kneecap with his right hand. This position helps expose more of the posterior lungs by exaggerating the separation of the scapulae. Do not attempt to percuss the chest of the patient who is lying on her side because the percussed sounds will be muffled. If necessary, ask someone to hold the patient in a sitting position by gripping the patient under the armpits or by gripping the patient's wrists from the foot of the bed. Alternatively, ask the patient to sit up in bed and hold on to the raised bedrails.

Start at the apices of the lungs and examine symmetrical areas of each lung at 5 cm intervals, moving from side to side and down the posterior chest. Do not percuss over bony surfaces. Place your plexor finger parallel to the ribs in the intercostal spaces and note the normal resonance of the air-filled lung tissue. Upon reaching the base of the lungs, ask the patient to raise both arms to the ceiling, and begin percussing from the upper mid axilla (armpit), down again to the base. Complete lateral percussion on one side before switching to the other.

Dullness over the lung is usually caused by the accumulation of fluid (e.g., pneumonia, pleural effusion) or by the presence of solid tissue (e.g., tumor). A **hyperresonance** sound is usually caused by hyperinflation of the lung (e.g., emphysema, asthma) or air in the pleural space (e.g., pneumothorax).

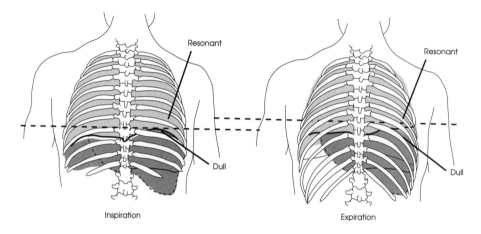

Fig. 9.10 To evaluate diaphragmatic excursion, compare the limits of resonance over the lung at inspiration and expiration.

To determine the location and height of each diaphragm (i.e., hemidiaphragms), ask the patient to "take a deep breath and hold it in." Then, starting from about the sixth rib in the midscapular line, percuss downward from normal resonance until a dull sound is heard. Mark the spot of dullness with a washable ink pen. Then instruct the patient to exhale fully without inhaling again. Percuss down the chest until the quality of tone changes and mark the point. Perform this procedure quickly and be sure to instruct the patient to resume normal breathing. Repeat these steps on both the left and right sides. The difference between the two marks made subsequent to inhalation and exhalation represents the range of motion of the diaphragm (or diaphragmatic excursion), which normally is about 3 to 5 cm in females and 5 to 6 cm in males (see Figure 9.10). The hemidiaphragms move equally; however, the diaphragm should be slightly higher on the right side because of the location of the liver underneath it (a normal variant). If the left side is higher, then something is abnormal (e.g., hemidiaphragm paralysis). With restrictive lung diseases or overinflated lungs (e.g., emphysema), the diaphragms move very little.

Posterior Chest: Auscultation

The movement of air through the respiratory tract produces vibrations that can be heard as sounds. These breath sounds have distinctive qualities associated with various pathophysiological processes and can best be evaluated when heard through a stethoscope. A stethoscope is an instrument that transmits sounds from body areas of the patient [e.g., heart, lungs, gastrointestinal (GI) tract] to the ears of the examiner. Contrary to popular belief, the stethoscope does not amplify sounds but rather, filters out extraneous sounds.

Before using the stethoscope, ask the patient to breathe normally through an open mouth to reduce the noise from the upper airways. Listen carefully near the patient's mouth for quiet breath sounds. Some abnormal sounds such as wheezing, "death rattle" (i.e., rhonchi), or stridor (i.e., a hiss, whistle or shriek) are easily heard even without a stethoscope. Allow the patient time to rest and to resume normal breathing to prevent hyperventilation.

Place the earpieces of the stethoscope pointing forward into your ear canals. Check to see that the diaphragm of the stethoscope is active by tapping on it to produce a sound. If no sound is heard through the earpieces, twist the head piece of the diaphragm a half turn until it clicks into position and try tapping on it again. During auscultation, keep the tubing of the stethoscope from rubbing against objects to minimize disruptive noise transmission through the stethoscope. Warm the diaphragm of the stethoscope before placing it on the patient by holding it in a closed fist for a few seconds or rubbing it vigorously on your palms. In temperate climates, carrying the stethoscope in a coat pocket may be adequate to warm it.

Ask the patient to fold his arms across his chest or to place his hands on his hips. This position spreads the scapulae laterally and enhances the posterior exposure of the lungs through the posterior chest wall. Place the stethoscope's diaphragm firmly, but not tightly, against the patient's chest wall. When examining a male with a thickly haired chest, dampen the hairy area to lessen artifactual sounds generated by dry hairs.

Close your eyes to prevent visual stimulation from interfering with the auscultatory examination and concentrate on listening to the breath sounds. Ask the patient to breathe through her mouth. Each time the diaphragm of the stethoscope is placed on the patient's chest, instruct the patient to "Take a deep breath in through your mouth. Now blow it all out." Occasionally, you may need to enlist someone to stand in front of the patient to coach the patient to breathe at the appropriate intervals. If a helper is not available, you can help the patient by saying, "Each time I tap your shoulder, take a deep breath then blow it out."

Auscultate from side to side and downward in a zigzag pattern across the posterior chest (i.e., the back). Begin the auscultation at the apex of the lung and move to the base from the posterior of the patient while concentrating on listening to the quality of the **breath sounds**. Listen through one complete inspiratory and expiratory breath for normal breath sounds which tend to rise in pitch during inspiration and fall in pitch during expiration. Evaluate the **pitch, intensity,** and **duration** of breath sounds and presence of adventitious sounds (i.e., those heard during auscultation of the lung but *not* coming from the lung).

Breath sounds result from the turbulence of air moving through airways. For example, a hollow blowing breath sound can be heard as air passes rapidly and freely through the trachea. As air passes into each subdivision of the bronchial tree, the air flow rate decreases because the diameter of the bronchial tubules becomes smaller and the character of breath sounds is changed. The intensity of breath sounds increases with diseased lungs and the characteristics of breath sounds change as well. The increased lung density from a diseased lung enhances the transmission of breath sounds because air-filled lungs normally filter and muffle sounds. The lungs act like the muffler on your car. When the muffler is working properly, engine sounds are quiet; but when the muffler is broken, the engine noise is loud and is clearly heard by everyone in town. Therefore, a pulmonary disorder such as lobar pneumonia leads to clearer transmission or intensity of breath sounds. The transmittance of breath sounds, however, is muted when a bronchus is obstructed (e.g., an asthmatic mucoid plug).

Diminished or so-called "distant" breath sounds occur with shallow breathing. Breath sounds may be diminished when air flow is decreased (e.g., restrictive lung diseases or neuromuscular weakness such as Parkinson's disease) and by pleural diseases (e.g., effusion or pneumothorax). The breath sounds also tend to be diminished in emphysematous patients breathing from a hyperinflated lung or in weakened, elderly patients, obese patients, or patients who have thick chest walls.

Table 9.2 provides a classification of normal breath sounds arranged in three categories according to their intensity, pitch, and duration of inspiratory and expiratory phases: vesicular, bronchial, and tracheal (see Figure 9.11). **Vesicular breath sounds** are heard as a whishing noise over most of the lungs, away from the trachea and main bronchi, during shallow quiet respirations. These sounds are soft, low-pitched, and best heard during deep inspiration. **Bronchial breath sounds** are best heard during expiration between the scapulae from the posterior chest and in the second intercostal

Normal Breath Sounds[a]

Table 9.2

Vesicular	Gentle, soft, low-pitched sounds heard over the lung peripheral areas; associated with air flow through the small airways. Is best heard on inspiration, especially deep inspiration.
Bronchial	Harsh, high-pitched sounds heard anteriorly in the second intercostal spaces and between scapulae on the back. They are heard equally well on either inspiration or expiration.
Tracheal	Loud, high-pitched, blowing sounds heard over the trachea with a brief pause between inspiration and expiration.

[a] Some clinicians report bronchovesicular breath sounds. They are considered transitional sounds between bronchial and vesicular sound.

spaces from the anterior chest (i.e., the front). These sounds are harsh, high-pitched, and about equally divided in duration between inspiratory and expiratory phases. Bronchial breath sounds are not generally heard in the normal lung and usually result from consolidation or congestion of pulmonary tissues. **Tracheal breath sounds** are heard directly over the trachea as loud, blowing, and high-pitched sounds. These sounds are continuous, with only a brief pause between inspiratory and expiratory phases, and are not associated with a pathophysiological abnormality. Practice identifying normal breath sounds by listening with a stethoscope on your own chest.

Bronchial or tracheal breath sounds heard in the peripheral lung tissue represent an abnormal finding. Under normal conditions, the various breath sounds are more clearly heard in specific areas of the lung and chest wall. For example, one of the first signs of lung congestion is the appearance of bronchial sounds in the lung bases, especially in the nonambulatory patient. Likewise, finding normal bronchial and vesicular breath sounds in the upper right lobe of the lung, but only bronchial breath sounds in the right lower lobe, suggests consolidation of the lower lobe.

Abnormal Breath Sounds

Abnormal breath sounds that can be superimposed on the normal breath sounds are called **adventitious** (i.e., **added**) **lung sounds** (see Table 9.3).

The adventitious sound known as "rales" (pronounced "rahls") has several different meanings and has gradually been replaced with the more precise term "crackle." **Crackles** are bubbly, **discontinuous** (i.e., intermittent) **sounds** in the lungs. They arise from the movement of fluid or exudate in the airways, or air through constricted spaces. Crackles are similar to the sound of rolling several strands of hair between your fingers next to your ear or listening to a bowl of Rice Krispies. Crackling sounds may be caused by the sudden opening of collapsed airways or the bubbling of air through secretions.

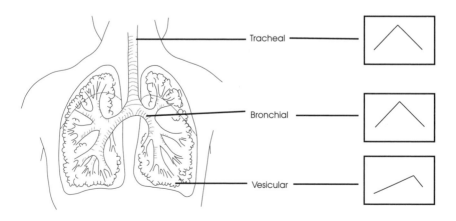

Fig. 9.11   Location and characteristics of normal breath sounds.

Remember, dampen any chest hairs on the patient to prevent a false positive finding of crackles made by the sound of chest hair touching the diaphragm of the stethoscope. Crackles are heard on either inspiration or expiration. If crackles are detected, ask the patient to cough, and note whether the sounds have different characteristics. If the crackles continue unchanged after coughing, they are true crackles representing pathology and not merely an artifactual finding. Some pulmonologists classify crackles as fine (i.e., soft, high-pitched), medium, and coarse (i.e., louder and lower in pitch). Crackles resulting from atelectasis (i.e., inadequate expansion of the lung) often disappear after a few deep breaths or a change in posture. Very sick or postsurgical patients normally have some crackly sounds.

Abnormal Breath Sounds

Table 9.3

Sound	Description	Timing	Cause	Example
Crackle[a]	Bubbly, discontinuous; coughing has limited effect	Inspiration	Small airway obstruction	Chronic bronchitis pneumonia
Wheeze	Whistle-like; coughing has variable effect	Expiration	Small-medium airway spasm	Asthma
Stridor	Loud shriek	Inspiration or expiration	Large airway or tracheal spasm	Epiglottis
Rub	Rough, creaky	Inspiration and expiration	Inflamed or fibrotic pleural membranes	Pleuritis
Rhonchi	Coarse rattle	Inspiration	Thick secretions in chest or nose	Bronchitis, upper respiratory infection

[a]Rales are considered as crackles.

Crackles are characterized by their number (i.e., few or many) and by their timing in relation to the breathing cycle. **Late inspiratory crackles** are associated with restrictive lung diseases such as asbestosis, pulmonary fibrosis, pneumonia, and congestive heart failure. Late inspiratory crackles resulting from atelectasis are common after surgery and clear with deep breathing or coughing. **Early inspiratory crackles** are clinically important findings heard with chronic bronchitis, asthma, and emphysema. Determining the precise location of crackles helps identify the underlying problem and provides a means to document the patient's response to therapy. For example, a patient with pneumonia and bilateral, diffuse crackles located two-thirds the height of the posterior chest should respond to several days of antibiotics with a decreased number or clearing of the crackles and a decreased area of involvement (i.e., about one-third the lung height). Similarly, a patient with congestive heart failure (CHF) and bilateral, basilar crackles should experience a clearing of the crackles if diuretic therapy is successful.

Wheezes and **rhonchi** are abnormal **continuous sounds**. Although some differentiate rhonchi from wheezes, most use these two terms interchangeably. When air flows rapidly through narrow airways, the lateral wall pressures decrease, and the wall briefly closes then quickly reopens. As a result, the walls vibrate and produce the whistling sounds of wheezes or rhonchi. To gain an understanding of this process, try whistling with your lips. By varying the airflow rate through your lips and the aperture between your lips, you can adjust the pitch and loudness of the whistling sound. These are the same principles controlling the quality of wheezing sounds.

Wheezes are heard as high-pitched musical sounds primarily upon expiration; inspiratory wheezes are more difficult to detect. Wheezes are associated with small airway diseases and can be heard without a stethoscope, especially during an acute asthma attack or chronic or acute bronchitis. Coughing may or may not significantly affect the sound of wheezes. When the wheezing clears subsequent to a cough, the airways probably contain considerable secretions. If wheezing is not clearly discernible, it can be accentuated by asking the patient to exhale rapidly. You may be able to make an expiratory wheeze yourself by taking a deep breath then quickly exhaling.

The timing of wheezes in the breathing cycle (e.g., early expiration or late inspiration) provides clues to the severity and location of the bronchospasm. Inspiratory wheezes usually are extrathoracic and associated with epiglottis or laryngospasm. Expiratory wheezes are more commonly heard and usually indicate intrathoracic diseases. Generalized wheezing suggests the presence of asthma or bronchitis, while a single or focal wheeze suggests a problem limited to a particular bronchus (e.g., a tumor). Wheezes heard over the trachea indicate a possible obstruction of the large bronchi.

The relative pitch of a wheeze is determined by the degree of airway obstruction and air flow rate. For example, during an acute asthma attack, the pitch of the wheeze rises as the airway narrows (i.e., worsening bronchospasm). However, the disappearance of wheezing does not necessarily indicate lessening bronchospasm. As the patient improves with bronchodilator treatment, the pitch becomes lower. A low-pitched wheeze, however, can also be encountered when severely ill patients become tired and are no longer capable of breathing vigorously. In this case, an apparent improvement actually is a worsening in the patient's condition because of decreasing ability to move air through the tracheobronchial tree.

The airway patency of a patient with obstructive airway disease can be measured with a simple bedside test used to assess forced expiratory time (FET). Place the diaphragm of the stethoscope on the patient's trachea. Ask the patient to inhale as deeply as possible through the mouth, not through the nostrils. Look at your watch and tell the patient, "Blow all the air in your lungs out through your mouth as quickly as possible." Be sure to listen for only the air flow, not vocal sounds which may occur after expiration. The length of time it takes the patient to exhale completely is a measure of FET. Normally, most adults can completely exhale in 3 seconds or less. An FET of 4 or more seconds suggests diffuse airway obstruction. This maneuver is helpful to assess post-treatment response to metered dose inhalation treatments. To improve the accuracy of the test, repeat the procedure three times and average the results.

A variant of the wheeze is known as a stridor. A **stridor** is a hiss, whistle, or shriek that is loud enough to be heard without a stethoscope. Best heard on expiration, it is a sign of bronchus or large airway obstruction (e.g., a situation in which a peanut has been aspirated and is lodged in a bronchus). Inspiratory stridor frequently signals a medical emergency of acute spasm of the trachea, larynx, or epiglottis that may require a tracheotomy.

Pleural **friction rubs** are rough, coarse sounds usually produced by inflamed or fibrous pleural surfaces rubbing together. Friction rubs are intermittent, discontinuous sounds, often described as creaky or like the sound of unoiled leather. These sounds are heard on either inspiration or expiration and are usually best heard at specific spots on the chest. Friction rubs detected over the heart are associated with pericarditis (i.e., pericardial friction rub), while rubs over the lung suggest pleurisy or fibrosis (i.e., pleural friction rub). The sounds of a pleural friction rub can be simulated by placing your palm over your ear and rubbing the back of the palm with the fingers of your other hand.

Voice Sounds

Voice sounds are not routinely assessed unless abnormal findings are noted and a more detailed examination is necessary. Listen over the lungs with the diaphragm of the stethoscope and ask the patient to whisper numbers or words. Speaking vibrates the respiratory tissue and transmits sounds to the chest wall. A normal air-filled lung transmits low frequency sounds (i.e., less than 200 cycles per second) while filtering out higher frequencies. Thus, when a patient speaks, low pitched mumbling should be heard over the lungs. To try this yourself, place the diaphragm on your larynx and whisper, "The cow jumped over the moon." Now, move the stethoscope to your chest and whisper the same sentence. Repeat this process several times. **Bronchophony** is a condition in which the words are heard as clearly over the lung as they are over the larynx (i.e., not the normal, muffled, or indistinguishable sounds).

Diseases can either increase or decrease transmission of voice sounds. The principles of sound transmission as described in the discussion of tactile fremitus also apply to the transmission of voice sounds or **vocal fremitus**. Pulmonary consolidation improves the transmission of sound waves; therefore, diseases such as pneumonia or atelectasis are associated with abnormally clear transmission of voice sounds (i.e., bronchophony). Transmission of these sounds is hampered by blocked airways or the presence of air in the pleural space (i.e., pneumothorax).

Abnormal consolidation of a lung can be indicated by the presence of either egophony or whispered pectoriloquy in the transmission of voice sounds. **Egophony**, which literally means "bleating of a goat," can be revealed by asking the patient to repeat the letter "e." Under normal conditions, a muffled, long "e" sound should be heard through the stethoscope. If egophony is present, the vocal sound will be transmitted through the lung with a nasal tonality and heard as the letter "a." To detect **whispered pectoriloquy**, ask the patient to whisper words that create high frequency vibrations (e.g., ninety-nine). These whispered sounds are heard faintly (if at all) through a healthy, air-filled lung. Loud and clear transmission of these high-pitched sounds suggests consolidation of the transmitting lung.

Anterior Chest

When examining the anterior chest, inspect the areas over the right middle lobe and both the right and left upper lobes of the lungs. Look at the skin, study the bony structures, and observe the retraction of lower interspaces during inspiration. Also, check the type, depth, and rate of breathing. Males generally use their diaphragms and abdominal muscles more, while females tend to use their intercostal muscles more during breathing. Visual inspection of these areas can often provide clues about underlying diseases of the lung [e.g., asthma, chronic obstructive airways disease (COAD)].

Anterior chest **palpation** includes checking for **tactile fremitus** and **respiratory expansion**. Tactile fremitus should be assessed in the same manner as outlined previously for the posterior chest examination. Assess respiratory expansion by placing both hands over the lower anterolateral chest along the costal margins with the thumbs pointing upward to the xiphoid process. Ask the patient to take a deep breath and watch your thumbs move equally apart as the chest wall expands during the inspiratory breath. Measure the circumference of the chest at the level of the nipple at complete expiration, and compare the measurement to that at full inspiration to assess respiratory expansion.

Percussion of the anterior chest should begin in the supraclavicular space. Percuss down the chest in a zigzag pattern, comparing each interspace with its contralateral side. With the patient's arms raised toward the ceiling, percuss the lateral chest, noting variations in percussive sounds when the anterior chest is percussed over solid tissues (e.g., dullness over the heart and liver) and over hollow organs (e.g., tympanitic over the stomach).

Auscultate the anterior chest as outlined for the posterior chest wall exam. While the patient breathes through an open mouth listen for breath sounds, adventitious sounds, and, if necessary, voice sounds. To minimize the potential for disease transmission, be sure to turn the patient's mouth to the side away from you.

Figures 9.12 and 9.13 show normal chest x-rays. Bony structures such as the clavicles, ribs, scapula, and vertebral bodies of the spine can be seen. In the mediastinum, the heart, aortic knob, and trachea can be seen. The diaphragm, which has been relatively flattened by the inspiration taken for the purposes of the x-ray, separates the abdomen below and the lungs above.

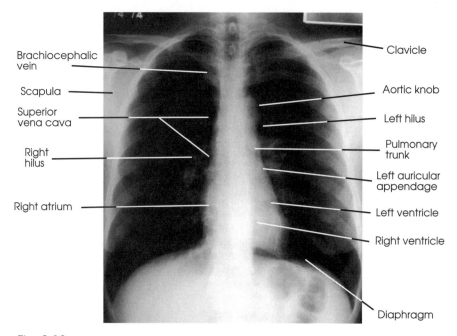

Fig. 9.12   A posterior-anterior view of a normal chest x-ray.

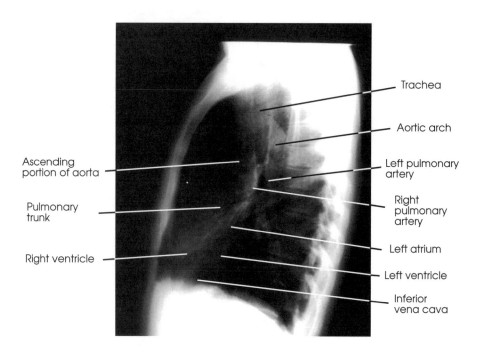

Fig. 9.13   A lateral view of a normal chest x-ray.

PHARMACOTHERAPEUTIC CASE ILLUSTRATION

History

A.K., a 24-year-old female, complained of "shortness of breath and cough." She said she experiences most of her breathing difficulty at night and describes the difficulty as a sudden tightening in her chest. These attacks sometimes occur at work. The shortness of breath (SOB) often dissipates quickly and recurs for no apparent reason. Past medical history (PMH) revealed that since childhood, A.K. has experienced asthmatic attacks that have been inadequately controlled. No other significant medical problems were noted. Her family history (FH) indicated that her father, 43, and mother, 42, are alive and in good health. She has two brothers ages 19 and 17. One brother had one episode of asthma that required emergency treatment. Her social history (SH) and medication history were non-contributory to the problem. The review of systems (ROS) was significant only as described in the history of present illness (HPI).

Physical Examination

Physical examination revealed a 24-year-old, alert, well-developed and well-nourished (WDWN) female who is 5'8" tall and weighs 135 lb. She was able to speak with moderate difficulty and was leaning forward in moderate respiratory distress. Her vital signs were as follows: blood pressure (BP) 135/85 mm Hg; pulsus paradoxus was not present; pulse 105 beats/min and regular; temperature was 38° C (oral); respiratory rate (RR) - 25 beats/min, shallow and regular. Examination of the thorax and lungs showed the following: breathing was labored at rest; accessory and abdominal muscles were being used to help breathing. There was slight decreased tactile fremitus with markedly reduced respiratory excursion. Normal lung resonance was present throughout the chest. Auscultation revealed diffuse wheezes heard on expiration. Average forced expiratory time (FET) was 4 seconds.

Laboratory Tests

Forced expiratory volume in 1 second (FEV_1) pre-bronchodilator was 68% of predicted; FEV_1 post-bronchodilator was 82% of predicted. A complete blood cell count (CBC) was normal except for eosinophilia. Oximeter testing showed hypoxemia.

Diagnosis and Management

The diagnosis was acute asthma attack. A.K. was administered aerosolized albuterol and she subjectively improved. For maintenance therapy, she was given a peak expiratory flow rate (PEFR) meter, an albuterol metered-dose inhaler, and a beclomethasone metered-dose inhaler. A.K. was given a diary to record symptoms, PEFR measurements, and frequency of episodes with a return appointment.

Discussion

Disease. Asthma is characterized by increased responsiveness of airways to a variety of stimuli (e.g., allergens, viruses, and chemical irritants) and manifested by narrowing of the airways that changes in severity either spontaneously or by therapeutic interventions. Although asthma is highly prevalent in children and is an alarming cause of childhood deaths, it can continue into adulthood. Occasionally, the first episode of asthma is experienced in adulthood.

The pathophysiology of asthma involves inflammation, obstruction, and hyperresponsiveness of airways. Inflammatory cells (e.g., mast cells) invade the airways and engage in complex reactions that result in mucosal edema, decreased mucus clearance, and increased mucus production, as well as marked hypertrophy and hyperplasia of bronchial smooth muscle. Obstructive signs and symptoms of asthma (e.g., dyspnea, coughing, and wheezing) are influenced by bronchial swelling, mucus production, airway spasm, and airway hypertrophy and hyperplasia.

A careful medical history, physical examination, and selected pulmonary studies are critical in the assessment of the asthmatic patient. A.K. first complained of dyspnea and cough, indicators of obstructive lung disease. She had a childhood history of asthma and another family member reported having experienced one episode. To assess the severity of her attack, note that she was alert and able to speak, all good prognostic signs. A severely hypoxic patient has fragmented speech, sits in an upright position to facilitate breathing, and is often confused. She said, "I have most of my difficulty at night." When she is supine at sleep, she develops a ventilation/perfusion mismatch. Her history showed a progressive dyspnea developing over time, finally to the point of seeking medical care. The history did not reveal a functional disability.

On physical examination, she was tachypneic and tachycardic, but her temperature and blood pressure were normal. Although a respiratory infection cannot be ruled out, an allergic or irritant etiology is more likely. Pulsus paradoxus was not detected (see Chapter 10: Blood Vessels). Because she did not have a 10 mm Hg or greater decrease in her systolic blood pressure (pulsus paradoxus), the airway obstruction probably was only of moderate intensity. She was "leaning forward," had "labored breathing at rest," and was using accessory muscles, all signs of obstructive breathing. When assessed for respiratory excursion, she was found to be "breathing off the top" of her lungs which were hyperinflated. The decreased tactile fremitus suggests that the breath sounds were not being transmitted to the chest wall which, in this case, reflected absent or decreased air flow through the bronchial tree. Generalized expiratory wheezes point to partially obstructed airways. A more severe obstructive sign is both expiratory and inspiratory wheezing. The most grave obstructive sign is the disappearance of wheezes when other findings indicate continuing hypoxemia (i.e., insufficient air flow to generate a wheeze). The bedside forced expiration time (FET) provides a quick estimate of obstructive breathing and her time of more than 3 seconds implies airway obstruction.

The forced expiratory volume in one second (FEV_1) is the volume of air expired in 1 second from a point of maximum inspiration. Obstructive lung disease prolongs the flow rate. A.K. had an FEV_1 value 68% of that predicted after adjustments for gender, age, height, and weight. Normally, A.K. should have expelled about 75% to 85% of her forced vital capacity in one second. Unless the patient is severely ill, has signs of infection, or does not respond to emergency treatment, other tests, such as a chest x-ray or arterial blood gases, are generally not needed.

Management. The treatment of an asthmatic patient may be quite complex and must be individualized. There are four components of management: objective measurements of lung function, various drug therapies, patient education, and environmental control of allergens and irritants.

In the emergency situation, aerosolized beta-adrenergic agents have become the standard treatment. Inhaled adrenergic drugs provide bronchodilation and have fewer severe side effects than systemic bronchodilators. A.K. was prescribed albuterol as jet nebulization in a dose of 2.5 mg every 20 to 30 min, if necessary, for 4 doses, and every 4 hours as needed to maintain bronchodilation. In severe cases, albuterol is administered every 2 hours. The dose is aerosolized in 3 mL of normal saline. The side effects of albuterol are extensions of adrenergic stimulation, primarily of the cardiovascular system. A.K. must be monitored for tachycardia and its related arrhythmias, especially excessive premature ventricular contractions (PVCs). Unless the patient has pre-existing cardiovascular disease or severe hypoxemia, cardiotoxic effects are generally not a problem.

Once A.K. was breathing comfortably, her lung function was retested. Her FEV_1 improved from 68% to 82% after bronchodilator inhalation therapy. If the patient is achieving maximal benefit, a 15% to 20% change after bronchodilator therapy should be expected. Despite the efficacy of treatment, more wheezing is often heard after treatment than before treatment because effective treatment opens previously blocked airways. An inhaled $beta_2$-adrenergic agent is the drug of choice for both emergency and maintenance therapy. Although albuterol was used, many $beta_2$-agonists work equally well. Compared to oral $beta_2$-agonists, the inhaled route offers direct delivery to the site of action and the advantages of smaller doses; therefore, side effects are fewer and the onset of action is quicker with equal duration of action. Inhalation can be administered as nebulization treatments or as a meter-dosed inhaler.

After the acute episode, A.K. was prescribed an albuterol metered-dose inhaler (MDI) for maintenance therapy and was instructed to use it routinely (QID) until her next appointment. She was instructed to monitor her peak expiratory flow rate (PEFR) twice a day. Her personal best percent PEFR was used to assess her response to treatment and the progression of disease. After the return visit, she would measure her PEFR and use her beta-agonist inhaler as needed to control symptoms.

The chronic nature of asthma is related to inflammatory cell damage. Generally, anti-inflammatory drugs (corticosteroids) manage the acute, and cromolyn sodium the long-term inflammatory response. Parenteral methylprednisolone (60 mg intravenously every 6 hours) is used in the acute attack, followed by metered-dose therapy (beclomethasone, triamcinolone, or flunisolide) two to four inhalations two to four times daily. Short-term and inhalation therapies are safe and have few toxicities. Oral corticosteroids are effective for acute flare-ups that are not responsive to usual treatment. For example, prednisone 60 mg orally followed by 60 mg in two to three divided daily doses would be given as a tapering dose over several days. PEFR monitoring helps guide the rate of dose tapering. Long-term (more than two to four weeks) or frequent use increases the risk of serious side effects.

Although not used for A.K., a long-acting theophylline could have been added to her bronchodilator regimen. Long-acting theophylline preparations provide a uniform release of the medication into the blood, decrease bronchospasm, are well tolerated, and may improve compliance. A maintenance dose could be prescribed without a loading dose which would lessen the chance for toxicities. Central nervous system (e.g., nervousness), cardiovascular system (e.g., various tachyarrhythmias), and gastrointestinal system (e.g., nausea) adverse effects of theophylline must be monitored by history and physical examination, and periodic blood levels when indicated. The maintenance dose in a young adult without complications is 12 mg/kg/day or 400 mg every 8 to 12 hours. Theophylline serum levels should be obtained initially and at periodic intervals to adjust dosage.

Thickened mucus secretions are a problem in asthmatic patients. Although the effectiveness of expectorant drugs is disputed, trying to free the bronchial passages of the blockage of such secretions is an important part of therapy and adequate hydration is essential to removing mucus. Percussion and postural drainage assist in the removal of mucoid plugs and in the treatment of atelectasis. Although not viewed as necessary for A.K., these physical therapy interventions are effective in removing the physical resistance to air flow. Whether using expectorants, percussion and postural drainage, or both, the goal is for the patient to expectorate the thickened sputum, allowing much easier breathing. To assess treatment response, measure the volume and color of the sputum. With adequate hydration and pulmonary expectoration, clear, copious sputum with clearing of wheezes should be expected.

A.K. said, "Sometimes my attack happens at work." The identification of environmental or occupational irritants or allergens should be a part of preventive treatment. An allergic etiology is more likely than an occupational irritant in most asthmatics; therefore, allergen identification and avoidance, if possible, are central to the management plan. A.K. did have an elevated eosinophil count, but this is not pathognomonic of asthma. A.K. should be evaluated by an allergist if her asthma continues.

Patient education is also important to helping A.K. adjust to a potentially chronic disease. A.K. needs to feel in control of her asthma. Confidence reduces anxiety and aids in management. An often missed drug education point is the proper use of metered-dose inhalers. The pharmacist, physician, or nurse needs to visit with A.K., teach her proper administration techniques, and watch her use the inhaler. Prescribing inhaled doses as "puffs" is misleading, they should be described on the labeling and during patient education as "inhalations."

Therapeutic Drug Monitoring Examples

PNEUMONIA (BACTERIAL)

The approach to therapuetic drug monitoring by clinicians varies depending upon many factors. Some of these include preferences among clinicians in a given community or region; concurrent medical problems which dictate that certain drugs be used or avoided; the patient's response to selected medication. The following outlines of therapeutic drug monitoring offer examples which may serve to stimulate discussion and further understanding of initiating and monitoring drug use. The drugs and dosages presented should not be applied to any clinical situation without proper medical supervision.

Drug Therapy

Cefazolin 1 gm IV Q 8 hr or antibiotics effective against the most common bacterial pathogens such as mycoplasma, *Streptococcus pneumoniae, Haemophilus influenzae*, and *Branhamella catarrhalis*.

Monitoring

Symptoms: Determine the patient's response to treatment by questioning about sputum color and amount, appetite, shaking chills, and lethargy. Ask about pleuritic chest pain, generalized fatigue/weakness, and dyspnea. Question about nausea and vomiting. Determine if the patient appears diaphoretic. Note whether the patient is coughing; ask if the patient's chest hurts when breathing or coughing?

Signs: *Gen:* Look for signs of respiratory distress such as tachypnea or labored breathing. *MSE:* Determine the patient's level of alertness and orientation (see Chapter 3: Mental Status Examination). *VS:* Check blood pressure, temperature, pulse, and respiration. *Skin:* Note skin color (e.g., hyperemia) and nail bed color (e.g., cyanosis). Check for excessive moisture (e.g., fever). Inspect fingernails for signs of clubbing. *Chest/Lungs:* Inspect respiratory rhythm and count rate. Look for guarding during quiet respiration. Observe for use of neck and abdominal muscles. Palpate for dullness over the

Therapeutic Drug Monitoring Examples

PNEUMONIA (BACTERIAL)
(continued)

Monitoring	consolidated area. Check for reduced respiratory excursion (i.e., splinting sign). Feel for the presence of increased tactile fremitus. Note the presence of abnormal egophony, whispered pectoriloquy, and bronchophony. Auscultate the breath sounds for signs of lobar consolidation, abnormal basilar crackles, and the possible presence of a pulmonary friction rub over the consolidation. *CVS:* Inspect the precordial area for pulsations or heaves. Palpate each valvular area. Feel for the location of the point of a maximal cardiac impulse (PMI) (see Chapter 11: Heart). Auscultate each valve for S_1, S_2 sounds; check for abnormal S_3 and S_4 sounds.
Laboratory Tests	The clinician may elect to order all, none, or some of these laboratory studies depending upon history and physical findings, as well as other specific clinical indications. Sputum gram stain, culture and sensitivity (C&S) of blood and sputum, chest x-ray, white blood cell (WBC) count.
Adverse Drug Event Monitoring	Examine the mouth for candidiasis (see Chapter 7: Mouth, Nose, and Sinuses). Ask if the patient has had diarrhea (e.g., antibiotic associated). Check for hypersensitivity reactions ranging from skin rash to anaphylaxis. Examine the IV infusion site for redness, tenderness, and heat (e.g., signs of phlebitis and possibly thrombophlebitis). If clinical status does not improve, consider the possibilities of an incorrect antibiotic selection, misdiagnosis, or bacterial resistance.

Therapeutic Drug Monitoring Examples

ASTHMA (ALLERGIC TYPE)

The approach to therapuetic drug monitoring by clinicians varies depending upon many factors. Some of these include preferences among clinicians in a given community or region; concurrent medical problems which dictate that certain drugs be used or avoided; the patient's response to selected medication. The following outlines of therapeutic drug monitoring offer examples which may serve to stimulate discussion and further understanding of initiating and monitoring drug use. The drugs and dosages presented should not be applied to any clinical situation without proper medical supervision.

Drug Therapy

Terbutaline aerosol 10 mg nebulizer every 20 minutes for 3 doses then Q 2–4 hr PRN wheezing. Theophylline SR tablet 400 mg Q 8 hr. Methylprednisolone 125 mg IV Q 6 hr.

Monitoring

Symptoms: Ask about difficulty breathing, coughing, and sputum production. Inquire about appetite, weakness, or fatigue. Question about feelings of "tightness in the chest" and shortness of breath (SOB). Note whether the patient can speak a complete sentence without respiratory difficulty. Determine if the patient breathes more comfortably in the upright position.

Signs: *Gen:* Look for signs of respiratory distress (e.g., the use of abdominal and neck muscles, nasal flaring, air hunger). Note whether diaphoresis (i.e., perspiration) is present. *MSE:* Note the patient's orientation, level of consciousness, agitation, and other signs of distress. Look for the presence of somnolence or severe agitation. *VS:* Measure the patient's breathing rate (e.g., tachypnea) and pattern (e.g., shallow). Record the pulse rate and rhythm. Note if it is greater than 120 beats/min or irregular. *Skin:* Check the skin and nail beds for cyanosis. Measure the skin turgor

Therapeutic Drug Monitoring Examples

ASTHMA (ALLERGIC TYPE)
(continued)

Monitoring	and mobility (see Chapter 4: Skin, Hair, and Nails). *Chest/Lungs:* Inspect the chest for accessory muscle breathing and interspace retraction. Note the skin color, texture, and moisture. Listen for breath sounds and wheezing; with severe attacks, breath sounds and wheezing may be diminished or absent. *CVS:* Measure the blood pressure for pulsus paradoxus (i.e., >10 mm Hg drop during inspiration; see Chapter 10: Heart). Auscultate for normal heart sounds. Count the apical pulse and note the presence of tachycardia or irregularity.
Laboratory Tests	The clinician may elect to order all, none, or some of these laboratory studies depending upon history and physical findings, as well as other specific clinical indications. Spirometry (especially if there is a 15%–20% FEV_1 improvement post-bronchodilator) and arterial blood gases (ABGs).
Adverse Drug Event Monitoring	**Terbutaline Inhalation:** Ask if the patient experiences any of the following symptoms after inhalation: unusual nervousness, anxiety, or restlessness; severe trembling; insomnia; fast or skipped heart beats; lightheadedness or dizziness; or severe headache. Measure the blood pressure for excessive elevation.
	Theophylline SR Tablet: Question about feelings of unusual nervousness, trouble sleeping, poor appetite, fast or pounding heart beats, and unusual headache. Check

Therapeutic Drug Monitoring Examples

ASTHMA (ALLERGIC TYPE)
(continued)

Adverse Drug
Event Monitoring
for rapid or irregular pulse and moderate blood pressure elevation.

Methylprednisone Injection: Check for signs of fluid retention (e.g., dependent edema).

Therapeutic Drug Monitoring Examples

CHRONIC BRONCHITIS/EMPHYSEMA

The approach to therapeutic drug monitoring by clinicians varies depending upon many factors. Some of these include preferences among clinicians in a given community or region; concurrent medical problems which dictate that certain drugs be used or avoided; the patient's response to selected medication. The following outlines of therapeutic drug monitoring offer examples which may serve to stimulate discussion and further understanding of initiating and monitoring drug use. The drugs and dosages presented should not be applied to any clinical situation without proper medical supervision.

Drug Therapy	Ipratropium bromide metered-dose inhaler, 2 deep inhalations QID. Prednisone tablet 20 mg PO Q a.m.
Monitoring	**Symptoms:** Inquire about any change in the amount, character, and color of sputum. Ask about episodes of shortness of breath (SOB) at rest and with exertion. Ask if the patient has difficulty breathing while sleeping or wakes up short of breath. Ask how far the patient can walk without SOB.

Signs: *Gen:* Observe the patient's physical appearance, and note any of the following signs of respiratory distress: use of accessory breathing muscles; sitting upright with elevated shoulders; hands propped on knees or table; pursed lips; nasal flaring. Note if the patient is overweight or underweight. Ask if the patient has experienced excessive belching (i.e., swallowing air). *MSE:* Measure the patient's alertness and orientation. *VS:* Check respiratory rate and rhythm (e.g., tachypnea), temperature, blood pressure (check for paradoxical pulse), and pulse rate and rhythm. *Skin:* Look for cyanotic appearance and finger clubbing (rare). *Chest/Lungs:* Inspect skin color (e.g., "blue bloater"). Look for interspace retraction, increased anteroposterior chest

Therapeutic Drug Monitoring Examples

CHRONIC BRONCHITIS/EMPHYSEMA
(continued)

Monitoring
diameter (i.e., "barrel chest"), or accessory muscle breathing. Percuss for normal resonance; hyperresonance is associated with mixed emphysema. Evaluate tactile and vocal fremitus, which are normally muffled. Ask the patient to inhale and exhale deeply through his mouth. Record total length of respiration; note the presence of a prolonged expiratory time (i.e., >4 seconds). Check respiratory chest expansion with a tape measure. Listen to breath sounds and note any of the following abnormalities: distant breath sounds; wheezes in the terminal phase of expiration; basilar crackles. *CVS:* Auscultate for normal heart sounds and abnormal sounds [especially S_3 and S_4 sounds associated with gallop rhythm (CHF)]. Examine for the following signs of right ventricle strain (i.e., cor pulmonale): PMI in the epigastric area; jugular vein distention (JVD); hepato jugular reflux (HJR); lower extremity edema; and hepatomegaly-splenomegaly.

Laboratory Tests
The clinician may elect to order all, none, or some of these laboratory studies depending upon history and physical findings, as well as other specific clinical indications. Spirometry, chest x-ray, electrocardiogram (ECG), arterial blood gases (ABGs).

Adverse Drug Event Monitoring
Ipratropium Bromide: Quiz for excessive nonproductive coughing or dry mouth. Ask if the patient has experienced any difficulty urinating, unusual nervousness, or stomach upset.

Therapeutic Drug Monitoring Examples

CHRONIC BRONCHITIS/EMPHYSEMA
(continued)

Adverse Drug
Event Monitoring

Prednisone: Query about epigastric pain or tarry stool (e.g., ulcer); decreased or blurred vision (e.g., diabetes mellitus, cataracts); unusual tiredness (e.g., hypokalemia); muscle weakness (e.g., myopathy); unusual weight gain (e.g., fluid retention); pain in bones (e.g., osteoporosis or fracture). Examine for the following signs of Cushing's Syndrome: striae, purpura, round face with telangiectasia (i.e., capillary dilation), extremity muscle weakness with back/abdomen fat build-up. Check for dependent edema in lower legs or feet. Examine the eyes for lens opacity.

Therapeutic Drug Monitoring Examples

TUBERCULOSIS

The approach to theraputic drug monitoring by clinicians varies depending upon many factors. Some of these include preferences among clinicians in a given community or region; concurrent medical problems which dictate that certain drugs be used or avoided; the patient's response to selected medication. The following outlines of therapeutic drug monitoring offer examples which may serve to stimulate discussion and further understanding of initiating and monitoring drug use. The drugs and dosages presented should not be applied to any clinical situation without proper medical supervision.

Drug Therapy

Isoniazid 300 mg tablet 1 PO QD.
Rifampin 300 mg capsule 1 PO BID.

Monitoring

Symptoms: Ask about the following: appetite, weight loss, productive cough, night sweats with low-grade fever, malaise/fatigue, and chest pain. Ask if the patient can breathe without difficulty or coughing up blood. Ask if the patient experiences chest pain when taking a deep breath; if so, ask if the pain is localized.

Signs: *Gen:* Assess the patient's degree of distress, weight, and body habitus. *MSE:* Measure the patient's alertness, orientation, physical appearance, and behavior. *VS:* Check the patient's respiratory rate for tachypnea and rhythm for shallowness. Measure pulse and blood pressure. Note whether the temperature is febrile. *Skin:* Examine the skin for excessive moisture and color (e.g., cyanosis). Also inspect the nail bed color. *Chest/Lungs:* Inspect for signs of respiratory distress. Look for splinting with deep inhalation. Palpate for abnormal tactile and vocal fremitus as well as crepitus. Explore the neck and axilla for lymphadenopathy. Check chest expansion via palpation or tape measure. Percuss lung fields for consolidation (i.e., dullness). Auscultate for breath sounds and

Therapeutic Drug Monitoring Examples

TUBERCULOSIS
(continued)

Monitoring	adventitious sounds. Listen in the apical areas for rales and distant breath sounds.
Laboratory Tests	The clinician may elect to order all, none, or some of these laboratory studies depending upon history and physical findings, as well as other specific clinical indications. Chest x-ray, TB skin test with anergy control, acid fast bacillus stain of sputum, culture and sensitivity (C&S) test, liver function tests (LFTs), ophthalmologic examination.
Adverse Drug Event Monitoring	**Isoniazid (INH):** Question about and examine for drug-induced (i.e., iatrogenic) hepatitis. Ask the patient about changes in appetite, any episodes of nausea or vomiting, and the presence of dark urine. Examine the skin and sclera for a yellowish hue (i.e., jaundice). Inquire about peripheral neuritis by asking if the patient has experience clumsiness or unsteady gait, numbness, tingling or pain in the feet or hands. Ask if the patient has had any problems with blurred vision or decreased eyesight (e.g., optic neuritis). Look for signs of a lupus-like syndrome such as skin rash, vasculitis, or joint pain (i.e., arthralgia).
	Rifampin: Ask if the patient has experienced any "flu-like" symptoms/signs such as shivering, muscle ache, fever, or headache. Examine carefully for iatrogenic hepatitis as described above. Ask if the patient is troubled by a reddish discoloration of body fluids.

Blood Vessels

B lood vessels transport nutrients to body tissues and carry waste from these same tissues to organs of elimination. The vascular system, like the heart, is dynamic and directly affected by many drugs.

ANATOMY AND PHYSIOLOGY

The vasculature is a continuous system composed of two types of blood vessels, arteries (see Figure 10.1) and veins (see Figure 10.2), with the heart imposed between them on one end and the organs and organ systems they supply on the other. The rhythmic pumping of the heart propels blood through the vessels resulting in hemodynamic changes. This vascular system can be viewed as consisting of a pulmonary circulatory component and a systemic circulatory component.

Pulmonary Circulation

In the pulmonary circulatory system, blood is pumped by the right ventricle and flows through the pulmonary arteries to the lungs (see Figure 10.3 on page 10–4). The circulation of blood through the pulmonary arteries is a low-pressure, low-resistance system, since these arteries are very distensible when they receive the right ventricular stroke volume. The distensibility of these arteries allows the pulmonary circuit to tolerate increases in blood flow without resultant changes in vascular pressure, this property is known as **capacitance**. Loss of these normal circulatory homeostatic changes can result in pulmonary edema, right-sided heart failure, and other adverse pathophysiologic events. After carbon dioxide is exchanged with oxygen in the right and left lungs, the oxygenated blood returns to the left atrium via pulmonary veins. Blood from the left atrium enters the left ventricle which contracts and expels blood into the systemic circulation.

Systemic Circulation

Oxygenated blood flows out of the left ventricle into the aorta and its great vessels. The coronary and aortic arch, carotid, intercostal, subclavian, brachial, radial, and

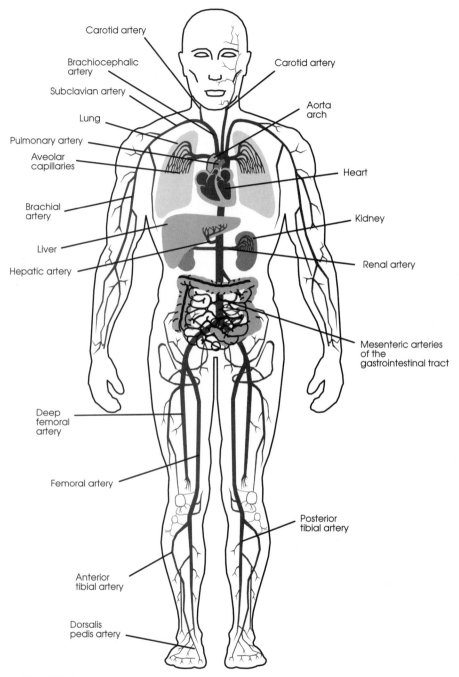

Fig. 10.1 The arterial system.

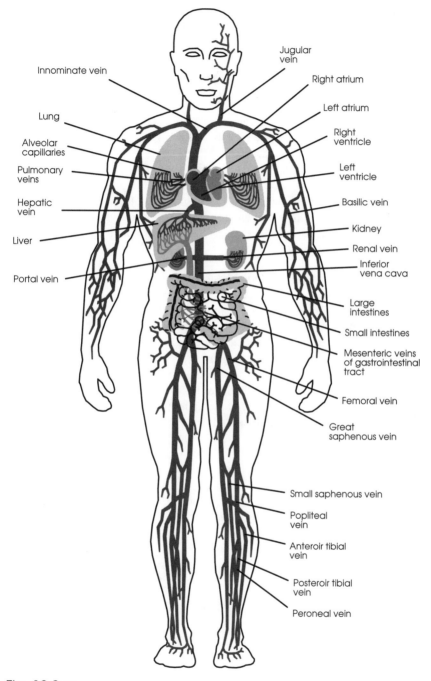

Jugular vein
Right atrium
Left atrium
Right ventricle
Left ventricle
Basilic vein
Kidney
Renal vein
Inferior vena cava
Large intestines
Small intestines
Mesenteric veins of gastrointestinal tract
Femoral vein
Great saphenous vein
Small saphenous vein
Popliteal vein
Anteroir tibial vein
Posteroir tibial vein
Peroneal vein

Innominate vein
Lung
Alveolar capillaries
Pulmonary veins
Hepatic vein
Liver
Portal vein

Fig. 10.2 The venous system.

ulnar arteries are the primary upper body (above the diaphragm) arteries. Below the diaphragm, the major arteries are the aorta, pancreatic, gastric, hepatic, renal, mesenteric, iliac, femoral, popliteal, dorsalis pedis, and posterior tibial arteries (see Figure 10.1). Vessels branching from the aorta supply blood to body organs and tissues. From the capillaries, deoxygenated blood and waste products enter into venules, which empty into larger veins that return blood to the heart.

The right and left common carotid arteries branch from the brachiocephalic artery and the arch of the aorta, respectively (see Figures 10.1 and 10.4). The common carotid arteries enter the neck just beneath the sternoclavicular joint. At the thyroid cartilage, the common carotid arteries divide into the internal and external carotid arteries. The carotid body, located at this bifurcation, senses blood gas changes and, through reflex control, decreases or increases respiration. The carotid sinus, located near the carotid body, senses blood pressure and, through neurogenic reflex arcs, changes blood flow and blood pressure by increasing or decreasing the heart rate and peripheral vasculature tone (see Figure 10.4).

The external carotid artery supplies blood to structures in the neck such as the thyroid gland. This artery extends one branch, the middle meningeal artery, to the meninges (covering) of the brain. The major blood supply to the brain proper is via the right and left internal carotid arteries. The right and left vertebral arteries branch off the aorta, which also supplies blood to the brain. These arteries are located one on each side of the vertebral column and pass through foramen in the transverse process of the cervical vertebrae. The two carotid and two vertebral arteries join near the base of the brain to form the "**Circle of Willis**" (see Figure 10.5). Because of this closed circuit, the brain can receive an adequate supply of blood through the vertebral arteries even if both internal carotid arteries are nearly occluded.

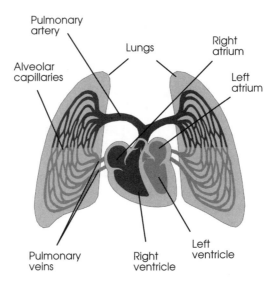

Fig. 10.3 Pulmonary circulation.

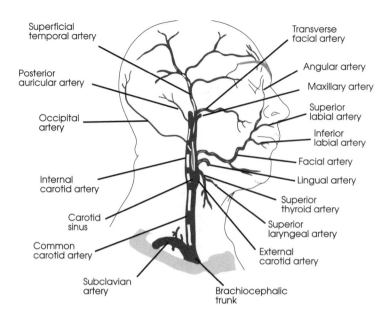

Fig. 10.4   Arteries of the head and neck.

Blood returns from the head and neck through several veins, but primarily through the external and internal jugular veins. The jugular veins receive blood from the superficial structures of the head and neck, and empty into the subclavian veins. They join to the subclavian veins to form the brachiocephalic vein before emptying into the superior vena and then into the right atrium.

Veins

Veins such as the external and internal jugular, right and left subclavian, axillary, and brachiocephalic, empty into the **superior vena cava** from the upper body (above the diaphragm; see Figure 10.6). Veins from the gastrointestinal (GI) tract and spleen empty into the portal vein. The portal vein carries blood to the liver and blood returns to the right atrium via the hepatic veins. All veins from the lower body (below the diaphragm) return blood to the inferior vena cava and then to the right atrium (see Figure 10.2).

The veins are under low pressure (i.e., 10 to 15 mm Hg), as compared to arteries (i.e., 90 to 100 mm Hg). As a low pressure system, the veins are capacitance vessels capable of holding in reserve about 50% of the total blood volume. This capacitance can either increase or decrease the volume of blood returning to the heart (i.e., preload) to control cardiac output (CO). Increasing sympathetic nerve tone increases the venous return to the heart and, therefore, increases stroke volume (SV) and cardiac output. As more blood is returned to the heart, left ventricular end diastolic volume (LVDV) increases. These adjustments in venous return to the heart reflect preload, a measure of cardiac work. Some antihypertensive or cardiovascular drugs are termed "preload drugs" because they primarily affect venous return to the heart.

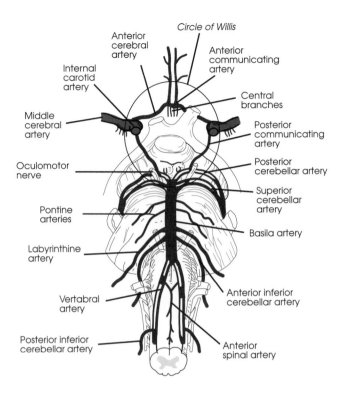

Fig. 10.5 A diagram showing the arteries of the base of the brain. Note the "Circle of Willis" at the upper portion of the illustration.

Arterial Pulse

When the heart rhythmically pumps blood into the arteries, the blood impacts against the arterial walls, causing them to expand and contract generating a pulse. Since each ventricular beat forces blood against the walls of arteries, the pulse rate is a measure of the ventricular heart rate and is expressed in cardiac (ventricular) contractions per unit time [i.e., beats per minute (BPM)]. The pulse rate is increased by sympathetic stimulation (especially of beta receptors) and decreased by parasympathetic input through the vagus nerve.

Blood Pressure, Cardiac Output

When a patient is at rest, the heart pumps about 4 to 7 L/min (i.e., cardiac output), or 80 to 90 mL/beat (i.e., stroke volume) per ventricle. The walls of the aorta and its branching arteries stretch; when they recoil they aid in the movement of blood through the arteries. The peak arterial pressure generated by ventricular ejection is known as the **systolic pressure**. When systole ends, the intra-arterial pressure slowly falls, but the next ventricular contraction begins before the arterial pressure reaches zero. The lowest intra-arterial pressure between ventricular beats is the **diastolic pressure** which closely mirrors the systemic vascular resistance (SVR). SVR is mostly determined by arterial and venous smooth muscle tone and is a measure of afterload. Blood pressure is reported in mm Hg with the systolic pressure in the numerator position and the diastolic blood pressure in the denominator position (e.g., 120/80 mm Hg). The pulse pressure is the difference between the systolic and diastolic pressures (e.g., 120 − 80 = 40 mm Hg). Stroke volume, heart rate, condition of the arterial circuit (e.g., hardening of the arteries, particularly the aortic arch), and arterial/venous tone all affect pulse pressure. A pulse pressure is considered as "widened" when it is more than 50% of the systolic pressure. A widened pulse pressure is associated with high stroke volume disorders such as hyperthyroidism, aortic insufficiency, anemia, or fever. A "narrowed" or low stroke volume can be experienced by the patient in cardiogenic shock.

The duration of left ventricular filling time (i.e., diastole) is longer than left ventricle emptying time (i.e., systole) when the heart rate is within the normal range; therefore, the mean arterial blood pressure must be greater than one-half the systolic pressure and diastolic pressure. The mean arterial pressure (MAP) is calculated as systolic pressure plus twice the diastolic pressure divided by three (MAP = [(SP − DP)/3] + DP). The normal MAP is 80 to 100 mm Hg; however, the mean arterial pressure can be increased by disorders such as pre-eclampsia.

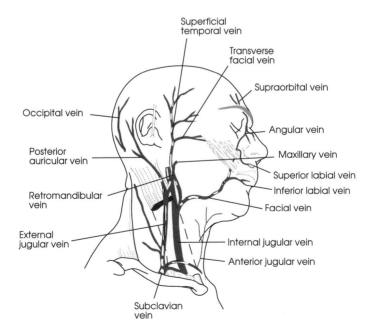

Fig. 10.6 Veins of the head and neck.

Blood pressure can be affected by cardiac output, systemic vascular resistance, or a combination of both. Cardiac output (L/min) is equal to the stroke volume (mL/beat) multiplied by heart rate (beats/min); and can be expressed as the mathematical formula of $CO = SV \times HR$. The major determinants of stroke volume are blood volume, systemic vascular resistance, and left ventricular function (i.e., healthy or diseased myocardium). Heart rate is regulated by the autonomic nervous system. Systemic vascular resistance is affected by blood viscosity, hematocrit, and all the variables that affect the diameter of arterioles (e.g., atherosclerotic plaques, vasomotor tone, vasoactive hormones, and sympathetic nervous system innervation).

The ventricular wall tension created during contraction (i.e., afterload) is determined by arterial resistance (i.e., or impedance), venous blood return (i.e., preload), and left ventricular function. As systemic vascular resistance decreases, cardiac output usually increases; and as systemic vascular resistance increases, cardiac output usually decreases.

The medullary center in the brain stem receives sensory input from baroreceptors, chemoreceptors, and peripheral vessel sensory receptors. Baroreceptors in the carotid sinus and aortic arch react to increased blood pressure and discharge impulses to the medullary center to reduce heart rate and relax arteriolar and venous tone. Chemoreceptors in the carotid sinus and aortic arch react to changing arterial oxygen tension and acid-base balance. Decreasing arterial oxygen concentration or increasing carbon dioxide concentration increases blood pressure, heart rate, and respiratory rate to provide more oxygen to the body.

Venous Pressure

The venous pressure primarily depends upon contraction of the left ventricle to empty the heart and generate intravascular pressure; and secondarily, on other variables such as blood volume and an effective right ventricle function. Decreases in blood volume (e.g., hemorrhage) reduce blood return to the right atrium and decrease cardiac output. When congestive heart failure (CHF) primarily results from the decreased ability of the right ventricle to pump blood to the pulmonary arteries (i.e., right-sided heart failure), right ventricular end-diastolic volume and venous pressure increase; this results in dependent edema, engorgement of the jugular veins, hepatomegaly, splenomegaly, fluid in the abdominal cavity, and bowel edema. In left-sided congestive heart failure, the inability of the left ventricle to pump effectively increases left ventricular end-diastolic volume which leads to increased venous pressure in the lungs. This increased venous pressure in the pulmonary vascular tree is clinically manifested as shortness of breath (SOB), wheezing (i.e., cardiac asthma), pulmonary venous engorgement, pleural effusion, and accumulation of fluid in the alveoli of the lung.

PHYSICAL ASSESSMENT

Blood Pressure

Measure the patient's blood pressure with an aneroid or mercury sphygmomanometer. The sphygmomanometer consists of a flat rubber bladder enclosed in a cloth cover (i.e., the cuff), a hand-held rubber bulb pump, and a pressure sensing gauge. The rubber pump inflates the bladder and the arterial impedance is read on the pressure gauge for an indirect measure for the intra-arterial pressure. Aneroid (i.e., spring-loaded) devices are more portable than mercury devices. However, the aneroid devices need to be periodically calibrated with a mercury

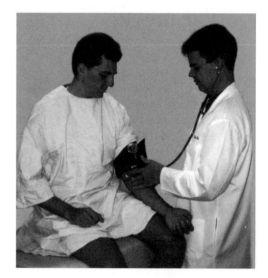

Fig. 10.7 Auscultation of blood pressure using an aneroid sphygmomanometer.

sphygmomanometer. The adult blood pressure cuffs come in two sizes: one for the arm and a larger one for the leg. The arm cuff should be at least 10 cm wide and the leg cuff 18 cm wide. The use of an incorrect rubber bladder size can result in inaccurate blood pressure measurements. An undersized bladder results in falsely high blood pressure readings and an oversized bladder may give a falsely low reading. The correct size bladder is judged by the circumference of the arm or leg. The width of the bladder needs to be about 40 percent of the circumference of the limb at its midpoint.

Instruct the patient to sit or lie down and hold her arm at about the level of the heart. If the patient has been smoking or engaged in vigorous physical activity, let the patient rest in a quiet, comfortable room for a few minutes before measuring the blood pressure. It is a good standard of care to check the blood pressure in both arms the first time you see a patient since the systolic pressure could show a 5 mm Hg difference between arms in adults. A difference of more than 10 mm Hg in the systolic pressure is a clinically significant finding. Depending upon the patient, a lower pressure in one arm may be caused by a sclerotic obstruction.

Wrap the deflated cuff snugly around the midpoint of the bared upper arm about 2.5 cm above the antecubital fossa. Avoid wrapping the blood pressure cuff over clothing which can affect the circulation of blood. To avoid extraneous noises, the bladder rubber tubing of the sphygmomanometer should not rub against the stethoscope. Before lightly applying the bell of the stethoscope, palpate either the brachial pulse at the elbow or radial pulse at the wrist. Then inflate the cuff about 10 mm Hg above the point at which the pulse can no longer be detected. This process provides a palpable rough estimate of the systolic blood pressure and decreases the possibility of underestimating the systolic pressure. Open the valve of the cuff and slowly deflate the cuff until the pressure gauge reads zero. Palpate the brachial artery which is medial to the brachial tendon in the antecubital fossa. Lightly apply the bell of the stethoscope over the brachial artery. After closing the valve of the blood pressure cuff, rapidly inflate the cuff to a pressure 10 mm Hg above the palpable pulse. Slowly open the valve and decrease the pressure in the cuff at a steady rate (neither too slow nor too fast). Watch the pressure gauge and listen for the first audible sound which identifies the systolic pressure. Keep watching and listening until no sounds are heard. The point of disappearance of the heartbeat indicates the diastolic pressure. These intra-arterial sounds are collectively called Korotkoff sounds. Occasionally, Korotkoff sounds are heard, disappear, and reappear (e.g., in a patient with atrial fibrillation). This may distort accurate recording of the blood pressure. The point of disappearance then reappearance of sounds is termed the auscultatory gap. Failure to recognize the auscultatory gap can result in underestimation of the systolic and overestimation of the diastolic pressures. This problem is avoided by inflating the bladder to a pressure that obliterates the palpable pulse.

Three consecutive elevated blood pressure readings, taken on three separate occasions, should be documented before the diagnosis of "hypertension" is applied to a patient. If the blood pressure is higher than normal, have the patient rest quietly and repeat the test. In the middle-aged or younger adult, normal diastolic blood pressure is 85 mm Hg or less, and normal systolic pressure is less than 130 mm Hg. Hypertension is defined as diastolic readings consistently greater than 90 mm Hg. With aging, the systolic pressure rises, and systolic hypertension is defined as a systolic pressure of more than 160 mm Hg with a normal diastolic reading. The

Table 10.1

Classification of Blood Pressures for Adults

Category	Systolic Pressure (mm Hg)	Diastolic Pressure (mm Hg)
Normal	<130	<85
High normal	130–139	85–89
Hypertension		
Stage 1	140–159	90–99
Stage 2	160–179	100–109
Stage 3	180–209	110–119
Stage 4	≥210	≥120

At Risk Blood Pressures[a]

Table 10.2

Age	Blood Pressure (mm Hg)	
Adults	**Men**	**Women**
under 45 y/o	>130/90	>130/90
over 44 y/o	>140/95	>160/95
Children		
3–5 y/o	>116/76	
6–9 y/o	>122/78	
10–12 y/o	>126/82	
13–15 y/o	>136/86	
16–18 y/o	>142/92	

[a] There is no critical level of blood pressure that appears to delineate excess risk. Therefore, definition of hypertension remains arbitrary.

blood pressure in adults generally responds to circadian variations and generally is highest in the mid-morning and lowest in the early morning around 2:00 a.m.

As shown in Table 10.1, some clinicians now classify hypertension in four stages. Besides blood pressure, one must specify the presence or absence of target-organ disease and other risk factors. For example, a patient with renal damage and hyperlipidemia and a blood pressure of 150/110 mm Hg should be classified as "Stage 3 with target organ damage (kidney failure) and with another major risk factor (hyperlipidemia)." When systolic and diastolic pressures fall into different categories, the higher category should be used to stage the person's blood pressure.

There is no critical level of blood pressure that appears to delineate excess risk. Therefore, definition of hypertension remains arbitrary. Morbidity and mortality are known to increase linearly with increased levels of either systolic or diastolic blood pressure. Even modest elevations in blood pressure carry substantial risk. When the diastolic and systolic blood pressures in Table 10.2 are exceeded, mortality in adults increases by more than 50%.

Any patient taking an antihypertensive medication and complaining of syncope, dizziness, or pre-syncope, should be evaluated for orthostatic hypotension. Although orthostatic hypotension is a common problem in the elderly, it can be caused by antihypertensive drugs or volume depletion (e.g., dehydration). Orthostatic hypotension can be evaluated by comparing the brachial blood pressure when the patient is in a supine position to the blood pressure obtained when the patient is in an upright position, either standing or sitting with his legs dangling over the side of the bed. Orthostatic hypotension is present if the systolic pressure drops (about 15 to 20 mm Hg) and diastolic pressure falls when the patient moves from a supine to an upright position. If the patient manifests orthostatic hypotension, be sure to take the patient's pulse. The heart rate should only increase minimally if the cause of the orthostasis is neurogenic in origin (i.e., caused by a disease such as diabetes mellitus or by sympatholytic medications). Orthostasis can be attributed to intravascular volume depletion if the decrease in blood pressure is accompanied by reflex tachycardia. It should be noted that beta blockers blunt or prevent the reflex tachycardia normally present on standing. Orthostatic hypotension is particularly important when accompanied by hypoperfusion symptoms (e.g., light-headed, fainting). The etiology of orthostasis should be determined and managed accordingly.

The decrease in systolic blood pressure of 15 to 20 mm Hg that accompanies orthostatic postural changes is a much more objective tool for evaluating volume depletion than the evaluation of skin turgor, dry mucous membranes, or "soft" eyeballs. Skin turgor is often difficult to assess in the elderly; the "moistness" of mucous membranes can be affected by anticholinergic medications; and pressure applied to "eyeballs" has the potential for iatrogenic injury.

Respirations can affect blood pressure. For example, systolic blood pressure drops slightly with inspiration as a consequence of negative intrathoracic pressure which reduces stroke volume and lowers cardiac output. This decrease in systolic pressure upon inspiration is exaggerated with some diseases. When the decrease in systolic pressure exceeds 10 mm Hg upon inspiration and when inspiratory venous pressure does not decrease, the term **pulsus paradoxus** or paradoxical pulse is applied (see Table 10.3). Pulsus paradoxus refers to the exaggerated see-saw or alternating pulse amplitude or volume associated with inspiration. The condition can usually be palpated or more precisely monitored with a sphygmomanometer. To measure this effect, slowly lower the cuff pressure and listen for the systolic pressure. Carefully watch the patient's breathing and note the first Korotkoff sound heard on expiration. You should hear first heartbeats during expiration. As the patient inhales and you continue to slowly lower the cuff pressure, the pulse rate will double; note the systolic pressure. The endpoint is attained when heartbeats are heard during both expiration and inspiration. The difference between these peak systolic pressure readings is the paradoxical pulse; a difference of more than 10 mm Hg is a sign of reduced cardiac output.

The respiratory effect on blood pressure can be explored by monitoring the blood pressure on a normal subject performing exaggerated, slow breathing or the Valsalva maneuver. A significant decrease in systolic pressure during inspiration can be encountered in patients with asthma, severe heart failure, pulmonary emphysema, tricuspid stenosis, pericardial tamponade, or shock.

Peripheral Arterial Pulses

Evaluation of peripheral arterial pulses provides valuable clinical diagnostic information. These peripheral arteries include the carotid, brachial, radial, ulnar, femoral, popliteal, dorsalis pedis, and posterior tibial arteries, the abdominal aorta, and

Abnormal Pulses

Table 10.3

Pattern	Description	Associated Cause
Paradoxical Pulse (Pulsus Paradoxus)	A variation in pulse amplitude with the respiratory cycle. The amplitude increases with expiration and decreases with inspiration. It is best detected by noting the systolic blood pressure which is best heard on expiration and grows faint on inspiration. As the cuff pressure is lowered, the sounds will be heard continuously throughout the respiratory cycle. When the systolic blood pressure falls more than 10 mm Hg during inspiration, and when inspiratory venous pressure does not decrease, a paradoxical pulse becomes evident as the pulse amplitude varies with respirations	Asthma, emphysema, pericardial effusion, constrictive pericarditis, mitral stenosis with right heart failure

Inspiration   Expiration   Inspiration

Pattern	Description	Associated Cause
Pulsus Magnus (Water Hammer, Collapsing)	A strong, bounding up stroke with a rapid descent. The peak is brisk and very brief.	Aortic regurgitation, hyperthyroidism, severe anemia, systolic hypertension, anxiety, exercise, fever, arteriovenous fistula, patent ductus arteriosus

Pattern	Description	Associated Cause
Small, Weak Pulse (Thready Pulse, Pulsus Parvus)	The ascending and descending strokes are small and weak. The pulse is difficult to palpate. The pulse contour is slow to form, has a sustained peak, and is slow to disappear.	Hypovolemia, severe aortic stenosis, acute myocardial infarction, constrictive pericarditis, shock

Table 10.3

Abnormal Pulses (Continued)

Pattern	Description	Associated Cause
Large, Strong Pulse (Hyperkinetic Pulse)	The stroke is full and bounding. The pulse is easily palpated. The amplitude is high and the contour moderately rapid, brief peak, and moderately rapid descend.	Exercise, anxiety, fever, hyperthyroidism, hypertension, aortic regurgitation, aortic rigidity

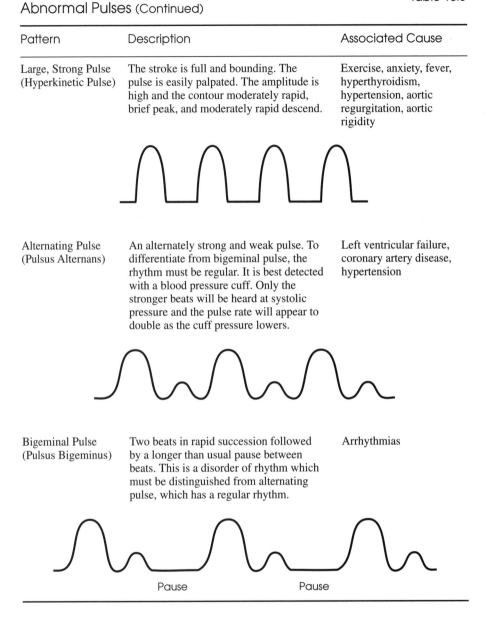

| Alternating Pulse (Pulsus Alternans) | An alternately strong and weak pulse. To differentiate from bigeminal pulse, the rhythm must be regular. It is best detected with a blood pressure cuff. Only the stronger beats will be heard at systolic pressure and the pulse rate will appear to double as the cuff pressure lowers. | Left ventricular failure, coronary artery disease, hypertension |

| Bigeminal Pulse (Pulsus Bigeminus) | Two beats in rapid succession followed by a longer than usual pause between beats. This is a disorder of rhythm which must be distinguished from alternating pulse, which has a regular rhythm. | Arrhythmias |

Pause   Pause

other abdominal arteries. The pulses should be measured for rate, amplitude, and rhythm and, with the exception of the carotid arteries, should be examined bilaterally and simultaneously for comparison. While feeling an arterial pulse, ask yourself the following questions: "Do I feel the pulse? How would I describe its amplitude? Does it feel the same as its contralateral counterpart?" Answering these basic questions will facilitate an understanding of arterial hemodynamics.

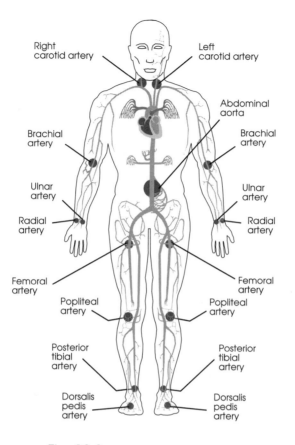

Fig. 10.8 Locations of peripheral pulses.

A pulse wave is described by its amplitude or strength as bounding, normal, diminished, or absent (see Table 10.4) and depends upon the pulse pressure. The pulse pressure relates to the elasticity of the arterial wall, stroke volume, and left ventricular force of ejection. The normal arterial pulse rises quickly, peaks, rapidly descends, then briefly turns upward and finally descends until the next ventricular contraction begins. Depending upon the particular artery, the exact wave form contour varies, but the general configuration is as described.

When possible, sit in a comfortable position to facilitate complete concentration on evaluating arterial pulses. Using your index and middle fingers or thumb, firmly compress a superficial artery. Ask yourself the following questions: "Do I feel the pulse? Am I pressing too hard and obliterating the pulse?" Explore the area to locate the artery. If the pulse is not felt, move to a larger, more proximal artery. Once located, note the amplitude of the pulse, taking into consideration the patient's age and presence or absence of vascular disease. For instance, in patients with a failing left ventricle or severe aortic stenosis, the pulse amplitude is diminished and is felt as a gentle impulse. A bounding pulse is felt as a brisk impulse; occasionally a throbbing

Table 10.4

Pulse Amplitude Rating Scale[a]

Grade	Amplitude
0	Absent
1	Weak
2	Normal
3	Strong
4	Bounding

[a]Compare arterial pulses simultaneously and bilaterally.

or pulsating artery is easily visible. In older patients, it is sometimes possible to identify a tortuous, pulsatile, inelastic beating pulse, known as Monckeberg's arteriosclerosis. Pulses may be very difficult to palpate behind the knee or in an edematous ankle or foot. In edematous tissue, apply constant pressure to gently express the excess interstitial fluid, exposing the pulsatile artery to touch. Table 10.4 presents a rating scale for comparing pulses. These bedside scores grade arterial pulses from absent to bounding.

The normal adult pulse rate ranges from 60 to 100 beats per minute. The cardiac exam (see Chapter 11: Heart) includes an evaluation of the radial and carotid pulses for rate and rhythm, as well as the carotid pulses for bruits and cardiac sounds. As a routine screening check, bilaterally examine the radial, carotid, and dorsalis pedis pulses. This provides a quick assessment of arterial flow to the head and extremities. If these are normal, other pulses need not be examined unless otherwise specifically indicated.

Lack of symmetry between pulses of the right and left extremities may be caused by unilateral arterial occlusion, a subclavian stenosis or a subclavian steal syndrome, or coarctation of the aorta (e.g., comparing upper extremity pulses with lower extremity pulses). Coarctation of the arch or aorta between the right brachiocephalic artery and the left subclavian artery can result in a weaker pulse and a lower blood pressure in the left upper extremity than in the right.

Having noted the amplitude and rate, next determine the rhythm of the pulse. Is the pulse regular with each beat equidistant from the other? Or is it irregular with skipped or dropped beats (i.e., heartbeats are heard with the stethoscope but the peripheral pulse is not felt)? Atrial fibrillation results in an irregularly irregular pulse (i.e., the pulse is irregular in rhythm and irregular in amplitude).

Carotid Pulse

The carotid arteries are particularly good sites for analyzing most of the various abnormal pulse patterns because of the close proximity of these vessels to the heart (see Table 10.3). Paradoxical pulses, however, are best analyzed while measuring the blood pressure. Avoid palpating the carotid sinus at the common carotid artery bifurcation located at the level of the thyroid cartilage (see Figure 10.9). Massaging the carotid sinus may slow the pulse rate and significantly decrease the blood pressure (see Chapter 11: Heart). These adverse cardiovascular responses are more common in the elderly or in patients who have heart disease. To examine the right carotid artery, relax the right sternocleidomastoid

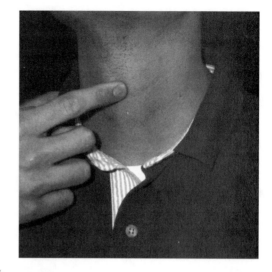

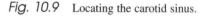

Fig. 10.9 Locating the carotid sinus.

muscle by turning the patient's head downward and to the left. On the patient's right side and with the middle and index fingers of your right hand wrapped around the lower anterior edge of the patient's sternocleidomastoid muscle, examine the right carotid artery by applying gentle but firm pressure. To examine the left carotid artery, reverse the method. In the elderly, diminution of cerebral blood flow is common because of carotid arteriosclerotic disease. For safety, do not simultaneously compress both carotid arteries.

Arteries with blood freely flowing through them are normally silent. As presented during the cardiac exam discussion, various cardiac and extracardiac sounds are referred to the neck from the heart via the aortic arch and carotid arteries. Using the bell of the stethoscope, listen for bruits in the carotid arteries above their bifurcation at the angle of the jaw; also note other neck sounds. A vascular bruit is a type of extracardiac murmur. Although the term bruit is frequently restricted to vascular sounds, it also applies to findings from other types of examinations (e.g., a venous hum or a thyroid bruit of a hyperactive thyroid). To hear a bruit, it may be necessary to ask the patient to hold her breath in mid-inspiration. Then listen carefully. Start at the angle of the jaw and inch downward to the precordium following the course of the carotid artery. Remember that some cardiac murmurs radiate to the neck. If the patient is having symptoms suggesting regional cerebral blood flow inadequacy, an artery can be "silent" because of a complete or almost complete obstruction (i.e., the artery may or may not be pulseless). Arteries with reduced flow and a palpable pulse may not have sufficient flow to create a bruit. A false bruit can be created by applying too much pressure with the stethoscope, causing a partial stenosis or obstruction of the artery. A carotid bruit may have accompanying symptoms. This may indicate a need for surgical correction and/or medical management. Besides the carotid area, remember to listen to the abdominal aortic, renal, and femoral arteries for bruits. An aneurysm (i.e., a weak, ballooning vessel wall) may also create a bruit. For example, patients at risk of atherosclerotic diseases need to be checked carefully for bruits. Anytime you hear a bruit, if possible, compress the proximal artery segment. If the distal bruit completely disappears, it is probably caused by stenosis.

Radial Pulse

To examine the radial artery, use the pads of your index and middle fingers to simultaneously compress the radial arteries at the wrists (see Figure 10.10). Make certain the patient is resting comfortably with both arms supported on a firm surface or the knees. Grade the pulses for their rate, regularity, and amplitude. The normal pulse wave begins with a swift upward stroke and a gradual, smooth descent. Note if the arterial wall is hard to compress. Sclerotic arteries tend to roll under your fingers, and generally suggest arteriosclerotic disease or possibly pseudohypertension. The effect of sclerotic arteries on blood pressure should be considered when checking the blood pressure.

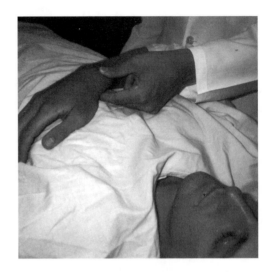

Fig. 10.10   Palpation of radial artery at the wrist.

If the radial pulse is absent, then palpate the brachial artery pulses in the groove between the triceps and biceps muscles medially just above the elbow. If the brachial pulses are patent and the radial pulse absent, check the ulnar artery patency by completing the Allen test as described below.

Allen Test. The Allen test evaluates the patency of the radial and ulnar arteries. To begin the test, ask the patient to sit with palms facing upward and resting on the knees. Occlude the right radial and ulnar arteries with your thumbs as the patient rapidly and firmly makes a fist to pump out the arterial blood. If the radial and ulnar arteries are occluded appropriately, the patient's fist should appear pale as it is slowly unclenched. Slowly release the pressure from your thumb on the patient's ulnar artery and look for a normal pink palmar skin flush as blood flows through the ulnar artery; maintain pressure on the right radial artery. Failure of the palm to flush suggests ulnar artery occlusion. Reverse these steps to check radial patency. Be sure to compare each hand for the length of capillary refilling time and flush intensity.

Pedal (Foot) Pulses

The patient should be in a supine or sitting position when you palpate the pedal pulses. Expose both feet to good lighting to examine for signs of poor circulation or edema. Using the backs of your hands, feel the skin temperature of each foot and lower leg comparatively and simultaneously. Examine the dorsalis pedis pulse using three fingers on the dorsum of the foot. Note the pulse just lateral to the extensor tendon of the great toes. Press lightly, then more deeply if needed to find the pulse. Pedal edema can obscure these pulses and posterior tibial pulses. In some patients, the dorsalis pedis or posterior tibia pulses are congenitally absent. However, both pulses should not be missing. Palpate the posterior tibial pulse by curving your fingers behind the medial malleolus of the patient's ankle. This pulse is located in the groove between the Achilles tendon and the tibia, just posterior to the medial malleolus. You may have to explore the area to find the pulse and it may not be palpable in a markedly obese patient or a patient with significant ankle edema. Again, note the presence and amplitude of the pulse.

Special Maneuvers to Enhance Arteriolar Assessments

If indicated, abdominal arteries can be examined by placing the patient in a supine position with knees flexed to relax the abdominal muscles. A pillow placed under the patient's knees will help relax the anterior abdominal wall muscles. The abdominal aorta is located to the left of the midline extending between the xiphoid process and the umbilicus. Apply gentle, but firm pressure in the epigastrium above the umbilicus. An aortic aneurysm, usually found at or above the level of the umbilicus, can complicate this examination when firm pressure is applied to the epigastrium, especially in susceptible patients (e.g., hypertensives). The aneurysm may be tender to palpation with pain radiating to the patient's back. Using the bell of the stethoscope, auscultate the iliac, renal, and aortic arteries for bruits that might be attributable to an aneurysm or stenosis (see Figure 12.11). Renovascular bruits, occasional findings in renal vascular hypertension, are high-pitched sounds formed by blood rushing past a partial occlusion. These bruits can be heard during systole and the sound can radiate laterally to the flanks. The finding of possible renal artery stenosis in a patient with renovascular hypertension is a relative contraindication to the use of angiotensin converting enzyme inhibitors (e.g., enalapril).

After examining the abdominal area for aneurysms and bruits, examine the femoral pulses while the patient remains supine with legs extended. Begin the examination of the femoral arteries by pressing below the inguinal ligament three to five centimeters lateral to the pubic symphysis, one third of the distance between the anterior superior iliac spine and the pubic tubercle. After you identify the femoral artery with palpation, gently press the bell of the stethoscope over the artery and listen for bruits. Be sure to apply gentle pressure because it is particularly easy to create a bruit in this artery with the head of the stethoscope.

Next, assess the popliteal pulses by slightly flexing the patient's knee and placing your hands behind the knee while compressing the popliteal fossa. Palpate slightly lateral to the midline and note the popliteal pulse. The popliteal artery is deep beneath the vein and often difficult to palpate, particularly in muscular or overweight individuals.

Evaluation of Arterial Insufficiency. Arterial insufficiency in the lower extremities can be estimated by evaluating the color remaining in the toes, feet, and legs when the patient's legs are elevated about 12 inches above the heart for approximately 60 seconds while the patient is in a supine position. With normal arterial circulation, slight pallor develops in the toes, feet, or legs. With arterial insufficiency, marked pallor appears. Next, have the patient sit with his or her feet over the side of the examining table. The color should return to the legs within 10 seconds if the arterial system is only minimally obstructed, because superficial veins generally fill under the influence of gravity within 15 seconds. With moderate to severe occlusive arterial disease in the lower extremities, it may take more than 40 seconds for the capillaries to refill and return color to the legs. In addition, look for the presence of other color changes in the legs suggesting arterial occlusive disease (e.g., a dusky red color or cyanosis). Evaluation of the lower limbs for signs of arterial insufficiency should include inspection of the feet and legs for skin atrophy, hair loss on the toes and legs, thickening or transverse ridges of the toe nails, ischemic ulcerations, and dry gangrene. The presence of **intermittent claudication** (i.e., symptoms characterized by absence of pain in a limb when at rest, commencement of pain after initiation of walking, intensification of pain until walking is impossible, and the disappearance of all these symptoms after a period of rest) usually indicates arterial insufficiency. Intermittent claudication can often be elicited by having the patient walk or exercise until pain develops; however, a good history and physical examination usually provide sufficient information. Pain at rest, particularly nocturnal pain, is a poor prognostic sign.

When arterial insufficiency of the lower extremities is suspected, use the dorsal surface of your fingers to symmetrically palpate the skin temperature of the extremities. With arterial occlusion, a cold line of demarcation is classic for chronic arterial occlusive disease and is also a common finding in acute arterial insufficiency.

When chronic arterial insufficiency is associated with intermittent claudication, measure the brachial systolic blood pressure by palpation when the patient is supine and compare it to the dorsalis pedis systolic pressure by palpation. The distal segment systolic pressure (e.g., at the ankles) should be equal to, or higher (sometimes 10 mm Hg higher) than the brachial systolic pressure; however, the distal segment systolic blood pressure decreases when arteries in the lower extremity become progressively occluded. The ankle to arm ratio for systolic pressure normally should be greater than 1.0. Patients with symptoms of exercise-induced ischemia have an ankle to arm ratio of systolic blood pressure between 0.5 and 0.9; patients with claudication at rest and ischemic necrosis usually have an ankle to arm ratio of less than 0.5.

Venous Pressures and Cardiac Action

The action of the heart produces changes in the venous system that can be observed during a physical examination. For example, by studying jugular venous pressure and analyzing pulse wave forms, the clinician can gather data about the pumping function of the right atrium and ventricle. Jugular vein wave forms also provide information about heart valve competence, cardiac arrhythmias, and heart conduction delays.

Depending upon the types of information sought, observe either the external or internal jugular vein. The right (rather than the left) external or internal jugular veins provide more meaningful data because of their anatomical relationship to the right atrium and ventricle. The **external jugular vein** mirrors the mean volume and pressure in the atria. The **internal jugular vein** also reflects volume and pressure changes in the atria and it usually is better for examining wave form. The right internal jugular is almost in a straight line anatomically with the right atrium, making the vein an excellent reflector of right heart function.

The jugular veins may be difficult to identify. Ask the patient to blow hard against closed lips and count to ten. This Valsalva maneuver causes venous blood to pool in the neck veins, allowing the internal jugular vein to be more easily identified. Having identified the veins, proceed with the examination. Caution: Do not confuse the jugular veins with the right carotid artery (see Table 10.5).

The **jugular venous pressure** (JVP) can be estimated by reclining the patient at various angles (see Figure 10.12). An adjustable bed is ideal for this purpose; however, frequently one has to improvise. Position the patient's head about 30° above the horizontal and adjust the position of the head until the gentle undulating pulsations of the right jugular veins can be seen. The higher the central venous pressure, the more perpendicular the patient can sit and still have venous pulsations observable. The

---

Table 10.5

Differentiating the Jugular Veins from the Carotid Arteries

The internal and external jugular veins are identified using the following criteria to distinguish them from the carotid artery.

1. Internal jugular vein is rarely palpable;

2. Venous pulsation descends on normal inspiration and rises on expiration;

3. Palpation stops the jugular venous pulse;

4. Height of venous pulse changes with body position;

5. The pulse is of soft, undulating quality; and

6. Venous pulse is easier to see when the patient is in a supine position.

lower the central venous pressure, the more supine the patient needs to be in order for the venous pulsations to be seen. Position the patient's head looking straight forward; do not turn the head to the left side because the right sternocleidomastoid muscle may mask the venous pulsations. Shine a pocket light tangentially across the neck to make the venous pulsations of the jugular veins easier to see. The pulsation of the jugular veins can be differentiated from arterial pulsations by being unable to be palpated because normal venous pressure is much less than that of arteries.

Using tangential light, note the position of the external jugular vein pulse. The external jugular vein can easily be found by applying gentle pressure with the right thumb at the base of sternocleidomastoid muscle near the clavicle. This gentle pressure occludes venous return and allows the vein to fill and bulge. Although the pulsations from the external jugular vein are not as visible as pulsations from the internal jugular vein, it is useful for evaluating volume and pressure changes in the right heart. In patients with congestive heart failure, the venous pressure increases as a result of increased preload, and distention of the jugular veins is more noticeable. Distended external jugular veins do not necessarily indicate an elevated mean right atrial pressure. In the patient with right ventricular congestive heart failure, as cardiac function improves and preload returns to normal, the jugular vein distention that was present with the patient sitting now is noted only when the patient reclines 30°.

Changes in the right internal jugular vein reflect pressure and volume changes in the right atrium; because of its anatomical location, it can be viewed as a manometer directly attached to the right atrium. When a patient is sitting or standing, the right atrium normally supports a column of blood in the superior vena cava to a height of about 10 cm above the level of the right atrium. When the patient is in the supine position, all peripheral veins become filled with blood. The right jugular vein distention, therefore, would collapse and disappear when the patient assumes a standing or sitting position. The jugular veins also collapse on inspiration and refill during expiration.

Directly estimate the venous pressure by measuring the height in centimeters of the column of blood in the external jugular vein at the sternal notch by using a ruler or straight edge (e.g., tongue blade). The venous pressure of a patient in the standing or sitting position should not be more than 3 to 4 cm vertically above the sternal angle or about 1 cm above the right clavicle. The higher that a column of blood rises above the sternal angle, the higher the right atrial filling pressure and the more severe the venous congestion. With increasing right atrial pressure, the height of the column of blood may rise to the angle of the jaw. When measuring and recording the venous pressure, also record the elevation of the head of the bed in degrees (i.e., 30°, 45°). This allows for more valid comparisons when venous pressure is checked later.

If the external jugular vein is abnormally distended, place both index fingers in the midpoint of the vein and milk it by moving your fingers 1 to 2 inches apart. While maintaining constant pressure on the vein from both separated fingers, release the pressure on the vein from the finger nearest to the clavicle and watch for venous filling from below (i.e., retrograde filling). Retrograde filling indicates a high central venous pressure. If the external jugular vein does not fill in a retrograde fashion, release the pressure on the vein from the remaining finger to watch for filling of the vein from above (i.e., antegrade filling).

Observation of the right internal jugular vein provides information not only about jugular venous pressure, but also about cardiac arrhythmias, cardiac conduction defects, and valvular murmurs. The interpretation of these physical examination findings involving the internal jugular vein is beyond the scope of this chapter and the reader is referred to a cardiology reference text for detailed information.

Venous pulse waves normally can be demonstrated in any superficial vein located near the heart. Analysis of pulse waves in the internal jugular veins can provide data that reflect the work of the right ventricle (see Figure 10.11). Since the action of the heart consists of several components, jugular venous pulse waves can consist of several components.

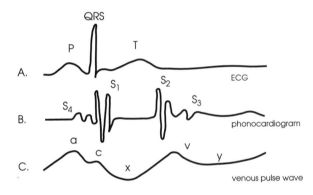

Fig. 10.11   Diagram illustrating the relationship between normal venous pulse patterns and cardiac action. A. A normal ECG reading. B. A normal phonocardiogram showing heart sounds. C. A normal jugular pulse tracing.

In the normal heart, right atrial pressure increases slightly just before ventricular contraction (i.e., the "a" wave). The "a" wave is reflective of the brief back flow of blood into the superior vena cava during right atrial contraction. Probably representing bulging of the tricuspid valve into the right atrium during early systole, the "c" wave occurs after the "a" wave. With right atrial contraction, blood enters the right ventricle, the atrial pressure drops, and the column of blood falls in the jugular veins as blood moves from the jugular vein into the right atrium. This action creates the downward slope of the "x" wave following the "a" wave peak. As the right atrium fills, the right atrial pressure rises because of the venous blood return, noted as the "v" wave. The tricuspid valve then opens and blood flows from the right atrium into the right ventricle; atrial pressure suddenly drops to form the downward "y" slope. This process repeats with each cardiac cycle.

With the patient still in the reclining position, place your right thumb on the left carotid artery while watching the right internal jugular vein. Be careful not to confuse the carotid pulse with the venous pulse. What is most noticeable are the two descent waves ("x" and "y"). Remember, the "x" descent is the antegrade flow into the right atrium heralding the beginning of systole (heard as the first heart sounds with the stethoscope). The "y" descent wave quickly follows, signaling the beginning of diastole. The examiner should identify a normal, strong rise, a brief collapse, and a slight rise, followed by a smooth downstroke. In other words, the internal jugular vein should be seen to collapse twice with each heartbeat.

Although normally silent, the sounds generated by blood flowing through the jugular veins can be heard with a stethoscope. A venous hum, for example, can be heard as a roaring sound that is a normal variant in many children and some adults. This extracardiac venous hum is loudest in diastole and is eliminated by compressing the jugular vein at the clavicle.

Special Venous Maneuvers

Hepatojugular Reflux is an early sign of systemic venous engorgement that is consistent with right-sided congestive heart failure, pericardial tamponade, or tricuspid valvular insufficiency. Hepatojugular reflux is observed as an increase in jugular vein distention (JVD) when venous blood is displaced to the jugular vein as a consequence of compression of the patient's midabdomen region at about the level of the liver. Hepatojugular reflux generally cannot be elicited in "pure" left-sided heart failure. Drugs that relax the venous bed [e.g., nitroglycerin (NTG)] or reduce venous return (e.g., diuretics) diminish or abolish hepatojugular reflux.

The hepatojugular reflux test begins with placement of the patient in a reclined position, bent at the waist with the upper body at about 30° to 45° above

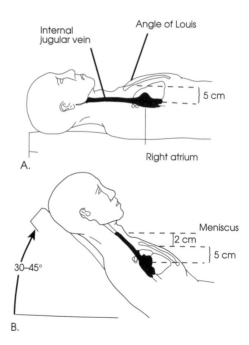

Fig. 10.12 Hepatojugular reflux. A. Jugular venous pressure cannot be measured in a supine patient. B. If the patient's head is inclined at a 45° angle, the patient' venous jugular pressure can be determined by measuring the distance from the Angle of Louis to the meniscus of the internal jugular vein and adding 5 cm (the distance from the mid-right atrium to the Angle of Louis).

the horizontal (see Figure 10.12). The patient's head, neck, and chest should be in a straight line, though this may vary depending on the severity of heart failure and patient comfort. Illuminate the jugular veins with tangential light and look closely for the venous oscillations. Tell the patient, "I want you to relax and breathe normally while I push on your stomach." Press with gentle, firm, steady pressure on the middle abdomen with the palm of your hand for 30 to 60 seconds. Avoid producing abdominal pain when compressing the middle abdomen. In the normal patient, look for a rise in the venous column of the right jugular veins followed by a drop in the column. It is not necessary to apply direct pressure on the liver or do anything that might cause the Valsalva effect. When systemic veins are engorged and systemic venous pressure is increased, the column of blood rises and remains elevated during the test. A sustained increase of more than 3 cm in the column of blood reflects venous engorgement and represents an abnormal finding. Venous pressure also is increased by high intra-thoracic pressure from chronic obstructive lung disease, large retrosternal goiter, or a venous obstruction distal to the right atrium. Nevertheless, the most common cause for an elevated jugular venous pulse is right-sided heart failure (see Figure 10.12).

Venous Incompetence. The return of blood from the extremities to the heart depends upon muscular contractions, patent veins, and competent valves that maintain the unidirectional flow of blood. To examine the leg veins for valvular incompetence, ask the patient to stand up from a sitting position. Observe venous filling in the feet and lower legs. Inspect for signs of venous stasis such as pitting edema, stasis-related hyperpigmentation, stasis ulceration, and varicose (i.e., dilated) veins.

To test vein competency of the patient in the supine position, drain the sapheno-femoral veins by elevating the leg 12 inches above the heart. Snugly apply a tourniquet or blood pressure cuff to compress the superficial thigh veins, but not the arteries. To confirm arterial flow, palpate a distal pulse. Ask the patient to stand with the tourniquet still in place and record the time it takes the veins to refill from below. Release the tourniquet within 60 seconds after application. When the saphenous and femoral veins are competent, the superficial veins fill from below within 30 seconds and no more filling should occur from above after release of the tourniquet pressure. The test is deemed to be positive when the saphenous vein fills from above within 10 seconds after compression release. This testing method is known as the **Trendelenburg-Brodie** test.

Edema is a sign of interstitial fluid accumulation. When edema is present, search for a systemic and/or local cause. Examples of systemic causes include congestive heart failure, nephrotic syndrome, severe malnutrition, renal failure, and liver disease. The mechanisms for systemic causes usually relate to an ineffective pumping of the heart, loss of vascular osmotic pressure (e.g., hypoalbuminemia), or retention of sodium and water. The mechanisms of local causes include blockage of venous flow (e.g., thrombophlebitis), postural stasis secondary to immobility, increased vascular permeability (e.g., allergic reaction, pre-eclampsia of pregnancy), and lymph vessel blockage.

Edematous fluid usually distributes by gravitational flow to the lower extremities while the patient is sitting or standing. Upon reclining, edema may also pool in the buttocks, sacrum, or calf. **Dependent edema** is a term used to describe the condition in which the fluid distributes by gravitational forces, and is usually associated with the legs. Dependent edema usually is observed as bilateral, pretibial pitting edema. In the bedridden patient, dependent edema may be manifest as presacral edema more often than pretibial edema.

Pitting and **non-pitting** are additional terms used to classify edema. Pitting edema is primarily caused by excessive interstitial fluid accumulation. It can be detected by firmly pressing your index finger over a bony prominence. An indentation (i.e., pit) remaining in the skin after you remove your finger signifies the presence of pitting edema. In comparison to pitting edema, non-pitting edema is a rare condition that results primarily from interstitial accumulation of nonaqueous fluid (e.g., myxedema) or blockage of lymph drainage (e.g., tumor).

A description of the location or distribution of edema is important in the assessment of its clinical significance. For example, in an ambulatory patient, bilateral edema that involves the whole leg to the level of the knees is more important than simple ankle swelling. The term **anasarca** is used to describe a severe condition of massive, generalized pitting edema involving the entire body. A rating scale of 1+, 2+, 3+, 4+ that denotes increasing severity of edema as the number increases (see Table 10.6) is used to provide a subjective assessment of the depth of the pitting. Edema may "shift" depending upon the patient's position. For example, an ambulatory patient presenting with 3+ pitting edema of the ankle and pretibial area may have only 1+ pitting edema in the same locations, solely because the edema has moved to a more dependent position (e.g., presacral area) when the patient assumes a recumbent position. With chronic edema, the skin becomes hyperpigmented, dry and scaly, and ulcers or dermatitis can develop. With acute edema, the skin appears tight, and sometimes erythematous and shiny.

Deep Vein Thrombophlebitis (DVT) is a term used to describe thrombosis (i.e., blood clots) involving the deep veins of the legs. The signs and symptoms of DVT are often insignificant or obscure; however, when the clot becomes dislodged from vessel walls, a fatal pulmonary embolism could result. A complaint of calf pain is suggestive of a blood clot (i.e., thrombophlebitis) in a calf vein; however, absence of calf pain does not exclude a venous thrombus. If a superficial calf vein is occluded (i.e., thrombosed), symptoms such as redness, tenderness, and a firm "cord-like" vein

Table 10.6

Edema Assessment

Grade	Pitting Depth
1+	0.5–1 mm
2+	2–3 mm
3+	4–5 mm
4+	>5 mm

usually are also apparent. In a deep calf vein thrombosis, the calf is swollen, tender, painful, and a tender cord-like vein can sometimes be palpated deep between the muscles of the calf. Acute dorsiflexion of the foot frequently elicits severe calf pain (i.e., Homans' sign). A positive Homans' sign also can indicate musculoskeletal disease, sacroiliac herniated disc disease, or shortening of the Achilles' tendon (e.g., from wearing high heels) rather than DVT. Homans' sign, therefore, is not a reliable indicator of deep vein thrombosis. With deep vein thrombosis, the superficial foot veins tend not to collapse when the affected calf is elevated above the heart. A more reliable bedside observation to assist with the diagnosis and to follow resolution is to objectively monitor calf swelling. With a pen, mark the top of each patella. Depending upon the leg length, measure 15 to 20 cm above the patella mark and make a second mark on the thigh, and 15 to 20 cm below the patella mark make a third mark on the anterior calf. At the two marks above and below the patella, measure the circumference of the thigh and calf. The affected calf and thigh will have a greater circumference than the contralateral normal calf and thigh. The gold standard for confirming diagnosis of deep vein thrombosis is the venogram (i.e., a radiogram of the veins).

PHARMACOTHERAPEUTIC CASE ILLUSTRATION

History

R.D., a 51-year-old white male (WM), was evaluated for hypertension because his blood pressure was noted to be high at a shopping mall screening program. He had no other complaints and has been in good health. His past medical history (PMH) includes childhood chicken pox, pneumonia, right knee surgery, and mild bronchitis. His social history (SH) notes that his father (age 81) has a history of coronary artery disease and experienced a myocardial infarction at age 61. His mother died at age 69 of diabetic complications. R.D. is the manager for an aerospace company. He drinks alcoholic beverages socially 3 to 4 times a week, and has smoked one pack of cigarettes per day for 30 years. He is divorced and remarried with three children. His present medications include diazepam 2 mg PO BID PRN nervousness, aspirin 325 mg 2 PO QD PRN headache, and magnesium-aluminum hydroxide 15 mL PRN heartburn. His review of systems (ROS) revealed: head, eyes, ears, nose, and throat (HEENT): occasional headaches; Respiratory: cough, especially in morning; gastrointestinal (GI): frequent indigestion.

Physical Examination

This 51-year-old WM appeared well-developed and well nourished (WDWN) and in no apparent distress (NAD). He weighed 210 lb and was 5 ft 11 in tall. He appeared to be in good state of health.

He had the following vital signs (VS): respiratory rate (RR) 16/min and regular; a temperature 97.8° F; pulse 78 beats/min regular; blood pressure (BP) in right arm 158/108 mm Hg (supine), 158/110 mm Hg (standing); left arm 154/104 mm Hg (supine), 155/108 mm Hg (standing). Eyes: arteriovenous (AV) nicking, retinal hemorrhages; chest and lungs were clear to auscultation. Heart: regular rate and rhythm, normal S_1, S_2 without gallop, murmur, or rub. Abdomen: normal bowel sounds. Extremities: normal without edema or cyanosis. Neurological: normal.

Laboratory

The following tests were normal: complete blood cell count (CBC), blood glucose, urinalysis (except proteinuria 1+), serum electrolytes (potassium, sodium, bicarbonate, chloride), serum triglycerides, and serum uric acid. The serum blood urea nitrogen (BUN) (30 mg/dL), serum creatinine (2.1 mg/dL), and serum cholesterol (258 mg/dL) were elevated. Chest x-ray (CXR) showed mild heart enlargement, and changes suggesting chronic lung disease. Electrocardiogram (ECG) showed left ventricular enlargement (i.e., hypertrophy). (See Figure 11.4 in Heart Chapter for an ECG showing left ventricular hypertrophy.)

Diagnosis and Management

R.D. was diagnosed as having stage 3 hypertension with target organ damage (i.e., left ventricular hypertrophy, renal failure, retinopathy) and multiple risk factors (i.e., hyperlipidemia, smoking, male, obesity, sedentary). He was referred to a dietitian for consultation to reduce his weight and lower dietary sodium and cholesterol. He was prescribed a regular walking program and told to reduce alcohol consumption. He will return for tobacco and stress management counseling. To control the elevated blood pressure, hydrochlorothiazide 25 mg PO QD and enalapril (Vasotec) 5 mg tablet PO QD were prescribed.

Discussion

Disease. Although high blood pressure is an important risk factor for coronary artery disease, myocardial infarction, stroke, renal failure, and blindness, hypertensive patients seldom have symptoms until end-organ damage is evident. Essential hypertension has no known cause (i.e., etiology). The vast majority of high blood pressure patients are determined to have essential hypertension.

Factors other than hypertension can increase the risk of developing cardiovascular disease. In R.D.'s case, male gender, stress, family history of diabetes and myocardial infarction, smoking, alcohol consumption, obesity, elevated cholesterol, and sedentary lifestyle increase his risk of developing a cardiovascular disorder. The decision to treat high blood pressure should be guided by the patient's risk factor profile and by the severity of the blood pressure elevation.

R.D. had some evidence of eye, kidney, and heart damage. His funduscopic (i.e., eye) exam showed retinal changes consistent with long-standing hypertension. With elevated blood pressure, the arterioles in the retina thicken, become less elastic, and compress the retinal veins leading to the physical finding known as "AV nicking" (see Figure 5.19 in Chapter 5: Eye). The deterioration of renal function in R.D. is manifested by increased serum concentrations of urea nitrogen and serum creatinine, as well as by the 1+ proteinuria. The CXR and ECG of R.D. noted left ventricular enlargement. If left untreated, the hypertension would predispose R.D. to retinal damage, renal failure, myocardial infarction, angina pectoris, or cerebrovascular disease. Hypertension must be treated, preferably before, but certainly when the high pressure already has begun to damage organs.

When the diastolic blood pressure is consistently lowered to less than 85 mm Hg, damage to retinal vessels may be halted and sometimes reversed. When cardiac afterload is reduced by antihypertensive medications, the workload on the heart is reduced, as is left ventricular hypertrophy. Long-standing renal damage may not improve with antihypertensives, but effective therapy may slow the development of further end-organ damage.

Management. The goals for the management of hypertension must be developed with the patient because drug treatment has risks and benefits, and hypertension is asymptomatic. A systolic/diastolic blood pressure of less than 140/90 mm Hg should be the goal; however, adverse drug effects have to be balanced against this goal.

The successful management of hypertension should not only reduce blood pressure, but also the other risk factors associated with cardiovascular disease. Therefore, programs such as weight reduction, salt restriction, exercise, alcohol/tobacco abstinence, change of dietary fat consumption, and stress reduction are also needed. These non-drug therapies should be initiated before drug therapy because they lower blood pressure and are important adjuncts to effective drug therapy.

Weight loss to no more than 15% above ideal body weight lowers blood pressure in the obese hypertensive. Although weight reduction is often unsuccessful, patients need encouragement and positive reinforcement because weight reduction can provide high benefits with small risks. Sodium restricted diets provide another non-drug therapy approach to hypertensive management because sodium intake expands vascular volume, especially in volume-sensitive hypertensives. In these hypertensives, diastolic blood pressure can be reduced by 5 to 10 mm Hg when salt is not added to food and when quick-fix, convenience foods (e.g., frozen entrees, canned soups) are avoided. R.D. should also be encouraged to stop, or at least restrict, tobacco and alcohol use because the use of these products can increase blood pressure and have other negative effects on health. Since R.D. has a high serum concentration of cholesterol and a family history of coronary heart disease, his dietary intake of saturated fats should be reduced. R.D. also should be encouraged to exercise regularly because the combination of these non-drug therapeutic interventions offers the patient benefits with small risk. Life-style changes are difficult because a strong support network and high personal motivation are needed for success.

Table 10.7

Suggested Therapy for Hypertension with Co-Existing Conditions

Condition	Non-Drug Therapy	Drug Therapy
Obesity with insulin resistance	Weight loss, physical activity	Diuretics, alpha blockers, ACE inhibitors
Sodium sensitivity (fluid retention)	Sodium restriction	Diuretics, calcium blockers
Hyperkinetic circulation	Physical activity, stress reduction	Beta blockers, alpha blockers, central alpha agonists
Renin activity: high normal levels	None	ACE inhibitors, beta blockers
Dyslipidemia	Low fat diet, physical activity	Alpha blockers, calcium blockers, ACE inhibitors
Coronary artery disease	Low fat and calorie diet, physical activity	Calcium blockers, beta blockers, ACE inhibitors, alpha blockers
Type II diabetes (non-insulin dependent diabetes mellitus)	Weight loss, diet control, physical activity	ACE inhibitors, calcium channel blockers, alpha blockers, central alpha agonists
Past myocardial infarction	Weight loss, diet control, measured physical activity	Beta blockers, peripheral alpha blockers

The decision to initiate drug treatment and the selection of an antihypertensive should be based upon risk factors, evidence of organ damage, and on potential drug-disease interactions. A diuretic and angiotensin-converting enzyme (ACE) inhibitor were selected for R.D.

Although diuretics have received considerable criticism because of their potential for disease interactions, they are effective in decreasing blood pressure and morbidity and mortality. Hydrochlorothiazide 25 mg/day was prescribed for R.D. because larger doses may increase the relative risk of side effects more than the incremental decrease in blood pressure. The thiazide diuretics are less effective when creatinine clearance is less than 25 mL/min; however, the creatinine clearance (56 mL/min) for R.D. is adequate. When evaluating the efficacy and toxicity of a diuretic as an antihypertensive, monitor the patient for reduced blood pressure, weight loss through diuresis, postural hypotension, and metabolic disturbances (e.g., hypokalemia, hyperuricemia, hyperglycemia, metabolic alkalosis, azotemia). The pulse also should be monitored to detect electrolyte-induced arrhythmias, especially since R.D. has an enlarged left ventricle which predisposes him to ventricular dysrhythmias. Although a slight decrease in serum potassium is expected, a potassium supplement is not generally needed and monitoring the serum concentration is adequate unless R.D. develops symptoms or receives a digitalis preparation.

The ACE inhibitor, enalapril, was added to the drug regimen for R.D. because the diuretic alone would not likely decrease the blood pressure from 155/108 mm Hg to the target diastolic pressure of less than 85 mm Hg. ACE inhibitors decrease blood pressure by decreasing the formation of the vasoconstrictor angiotensin II, decreasing the metabolism of the vasodilator bradykinin, and by blocking renin-controlled sodium and water retention. The choice of antihypertensive therapy must take into consideration co-existing medical problems. Table 11.5 outlines some approaches to antihypertensive drug therapy when there is co-existing disease.

R.D. was asked about symptoms such as dizziness, fatigue, altered taste sensations, headache, nausea, skin rash, and nonproductive cough because these have been associated with ACE inhibitors such as enalapril. Urinalyses and renal function tests should be monitored periodically because of R.D.'s history of proteinuria and azotemia. A CBC also should be monitored in the first three months of enalapril therapy because of a small potential for drug-induced neutropenia. If R.D. successfully responds to the non-drug therapeutic interventions, the drug therapy can be modified and perhaps even discontinued if the blood pressure remains within the targeted range. The hypertensive patient should take frequent blood pressure readings at home and record them in a diary for review with a health care provider.

Therapeutic Drug Monitoring Examples

HYPERTENSION (PRIMARY)

The approach to therapeutic drug monitoring by clinicians varies depending upon many factors. Some of these include preferences among clinicians in a given community or region; concurrent medical problems which dictate that certain drugs be used or avoided; the patient's response to selected medication. The following outlines of therapeutic drug monitoring offer examples which may serve to stimulate discussion and further understanding of initiating and monitoring drug use. The drugs and dosages presented should not be applied to any clinical situation without proper medical supervision.

Drug Therapy | Hydrochlorothiazide 25 mg tablet 1 PO QD. Enalapril 20 mg tablet 1 PO QD.

Monitoring | **Symptoms:** Hypertension is usually asymptomatic. End-organ damage to the eyes, heart, brain, and kidneys becomes evident as the disease progresses.

Signs: *Gen:* Measure the patient's body weight and determine the ideal body weight. *VS:* Check the pulse (rate/rhythm). Carefully measure the blood pressure in both arms (routinely check the arm with the higher reading) in the supine and upright (i.e., sitting or standing) positions. *Eyes:* Test the visual acuity separately in each eye by asking the patient to read. Examine the retina and vessels for damage (see Chapter 5: Eye). *Heart:* Listen for normal and abnormal sounds, especially note S_3 or S_4. *Ext:* Examine the legs and feet for pitting edema and blood circulation (e.g., pulses).

Laboratory Tests | The clinician may elect to order all, none, or some of these laboratory studies depending upon history and physical findings, as well as other specific clinical indications. Electrocardiogram (ECG), serum electrolytes, serum creatinine, serum uric acid, serum cholesterol and triglyceride, serum glucose, white blood cell (WBC) count.

Therapeutic Drug Monitoring Examples

HYPERTENSION (PRIMARY)
(continued)

Adverse Drug
Event Monitoring

Hydrochlorothiazide: Ask about muscle weakness, fatigue, or leg cramps (e.g., electrolyte loss: potassium/calcium). Ask if the patient has experienced dizziness upon standing. Ask about increased thirst, irregular heartbeats, joint or abdominal pain. Check the skin turgor for dehydration, blood pressure for hypotension, and pulse.

Enalapril: Does the patient report coughing, skin rash (e.g., maculopapular or urticarial); swelling of the feet, face, or hands; sore throat; dizziness; or loss of taste? Ask about symptoms of hyperkalemia: (i.e., irregular heartbeats, numbness, confusion, weakness or heaviness of legs). Measure the blood pressure and pulse. Inspect the skin and extremities.

Therapeutic Drug Monitoring Examples

PERIPHERAL VASCULAR DISEASE (PVD; ARTERIOSCLEROSIS OBLITERANS)

The approach to therapeutic drug monitoring by clinicians varies depending upon many factors. Some of these include preferences among clinicians in a given community or region; concurrent medical problems which dictate that certain drugs be used or avoided; the patient's response to selected medication. The following outlines of therapeutic drug monitoring offer examples which may serve to stimulate discussion and further understanding of initiating and monitoring drug use. The drugs and dosages presented should not be applied to any clinical situation without proper medical supervision.

Drug Therapy — Pentoxifylline 400 mg tablet 1 PO TID.

Monitoring — **Symptoms:** Ask about the distance the person can walk before having to stop because of leg cramping (e.g., intermittent claudication). Ask if the patient has experienced any other leg-related symptoms (e.g., numbness, heaviness, weakness, or coldness). Does the patient awaken at night with leg pain? Ask how the patient relieves the pain. (e.g., stops activity, takes medicine). How often do the attacks happen? Does the patient have swollen feet? Any poorly healing sores on the feet? Question about loss of feeling or tingling sensation in the feet (e.g., neuropathy). Determine if the patient is diabetic or has other arteriosclerotic diseases.

Signs: *VS:* Measure the patient's blood pressure. *Skin:* Inspect the feet for signs of infection, ulcers, scaling, and edema. Continue to look for other skin changes such as pale elevated areas, and dependent, dusky red patches. Also note whether the skin is thin, shiny, or atrophic. *Abd:* Palpate the abdominal aorta and auscultate for bruits over the renal and iliac arteries and the aorta. *Ext:* Palpate the femoral,

Therapeutic Drug Monitoring Examples

PERIPHERAL VASCULAR DISEASE
(PVD; ARTERIOSCLEROSIS OBLITERANS)
(continued)

Monitoring	popliteal, dorsalis pedis, and posterior tibial pulses. Place the patient in a supine position and elevate both of the patient's legs. Observe any changes in color (e.g., from pale to dusky red) and note arterial and venous fill time. Auscultate the femoral pulses for bruits. Palpate the carotid arteries and listen for bruits.
Laboratory Tests	The clinician may elect to order all, none, or some of these laboratory studies depending upon history and physical findings, as well as other specific clinical indications. Serum cholesterol and triglycerides, Doppler segmental limb blood pressures, complete blood count (CBC), electrocardiogram (ECG), chest x-ray, and treadmill walking.
Adverse Drug Event Monitoring	**Pentoxifylline:** Quiz about adverse gastrointestinal reactions such as nausea and dyspepsia. Check for troublesome cardiovascular problems including dizziness, headache, and flushing. If the patient is taking antihypertensive drugs, measure the blood pressure for hypotension.

Heart

P hysical examination of the cardiovascular system, as with all organ systems, requires a thorough working knowledge of both normal and abnormal anatomy and physiology. Experience with medically-managed patients in common disorders such as congestive heart failure (CHF), angina pectoris, and myocardial infarction (MI), is especially important in learning to assess a patient's response to cardiovascular drugs.

ANATOMY AND PHYSIOLOGY

Heart

The mediastinum is divided into anterior, middle, posterior, and superior regions, and contains the heart, aorta, trachea, esophagus, venae cavae, thymus, lymph nodes, vagus nerve, and other tissues (see Figure 11.1). The heart is located in the lower middle mediastinum, just behind the sternum and resting primarily on the anterior left diaphragm. The top of the heart (i.e., atria) is termed the **base**, and the tip (i.e., left ventricle) is the **apex**. The anterior surface of the chest closest to the heart (i.e., the chest wall surface overlying the heart) is called the **precordium** and extends from the third to the fifth intercostal space. Major structures found behind the heart in the posterior mediastinum include the aorta and the esophagus. The principal structures in the superior mediastinum are the trachea, esophagus, and superior vena cava. The phrenic nerves that innervate the diaphragm pass on each side of the heart, between the pericardial sac surrounding the heart and the parietal pleura of the lungs. The heart is innervated by both sympathetic and parasympathetic (i.e., vagus) nerves. It has its own blood supply, two coronary arteries, which arise from the ascending proximal aorta just distal to the aortic valves.

Cardiac Muscle

The **pericardium** or pericardial sac is a membranous structure that surrounds the heart and separates it from the rest of the thoracic viscera (see Figure 11.2). The pericardium consists of two layers: fibrous pericardium and serous pericardium. The **fibrous pericardium** suspends the heart from the great vessels and anchors it below to the diaphragm. The **serous pericardium** lines the pericardial sac and is composed

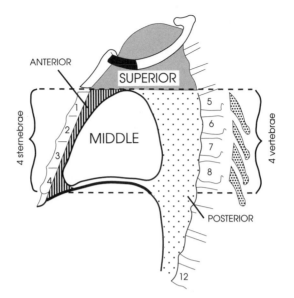

Fig. 11.1 Mediastinal compartments. The mediastinum of the chest (thorax) is divided into compartments, each containing central vital structures. For example, the heart is in the middle mediastinum; the thymus in the anterior mediastinum; the esophagus in the posterior mediastinum; and the trachea in the superior mediastinum.

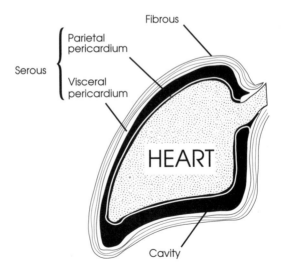

Fig. 11.2 The pericardial sac surrounds the heart and is composed of two layers. The portion of the serous layer that covers the heart is termed the visceral pericardium and the portion covering the thickened fibrous pericardial sac is termed the parietal pericardium.

of a visceral layer (i.e., visceral pericardium) that encases the heart and a parietal layer (i.e., parietal pericardium) that lines the inner surface of the pericardial sac. The space between the visceral and parietal layers is a thin, fluid-filled cavity known as the **pericardial cavity**. The heart is composed of three layers, a thick muscular layer, or myocardium, which is lined by an inner endocardium and an external epicardium. The **epicardium** or visceral pericardium is made up of the squamous mesothelial cells. The **endocardium** is the membrane lining the interior surface of the four chambers of the heart and is contiguous with the endothelial lining of the blood vessels.

Cardiac Chambers and Work

The heart has four chambers. The upper chambers are the right and left atria, and the lower chambers are the right and left ventricles (see Figure 11.3). The right side of the heart pumps venous blood through pulmonary circulation and the left side pumps oxygenated blood from the pulmonary circulation to all tissues and organs through the systemic circulation. The right atrium and right ventricle form the anterior surface of the heart nearest to the chest wall with the right ventricle touching the sternum. The left ventricle points left laterally and posteriorly and lies primarily behind the left, anterior rib cage (i.e., the left ventricle lies behind and to the left of the right ventricle).

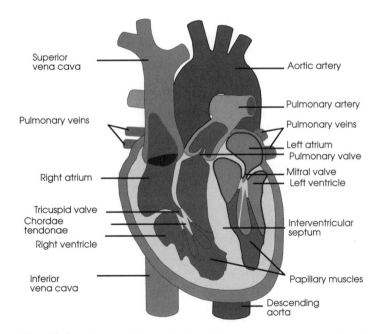

Fig. 11.3 The heart. The right side of the heart receives venous blood and pumps it to the lungs to be oxygenated. Oxygenated blood returns to the left side of the heart and is pumped to the systemic circulation through the aorta. Heart valves that do not open or close properly or holes in walls between the chambers (e.g., a defect in the interventricular septum) can result in abnormal function of the heart and heart failure.

The right and left ventricles discharge 80 to 90 mL of blood per heart beat [i.e., stroke volume (SV)]. The residual blood in each ventricle after contraction is about 50 mL at rest (i.e., the end-diastolic volume) and is affected by both venous return and ventricular emptying. At rest, the heart normally pumps 4 to 7 L/min [i.e., cardiac output (CO)]. To increase cardiac output, the stroke volume and/or heart rate must increase. When cardiac output (i.e., stroke volume x heart rate) must be increased to meet increased demand, the ventricles can pump up to 12 to 15 L/min/m^2 [i.e., cardiac index (CI)]. Cardiac preload and afterload directly affect the force of contraction and the cardiac output. The degree to which the myocardium is stretched before contraction is known as preload. The resistance against which blood is expelled is known as afterload. Factors affecting afterload and preload are noted in Table 11.1.

Cardiac Innervation

The right **vagus nerve** innervates the heart through its branches, known as the **cardiac nerves**. The cardiac nerves innervate both atria, but primarily influence the heart through actions on the sinoatrial (SA) node and atrioventricular node (AV). Normally, vagal stimulation decreases the rate of SA nodal discharge and slows impulse conduction through the AV node, resulting in a slower heart rate and reduced cardiac output. Sympathetic nerves from the sympathetic trunk innervate both the atria and ventricles and exert an opposite effect on the heart. This adrenergic stimulation increases SA nodal discharge, cardiac tissue excitability, and force of contraction, resulting in increased heart rate and increased cardiac output.

Table 11.1

Factors Affecting Afterload and Preload

Afterload

Definition:	forces against which blood must be ejected from the left ventricle
Factors:	1. Resistance of peripheral vessels 2. Degree to which wall of left ventricle distended (preload) 3. Elasticity of vessels (e.g., declines with increasing age) 4. Presence of obstruction to outflow from left ventricle (e.g., aortic valve stenosis)

Preload

Definition:	volume of blood in left ventricle during diastole; degree to which myocardium is stretched before contraction
Factors:	1. Blood volume total 2. Sympathetic tone of venous system 3. Effectiveness of atrial contraction 4. Position of body (e.g., erect, supine, sitting) 5. Pressure within chest (e.g., breathing, emphysema, pneumothorax, pericardial effusion) 6. Return of blood to heart through pumping action of skeletal muscle

Respirations and physical interventions (e.g., carotid sinus massage, Valsalva maneuver) can affect cardiac function. For example, deep inspiration slows venous return to the right side of the heart chambers and prolongs cardiac filling time. The Valsalva maneuver (i.e., the voluntary increase of intrathoracic pressure caused by forced exhalation against a closed glottis) slows the heart rate and is useful when studying heart sounds. Carotid sinus massage, like the Valsalva maneuver, is another physical intervention that can slow the heart rate through vagal stimulation but carries added risk to certain patients.

Heart Valves

The coordinated movements of the heart and the tricuspid, pulmonic, mitral, and aortic valves, cause blood to flow unidirectionally through and away from the heart. Blood flows from the right atrium through the **tricuspid valves** into the right ventricle. It then leaves the right ventricle, passing through the **pulmonic valves** into the pulmonary artery and then through the pulmonary tree and alveoli to exchange gasses. The oxygenated blood is returned to the left atrium and flows past the **mitral valves** into the left ventricle. Blood then flows from the left ventricle past the **aortic valves** that separate the left ventricle from the ascending aorta, thereby preventing blood from flowing back into the left ventricle during diastole (i.e., ventricular filling).

Coronary Arteries

The coronary artery system supplies the heart itself with blood (see Figure 11.4). The coronary arteries come off the ascending aorta just distal to the aortic valves as separate right and left coronary arteries. The **left coronary artery** further divides into circumflex and anterior interventricular branches. The **circumflex coronary artery** supplies the left posterior atrial and ventricular myocardium with oxygenated blood. The **anterior interventricular** branch supplies blood to both ventricles and the septum. The **right coronary artery** passes along the coronary groove between the right atrium and ventricle, and sends blood to these chambers. The right coronary artery also brings oxygen to the AV node and, sometimes, the SA node.

Blood flow through the coronary arteries increases during diastole, facilitated by relaxation of the myocardium and reduced obstruction to blood flow through the coronary vessels. During systole, blood flow to the myocardium is at its lowest because the ventricles contract and limit flow through the coronary arteries.

Cardiac Cycle

During diastole the ventricles relax and blood flows into them from the atria through the opened atrioventricular (i.e., tricuspid and mitral) valves. In late diastole, the ventricles fill more rapidly when the atria contract (i.e., "atrial kick") to expel their

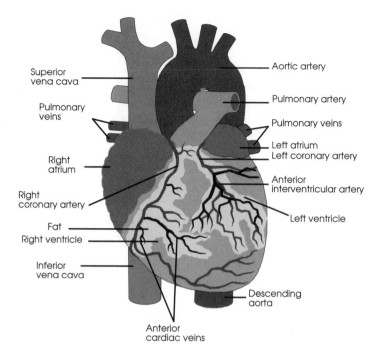

Fig. 11.4 Blood flow to the heart. Not seen is the first branch or the left coronary artery, the circumflex, as it circles the heart between the left atrium and left ventricle.

residual blood volume. This extra blood volume stretches the ventricles for maximal contraction (i.e., end-diastolic pressure). When the ventricles are relaxed during diastole, the pressure in the ventricles is less than that within the atria. When the ventricles fill with blood and start to contract, pressure in the ventricles exceeds that in the atria and the tricuspid and mitral valve leaflets quickly close to prevent regurgitation (i.e., backflow) of blood into the atria. The leaflets of these valves are prevented from being forced up into the atria during systole by tendinous chords attached to the wall of the ventricles known as the chordae tendineae.

During systole, blood leaves the ventricles through the semilunar (i.e., pulmonic and aortic) valves which have pocket-like leaflets that prevent the backflow of blood from the pulmonary and aortic arteries into the ventricles during diastole (ventricular filling). After systole, the ventricles relax and the pressure in the ventricles again falls below the pressure in the pulmonary artery and aorta and, thereby, allows the pulmonic and aortic valves to float shut preventing backflow. The leaflets of the pulmonic and aortic valves are not restricted by chordae tendineae and move solely in response to backflow pressure gradients between the ventricles and arteries.

In summary, the cardiac cycle begins with the right and left ventricles passively filling with blood that passes through the mitral and tricuspid valves separating the atria from the ventricles. The atria then contract to increase ventricular end-diastolic pressure and initiate systole. At the beginning of systole, the tricuspid and mitral valves between the atria and ventricles close. The blood is then expelled through the opened pulmonic and aortic valves of the ventricles into the pulmonary artery and the aorta. As the pressure in these vessels exceeds ventricular pressure, the aortic and pulmonic valves close and the mitral and tricuspid valves open to begin another cycle.

PHYSICAL ASSESSMENT

The heart is examined with the patient unclothed to the waist, and seated or in a supine position. The room should be adequately illuminated, warm, and quiet. If the patient cannot sit in an upright position, elevate the upper body to a 30° angle, especially during neck vessel examination (see Chapter 10: Blood Vessels). The right-handed examiner should stand at the patient's right side.

The sounds of the opening and closing of the heart valves can best be heard at specific locations on the chest (see Figure 11.5). These are not the true anatomical sites of the valves, but points where the valves maximally project the sound of their hemodynamic action. The second right intercostal space (ICS) next to the sternum is the preferred location for listening to the actions of the aortic valve; the second left intercostal space next to the sternum is best for listening to the pulmonic valve. Moving

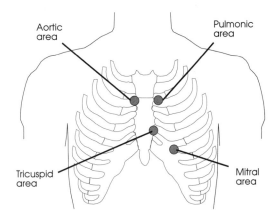

Fig. 11.5 Location of sites for ausculating the heart

down along the left sternal border, the tricuspid valve is best heard in the fourth ICS; and the mitral valve at about the fifth ICS just medial to the midclavicular line (MCL) at the point of maximal cardiac impulse (i.e., apical impulse).

Inspection and Palpation

Inspect the surface of the anterior chest for skin color, pulsations, and heaves. **Cyanosis** or **pallor** may reflect insufficient cardiac output. In the thin patient with a small chest wall, normal **pulsations** often are visible in any of the valvular areas, especially at the cardiac apex. In a patient with an enlarged (i.e., hypertrophic) left ventricle, the pulsations can be seen as far lateral as the left anterior axillary line. In the patient with an enlarged right ventricle, the point of maximal cardiac impulse (i.e., PMI) may be seen near the xiphoid process. These pulsations sometimes can best be seen by looking horizontally across the chest surface illuminated by tangential lighting.

Palpate the apical pulse (i.e., PMI) with your palms and fingertips. Be alert for any vibrations such as **heaves** or lifts (i.e., an uplifting of the chest wall during vigorous ventricular contractions). Test your ability to detect vibrations by alternately placing a vibrating tuning fork on your fingertips and palmar-carpal surface. Palpate and identify each valve area. In the fourth ICS medially to the left MCL, check for the apical impulse by finding the point of maximum impulse (PMI). The PMI is the point where the apex of the heart (i.e., left ventricle) comes into contact with the chest wall (see Figure 11.6). Palpation of the PMI can provide a rough approximation of heart size and an accurate determination of the heart rate. Note the PMI's location, surface area involved (i.e., diameter), duration (i.e., lift), and timing in the cardiac cycle. Normally, the PMI is 2 cm in diameter and heralds the onset of systole. Systole coincides with the first heart sound (S_1) and is gentle and brief. The amplitude and duration of the PMI increases in patients with anemia, hyperthyroidism, fever, anxiety, or a thin chest wall. When the PMI is shifted laterally to the left, left ventricular enlargement should be suspected; however, any disease that shifts the mediastinum to the left (e.g., massive pleural effusion in the right chest) could move the PMI laterally to the left of the midclavicular line. In chronic obstructive lung disease, the PMI is displaced inferiorly as the diaphragm flattens and lungs are hyperinflated.

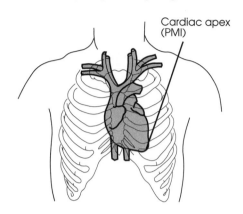

Cardiac apex (PMI)

Fig. 11.6 Surface topography of the heart.

Sometimes a murmur, or thrill, may be palpable on the chest surface. A murmur is felt as a fine vibration that usually is detected in the right or left second ICS when blood flows through a narrowed opening (e.g., aortic or pulmonic stenosis, or atrial septal defect).

When present, a pericardial friction rub may be palpable on the chest as a grating, sandpaper-like sensation. This condition is caused by the rubbing of "roughened" visceral and parietal pericardial surfaces that have become inflamed or fibrinous. To differentiate a pericardial rub from a pulmonary rub, ask the patient to hold his breath. The vibrations of a pulmonary rub will disappear, while those of a pericardial rub will continue.

Percussion

Since the fluid-filled heart is more dense than air-filled lung tissue, percussion can be used to outline the left cardiac border (LCB), which correlates closely with the PMI.

The apical impulse (i.e., the PMI) may be difficult to detect merely by inspection and palpation of the chest wall, especially in muscular or overweight patients. Percussion is another method used to approximate cardiac size and PMI location.

With the patient in a supine position, lightly percuss the chest and listen for the change of sounds over the lung (i.e., a resonant sound) and the heart (i.e., a dull sound). Outline the heart with the pleximeter finger parallel to the ribs in the third left ICS. Percuss medially at 1 cm intervals until the percussive sounds become dull over the area of the heart; repeat this procedure in the fourth and fifth left ICS. The left cardiac border should be at, or medial to, the MCL in the 4th to 5th intercostal space. When the left ventricle is enlarged or displaced, the LCB shifts laterally to the left. The left cardiac border cannot be accurately located by percussion in patients with emphysema or pericardial effusion. Emphysema causes a hyper-resonant chest (understates the cardiac border) and pericardial effusion overstates the true cardiac border.

Auscultation

Accurate auscultation of the various heart sounds demands practice and concentration. "Active listening" is crucial to appropriate understanding of the language of the heart. Close your eyes to decrease distractions and listen to each heart sound with undivided attention.

Heart sounds are described by their pitch, loudness, and duration. **Pitch** is a measure of frequency of vibrations [i.e., cycles per second (cps)]. The more cycles per second, the higher the pitch of the sound. **Loudness** or intensity reflects the energy or force expended to create the heart sound. Loudness is also determined by the distance the sound travels and the material (e.g., fat, muscle, air, or water) through which it passes. **Duration** is the length of time the heart sound can be heard. Short sounds are described as snaps and clicks, while murmurs are heard as longer sounds.

Practice listening to the differences in auscultatory sounds by using a stethoscope and various tuning forks (e.g., 128 cps, 512 cps, and 1034 cps). Place the diaphragm of the stethoscope on the cover of a book, then strike a tuning fork and place it on the opposite side of the book's cover. Listen for the pitch, loudness, and duration of the tone. Each of the sound qualities can be varied by changing tuning forks, adjusting the thickness of material between the stethoscope and tuning fork, or altering the distance between the stethoscope and tuning fork. Now, try this experiment using the bell chest piece of the stethoscope to gain an understanding of the differences in sounds heard through the bell versus the diaphragm. Unlike the tuning fork, heart sounds are not of a single frequency, but are composed of mixed frequencies.

Be systematic in your analysis of heart sounds. Focus your attention and actively listen to each cardiac sound individually. Do not allow dramatic sounds (e.g., a murmur) to distract your attention from other important heart sounds. In your mind, visualize each phase of the cardiac cycle, listen to each phase separately, then move on to the next phase. If the heart is beating too rapidly to distinguish each phase (i.e., greater than 100 beats per minute), decrease the heart rate momentarily using one of the following techniques. Cautiously massage a single carotid sinus, or ask the patient to perform the Valsalva maneuver by increasing intrathoracic pressure against a closed glottis while pushing down on the diaphragm. Because of the potential for cardiac arrest, do not massage the carotid sinus if a carotid bruit is heard or an electrocardiogram (ECG) machine is not recording the patient's cardiac activity. Likewise, the Valsalva maneuver is contra-indicated in patients with a recent myocardial infarction (MI), recent cerebrovascular accident (CVA), or uncontrolled hypertension. When the heart rate must be slowed during the auscultatory examination, the safest approach is to have the patient with a history of cardiac disorders to merely take a deep breath. This, by itself, sometimes slows the heart rate. Listen carefully to the first heart sound, the second heart sound, the events in the systolic interval, and, finally, to extra heart sounds during diastole.

When auscultating heart sounds, learn to mentally block out extraneous background noises from the surrounding environment. Listen to only one part of the cardiac cycle at a time. For example, to hear the systolic interval (i.e., systole) listen to the interval that begins just after the first heart sound and ends just before the second heart sound. Heart sounds can be better heard by listening at specific locations on the surface of the chest, by manipulating respiration efforts, and by placing the patient in a different position.

During auscultation, the experienced clinician must always be alert for the detection of specific sounds. A useful story illustrating cardiac auscultation involves the visit of a country cousin to the city. One day while walking on a noisy sidewalk in the city, the country cousin asks his city cousin, "Do you hear that cricket?" The city cousin responds, "What are you talking about? You hear a cricket with all the cars passing?" "Yes," replies the country cousin. Searching the nearby grass, the country cousin finds and picks up a small cricket. With experience, you too will learn how to selectively listen for various heart sounds.

To auscultate heart sounds effectively, practice listening to both normal and abnormal hearts with a stethoscope that has a bell piece and a diaphragm. The flat diaphragm picks up high-pitched sounds and some murmurs better than the bell piece. The bell piece, when held lightly against the chest wall, detects low-pitched sounds and some murmurs better than the diaphragm. Press the diaphragm of the stethoscope to the chest wall with a firmness sufficient to leave an indentation of its outline when removed. When using the bell piece, apply very light pressure on the chest wall surface (i.e., pressure that merely blanches the skin). When the bell piece is placed too firmly against the chest, it transmits sounds in a manner similar to that of the diaphragm (i.e., filtering out low-pitched sounds).

A good bell should have a soft rubber rim to make a good seal with the chest and should not be more than 1 inch in diameter. The ear plugs should fit comfortably into your ear canals. The tubing may be single or double, should have a thick wall, and be about 15 inches long. If the tubing is too long, the sounds may be too faint.

Standing at the patient's right side, begin with the patient sitting up or at least inclining about 30°. Some abnormal and normal heart sounds are best heard with the patient sitting upright or sitting in a leaning forward position. Other sounds are better heard with the patient supine. The discussion on positioning the patient will be presented later in this chapter.

Before auscultating the chest for heart sounds, inform the patient that the process will take some time. This can avoid creating undue anxiety in a patient who might be worried that something is abnormal because of the length of the examination.

Rate and Rhythm

Using the diaphragm of the stethoscope, listen at the apex of the heart (i.e., at PMI) for the rate and rhythm of the heart. First, listen to determine if the beat is regular or irregular (see Figure 11.7). If the rhythm is regular, count the beats for 15 seconds and multiply by 4 to obtain the ventricular rate per minute. A heart rate greater than 100 beats per minute indicates tachycardia, and a rate less than 60 beats per minute indicates bradycardia. When the ventricular rate is bradycardic, determine the heart rate over a period of a minute or more. If the heart beat is irregular, listen to the apical

Table 11.2

Classifying Heart Rhythms and Rates

	Rhythm					
	Regular			**Irregular**		
<60	60–100	>100		<60	60–100	>100
[g]Sinus Brady	[b]Sinus Rhythm	[b]Sinus Tach		AV Block	[d]Sinus Arr.	[e]A Fib
[a]3° AV Block	[b]A Flutter w/3:1	[c]PAT		[f]PAC/PVC	V Tach	
A Fib w/ dig toxicity		[c]PVT				
A Fib w/ AV Block		[b]A Flutter				

[a]Exercise does not increase rate.
[b]Holding breath slows rate.
[c]Rate does not slow when holding breath.
[d]Rate decreases with inspiration and decreases with expiration.
[e]Rhythm remains irregular with exercise to rate >120 bpm.
[f]Each beat not evenly spaced with a silent pause following the early beat. Exercising to increase the rate to >120 bpm changes to regular rhythm.
[g]Exercise increases rate.

Sinus Brady = sinus bradycardia; 3° AV Block = third degree AV block; A Fib w/ dig toxicity = atrial fibrillation with digoxin toxicity; A Flutter w/ 3:1 = atrial flutter with 3 to 1 block; Sinus Tach = sinus tachycardia; PAT = paroxysmal atrial tachycardia; PSVT = paroxysmal ventricular tachycardia; AV Block = atrioventricular nodal block; Sinus Arr = sinus arrhythmia; PAC/PVC = premature atrial contraction or premature ventricular contraction; A Fib = atrial fibrillation; V Tach = ventricular tachycardia pulse rate for several minutes to determine the pattern. At slow heart rates, irregular patterns are more difficult to identify. If the rhythm is irregular, try to determine whether the beat is regularly irregular (i.e., the irregular pattern repeats) or irregularly irregular (i.e., the irregular pattern is random both in stroke volume and frequency of beat). Simultaneous auscultation of the heart and palpation of the pulse will help differentiate these patterns. By determining the rhythm and rate, normal and abnormal cardiac rhythm patterns can be discerned.

First and Second Heart Sounds (S_1 and S_2)

The opening and closing of the mitral and tricuspid valves, the movement of the ventricular walls, and the movement of the aortic and pulmonic leaflets transmit vibrations to the chest wall that are heard as heart sounds. The first two heart sounds are heard as the syllables "lub-dub." The "lub" sound is the first heart sound (S_1) and represents the closure of the mitral and tricuspid valves, as well as the movement of

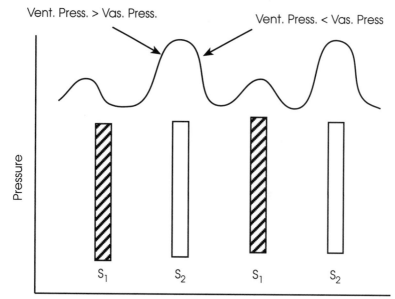

S_1 = closure of tricuspid and mitral valves; the beginning of systole

S_2 = closure of pulmonic and aortic valves; the beginning of diastole

Vent. press. = ventricular pressure

Vas. press. = vascular pressure

Fig. 11.7   The relationship between heart sounds and changes in ventricular and vascular pressure.

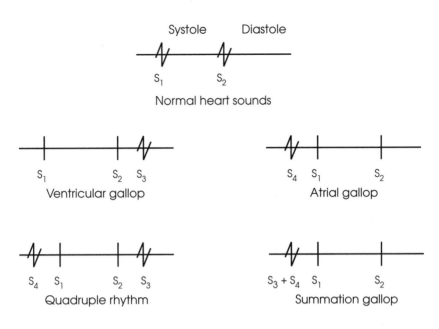

Fig. 11.8 Normal Heart sounds and presystolic sounds.

the left ventricle (see Table 11.3 and Figure 11.7). The sounds heard on the surface of the chest, however, also can be made by vibrations of the right ventricular wall and by the flow of blood. Nevertheless, movement of the left ventricle and closure of the mitral valve are the primary contributors to the first heart sound. Movement of the tricuspid valve and right ventricle contribute to a lesser degree to S_1.

Use the diaphragm of the stethoscope to listen for S_1. Although this sound generally is heard over the entire chest, it is loudest at the cardiac apex in the left 5th intercostal space just to the right of the midclavicular line (i.e., in the mitral area). S_1 is less intense than the second heart sound (S_2) at the base of the heart. In the 5th ICS to the right of the MCL, most of the sounds are made by the left ventricle and mitral valve (M_1). Next to the sternum in the fifth ICS (i.e., the tricuspid area), the right ventricle and tricuspid valve (T_1) components of the first heart sounds are believed to be heard best.

To identify the first heart sounds, listen at the mitral area for the softer, lower-pitched sound ("lub") that has a frequency of about 110 to 120 cps. Simultaneous palpation of the carotid pulse or apical impulse can help to determine the onset of S_1. If the heart rate is too rapid, ask the patient to take a deep breath and hold it because vagal stimulation by this process should somewhat decrease the heart rate. After an initial pause, S_1 is followed by S_2.

Following the first heart sound (i.e., the sound of the closure of the mitral and tricuspid valves), and early in systole, the ventricular pressure increases until it exceeds aortic and pulmonary artery pressures and forces open the aortic and pulmonic valves without creating any audible sounds. When the pressure in the aorta and pulmonary arteries exceeds left and right ventricular pressure, the aortic and pulmonic valves close, creating the second heart sound (S_2). Clinically, S_2 is believed to represent closure of the aortic (A_2) and pulmonic (P_2) valves. Some clinicians believe S_2 is also caused by vibrations in the great vessels, rapid outflow, acceleration, and deceleration. Normally, the intervals between S_1 and S_2 and between S_2 and S_1 are clinically silent.

S_2 can best be heard in the aortic area of the chest surface in the second right ICS, 2 cm from the midsternal line (MSL). At the aortic area, S_2 ("dub") is louder than S_1. S_1 and S_2 must be correctly identified, otherwise events in the cardiac cycle cannot be identified and described properly. Focus and concentrate on each heart sound separately, then focus on the systolic period and lastly the diastolic period.

Move the stethoscope to the pulmonic area on the surface of the chest, 2 cm from the MSL in the second left ICS. In this area, normal physiologic separation (splitting) of the S_2 sound into its two parts (i.e., A_2 = aortic valve and P_2 = pulmonic valve) can be heard. Normal splitting of S_2 occurs during inspiration and sounds as though S_2 pulls apart with each inspiration and comes back together on expiration. Listen for the pitch, loudness, and duration of S_2 sounds.

Inch the stethoscope down the chest wall surface to the mitral and tricuspid areas. Now, identify S_1, systole, S_2, and diastole. Splitting of the first heart sound may be heard with deep concentration in the tricuspid area on inspiration; but S_1 splitting is

Heart Sounds

Table 11.3

Sound	Location Best Heard	Listen With	Occurs During	Patient Position	Effect of Breathing	Comment
First (S_1)	Apex, especially mitral area	Diaphragm	Beginning of systole	Sitting, lying	No significant effect	Normal sound caused by closure of tricuspid (T_1) and mitral valves
Second (S_2)	Base, especially aortic area	Diaphragm	End of systole	Sitting, lying	Inspiration accentuates normal splitting	Normal sound caused by closure of pulmonic (P_2) and aortic (A_2) valves
Third (S_3)	Apex, especially mitral area	Bell	Early diastole	Left lateral lying	Inspiration may accentuate if pathologic	Normal sound in young patients, caused by rapid ventricular filling, not usually heard in adults. If other cardiac signs and symptoms are present, an S_3 would be abnormal
Fourth (S_4)	Apex, especially mitral area	Bell	Late diastole	Left lateral lying	Inspiration may accentuate	Normal sound caused by forceful atrial contraction into the ventricle; not usually heard. If other cardiac signs and symptoms are present, an S_4 would be abnormal

more difficult to hear than S_2 splitting. Many disease states change the loudness, pitch, or duration of the normal heart sounds (for more detailed information, consult a medical textbook).

Splitting of the Heart Sounds

Sometimes, variant sounds can be heard that may be normal. For example, delay in closure of one of the heart valves can separate or split a heart sound into two components. Normal splitting of heart sounds can result from mitral valve closure preceding tricuspid closure or when the aortic valve closes slightly ahead of the pulmonic valve. "Physiologic splitting" of heart sounds is normal and can be heard when the patient takes a deep breath; the splitting then disappears with deep expiration. The closure of the aortic (A_2) and pulmonic (P_2) valves creates the S_2 sound. Normal splitting of S_2 can best be heard in the pulmonic area of the chest surface. Normal splitting of S_2 occurs when ejection of blood from the right ventricle is delayed. Deep inspiration, with a resultant increase in return blood flow to the heart, further delays the ejection time. On expiration, the A_2 and P_2 sounds merge into one sound (see Figure 11.4). Normal S_2 splitting is best heard with the patient in a sitting or standing position since this lessens venous return to the heart. Normal splitting of S_2 is common in children.

Although the splitting of S_2 can be normal, mitral insufficiency and other cardiac abnormalities also can cause S_2 splitting (see Figure 11.9). The relationship of the split pattern to the respiratory cycle can help to differentiate abnormal from normal splitting of heart sounds. A **fixed split pattern** can be encountered when the A_2 and P_2 are heard on both inspiration and expiration; it is caused by a delay in the closure of the pulmonic valve or premature closure of the aortic valve. This fixed split pattern is heard with right bundle branch block, right ventricle failure, or mitral insufficiency. Paradoxical splitting occurs when the normal pattern reverses (e.g., with left bundle branch block).

Presystolic Sounds

In normal sinus rhythm, the ventricles receive blood during diastolic filling periods. The first phase of ventricular filling begins immediately after ventricular emptying, when blood rapidly empties out of the atria into the ventricles. This rapid ventricular filling causes vibrations in the heart wall that can be transmitted as audible third heart sounds. The third heart sounds (S_3) and fourth heart sounds (S_4) generally are inaudible in most adults and when heard could suggest an abnormality. For example, the S_3 sound (see Table 11.3) can be heard in a patient with a stiff, failing heart. S_3 is a low-pitched (i.e., 70 to 90 cps) sound heard best as a normal variant in healthy children and young adults at the beginning of expiration. It usually disappears with advanced age. Pathologic S_3 heard with myocardial failure or AV valve incompetence becomes much louder on inspiration and is sometimes best heard with the patient turning or turned to the left side. Left-sided third heart sounds (S_3) are heard more

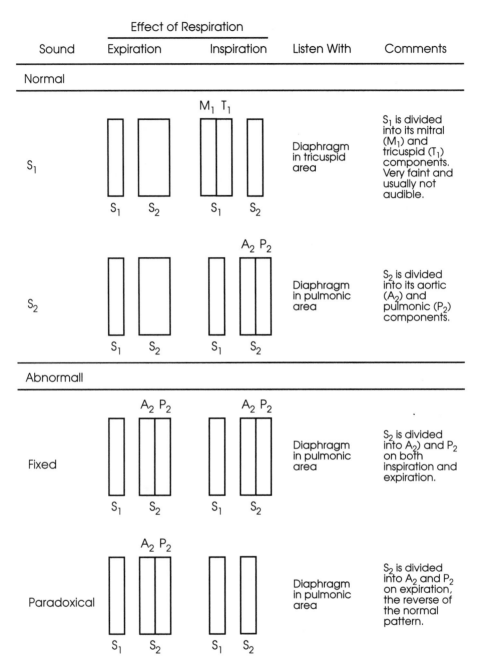

Fig. 11.9 Splitting heart sounds.

easily with the bell piece than with the diaphragm of the stethoscope and when the patient lies in the left lateral position. Right-sided third heart sounds (S_3) are best heard at the xiphoid process or the left lower sternal border.

Both S_3 and S_4 are low-pitched sounds that can be enhanced by some physical maneuvers. For example, the patient can exercise, increase intra-abdominal pressure, maintain a sustained handgrip, flex the knee to the chest, or elevate the legs to increase venous return to the heart. Deep inspiration by the patient also accentuates right-sided S_3 sounds and S_4 sounds and can assist in the differentiation of right-sided from left-sided presystolic sounds.

S_3 is best heard at the apex area of the chest wall surface when it comes from the left ventricle and S_4 in the tricuspid area if it originates in the right ventricle. The presence of S_3 is normal in children, young adults, and women during the third trimester of pregnancy. S_3 is abnormal after age 40, except in some women. A pathologic S_3 (i.e., ventricular gallop) can develop with myocardial failure.

Atrial systole (i.e., "the atrial kick") concludes the ventricular filling phase by squeezing the remaining 10% to 15% of blood from the atria into the ventricles. The ventricles are thus stretched and ready for subsequent maximal contraction. When audible, the sounds made during this late ventricular filling phase of atrial systole are the fourth heart sounds (S_4). The S_4 (i.e., atrial gallop) is more easily heard with the bell piece of the stethoscope that is applied with very light pressure to the chest wall surface and is usually heard as a very low-pitched (i.e., 50 to 70 cps) sound in late diastole (see Table 11.3). When originating from the left ventricle, S_4 is loudest at the cardiac apex in the left lateral position. Right-sided S_4 is heard best near the xiphoid process with the patient in a supine position. Although S_4 sometimes can be heard in a healthy elderly patient or after a period of physical exertion, audible fourth heart sounds are more commonly encountered in a patient with hypertension, pulmonary hypertension with cor pulmonale, pulmonic stenosis, acute myocardial infarction, coronary artery disease, during an angina attack, cardiomyopathy, or aortic stenosis.

At a rapid ventricular rate, S_3 or S_4 may sound like the cadence of a galloping horse, the so-called triple or **gallop rhythm** (see Figure 11.10). If S_1, S_2, S_3, and S_4 occur simultaneously, these sounds produce an abnormal **quadruple rhythm** (see Figure 11.8). At rapid heart rates, S_3 and S_4 merge into a loud single sound called a **summation gallop** (see Figure 11.8). Physical maneuvers (e.g., deep breathing) can slow the heart rate to separate the summation gallop into S_3 and S_4.

Murmurs

Murmurs are vibratory sounds caused by the turbulence of blood flowing past an incompetent, constricted, or irregularly shaped valve, a septal defect, a dilated vessel, or a partially obstructed vessel (i.e., stenosis). The presence of murmurs generally suggests a structural defect (e.g., valve or septum), or a functional defect (e.g., anemia or hyperthyroidism), although benign murmurs sometimes can be heard in children, adolescents, and pregnant women.

Systolic Murmurs

Table 11.4

	Location	Radiation	Loudness (Intensity)	Shape	Quality (Timbre)	Other Possible Findings
Holosystolic Murmurs						
Mitral Regurgitation	Mitral area; heard with the bell at the apex; if faint, listen immediately after exercise with patient in left lateral position or sitting up, leaning forward and to the left	Left axilla	Very loud; apical thrill present when very loud; sometimes, S_3 present; does not vary with respiration; grade 2–4	Holosystolic or diamond. If loud, may replace first heart sound	Pure to coarse, blowing character	S_1 diminished; S_2 louder; S_3 often heard; in late disease, ventricular gallop heard with other LVH findings
Tricuspid Regurgitation	Tricuspid areas; heard with the bell at the left lower sternal border	Right side of sternum or left MCL; does not radiate well to left axillary region	Variable; increases during early inspiration and fades during early expiration	Holosystolic or diamond.	Pure to coarse	May see systolic retraction of apical impulse
Midsystolic Murmurs						
Aortic Stenosis	Aortic areas; patient sitting up and leaning forward with held expiration	Widely into neck and along great vessels, apex (higher pitch than more proximal radiation)	Variable; if loud, thrill in aortic area and neck; loudest in early to midsystole; grade 2–4	Diamond	Coarse to pure	S_4; thrusting PMI of LVH; narrow pulse pressure; with increasing aortic stenosis, S_2 diminished; paradoxical splitting of S_2 (severe cases)
Pulmonic Stenosis	Pulmonic area; best heard in sitting position	Left shoulder; left neck	Variable; if loud, thrill in pulmonic area; very similar to aortic stenosis; grade 2–4	Diamond	Coarse	S_4; thrusting PMI of RVH; P_2 lengthens and blends with A_2
Mid to Late Systolic Murmurs						
Mitral Valve Prolapse	Mitral area (apex)	Negligible	Begins soft and increases (crescendo effect); moving from standing to squatting position increases loudness; Valsalva maneuver or moving from squatting to standing prolongs sound but softens it	Crescendo	Similar to mitral regurgitation; physical maneuvers may change murmur to "whoop" or "honk"	Early systolic click often heard. Moves closer to S_1 with Valsalva maneuver

Table 11.5

Diastolic Murmurs

	Location	Radiation	Loudness (Intensity)	Shape	Quality (Timbre)	Other Possible Findings
Mitral Stenosis	Apex; heard with bell in light skin contact at the PMI	Very little	Variable; louder in left lateral decubitus position or with exercise; grade 1–4	Decrescendo-crescendo	Rumble	Opening snap following P_2; palpable thrill at apex; increased S_1; loud split S_2 with accentuated P_2 componnt; with lift or RVH palpable in right parasternal area
Tricuspid Stenosis	Tricuspid areas; listen with bell in lower left sternal border in the xiphoid area	Very little	Similar to mitral stenosis; loudest during inspiration; grade 1–2	Decrescendo-crescendo	Rumble	Diastolic thrill palpable over right ventricle; S_2 may be split during inspiration
Aortic Regurgitation	Aortic areas; use diaphragm; have patient sit and lean forward; exhale completely	Sternal borders	Faint; grade 1–2	Decrescendo	Coarse to pure	Sometimes early ejection click; soft S_1; S_1 split with intense A2 component; ventricular gallop; PMI in left axilla with LVH; wide pulse pressure with water hammer pulse; Austin-Flint murmur (i.e., low-pitched rumbling at apex) is common
Pulmonic Regurgitation	Pulmonic area; use diaphragm; have patient sit and lean forward	Left sternal border	Faint; grade 1–2	Decrescendo	Coarse	With split S_2, murmur begins after P_2 component

Listen for murmurs on the precordium. If a murmur is heard, characterize the sound in terms of its **timing** in the cardiac cycle (i.e., systolic versus diastolic, both systole and diastole), **loudest location**, intensity of sound, **shape** (i.e., crescendo, decrescendo, or combination), **radiation** to other locations, **quality**, and other unique characteristics (see Tables 11.4 and 11.5).

First, determine the **timing** of the murmur in the cardiac cycle. If the murmur is heard between S_1 and S_2, it is described as a **systolic murmur** If the murmur begins after S_2 but ends before S_1, it is characterized as a **diastolic murmur**. If the murmur is heard throughout the cardiac cycle, it is a **continuous murmur**. Systolic and diastolic murmurs can be further delineated relative to the time of systole or diastole (i.e., early, middle, or late in the interval between the first and second heart sounds). The term holosystolic or pansystolic describes a murmur that occupies the entire systole (see Figure 11.11). Systolic murmurs may be pathologic or innocent; diastolic murmurs are almost always pathologic.

If the murmur is the result of a valvular defect, it should be loudest in the valvular area with the defect. Listen in each valvular area with the diaphragm and then the bell of the stethoscope. When the patient is lying down, a change in the patient's position can enhance or attenuate the audibility of some murmurs. The sound of a murmur can also radiate to a distant location (e.g., the murmur of mitral regurgitation radiates sound to the left axilla).

The **loudness** or **intensity** of a murmur is graded on a subjective scale of 1 to 6 based upon the ease of hearing the murmur (see Table 11.6). Systolic murmurs of grade 3 or more, or those that tend to occur late in systole are clinically significant.

Next, note the so-called **shape** or **configuration** of the murmur (i.e.,

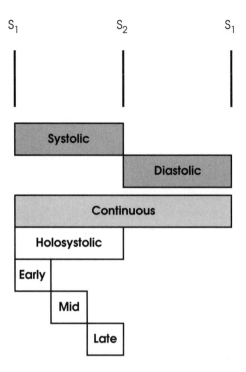

Fig. 11.10 Timing murmurs.

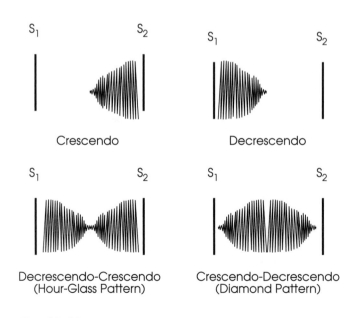

Fig. 11.11 Murmur wave patterns.

whether the murmur is uniform in intensity or pitch throughout the cardiac cycle). These shapes are described as decrescendo, crescendo, the combination of crescendo-decrescendo (i.e., **diamond pattern** because of the shape made when the murmur is graphically depicted on phonocardiography), or the combination of decrescendo-crescendo (i.e., **hourglass pattern**). A crescendo murmur begins quietly and increases in loudness; a decrescendo is loud initially and then fades (see Figure 11.11).

Quality describes the pitch of the murmur. Low pitched or rumbling murmurs have a frequency of 60 to 100 cps. Medium (i.e., rough, harsh, coarse) pitch murmurs are 100 to 250 cps. Pure or high pitch murmurs are 300 to 400 cps.

Depending upon the severity and type of the murmur, additional unique characteristics can be associated with specific murmurs. For example, with advanced aortic stenosis, the S_4 is displaced to the left of the PMI and S_2 is split more during expiration than inspiration (i.e., **paradoxical splitting**).

Murmurs heard during diastole usually are pathologic; however, **cervical venous hum** and **mammary souffle** are benign extracardiac murmurs also heard during diastole. A cervical venous hum is audible in most children, and also can be heard in young adults, pregnant women, and patients with anemia or thyrotoxicosis. Using the bell of the stethoscope with the patient in the sitting position, the cervical venous hum can be heard in the supraclavicular spaces over the right internal jugular vein next to the sternal end of the clavicle. Turning the patient's head to the left accentuates the hum, while applying gentle pressure on the internal jugular vein stops the hum. When the patient assumes a supine position or initiates the Valsalva maneuver, the cervical venous hum is diminished. The mammary souffle is heard in some pregnant or lactating women as a continuous murmur over the breast. Gentle pressure with the stethoscope stops the sound of the mammary souffle.

Rating Murmur Loudness

Table 11.6

Grade	Ease of Hearing
1	*Very faint:* heard only with intense listening
2	*Faint:* heard without difficulty
3	*Intermediate:* heard without difficulty; louder than grade 2
4	*Loud:* associated with a thrill
5	*Very loud:* heard *with* edge of stethoscope touching chest
6	*Very, very loud:* heard *without* stethoscope touching chest

PHARMACOTHERAPEUTIC CASE ILLUSTRATION

History

R.F., a 67-year-old male, complained of "weakness, cough, and difficulty breathing, especially if I walk." R.F. said he had visited his physician two weeks ago and had his blood pressure medication changed. The shortness of breath has been awakening him at night. He stated that he felt better when he sat up in bed. He had occasional nausea and loss of appetite.

Past medical history (PMH) revealed appendectomy at age 15, myocardial infarction at age 59, history of (H/O) peptic ulcer disease (PUD), angina pectoris, and hypertension. The family history (FH) disclosed that his father died of a stroke at age 71, his mother died of pneumonia at age 82, and two brothers are alive (one has diabetes mellitus). Two sons are in good health. He has smoked cigarettes 1 to 2 packs per day for 35 years. Furosemide 40 mg PO QD, propranolol 80 mg PO BID, and hydralazine 50 mg PO TID are his current medications. He has no known drug allergies. No significant findings except as outlined in present complaint are reported in the review of systems (ROS).

Physical Examination

R.F. appeared to be a 67-year-old (YO), well-developed and well-nourished (WDWN) male in moderate distress. His vital signs (VS) were as follows: blood pressure (BP) 180/128 mm Hg (supine); pulse 120 beats/min and regular; respiratory rate (RR) 20/min with Cheyne-Stokes pattern; temperature 97.8° F (oral). Examination of the heart revealed: apical impulse (PMI) at the 6th intercostal space at the anterior axillary line; S_3 gallop heard at apex, accentuated with inspiration; no murmur or rubs. Auscultation of the lungs revealed the following: bilateral diffuse, moist crackles with a wheeze in the left lung. Examination of the abdomen revealed the following: nontender, normal bowel sounds, hepatomegaly, jugular vein distention (JVD), and positive hepatojugular reflux (HJR). R.F.'s extremities were cyanotic, and he displayed pitting, pretibial edema to knees.

Laboratory

Chest x-ray presented in Figure 11.13 revealed hilar congestion and increased vascular markings with cardiomegaly (compare with normal chest x-ray in Figure 9.12 on page 9–22). Electrocardiogram (ECG) in Figure 11.14 showed sinus tachycardia with left ventricular hypertrophy. Serum chemistries were normal except for elevation of liver enzymes.

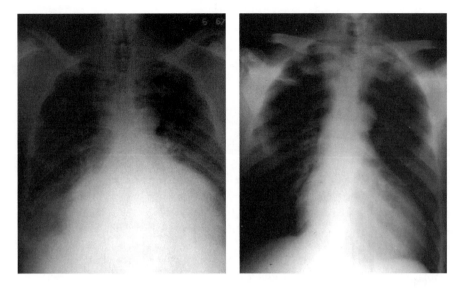

Fig. 11.12 A. Chest radiograph, taken at the time the patient was first seen, demonstrating marked cardiomegaly, pulmonary congestion, pleural effusion (e.g., pleural fluid in the costophrenic angles), and vascular engorgement. B. Chest radiograph of the same patient taken several days after therapy was initiated. Pulmonary congestion is gone, as is pleural effusion (i.e., no fluid in the costophrenic angles). Cardiomegaly remains, but is greatly reduced.

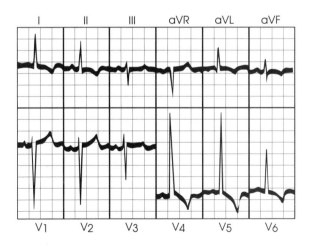

Fig. 11.13 Electrocardiogram (ECG) demonstrating normal sinus rhythm with evidence of left ventricular hypertrophy.

Diagnosis and Management

R.F. was diagnosed as having congestive heart failure (CHF) and was admitted to the hospital. His orders were bed rest, a salt restricted diet, and oxygen per nasal cannula at 2 L/min. His medications were digoxin 0.25 mg PO Q 6 hr times four doses then 0.25 mg PO QD, furosemide 40 mg PO TID, and potassium chloride 20 mEq PO BID.

Discussion

Disease. The syndrome of congestive heart failure arises when the heart cannot supply sufficient oxygen to meet the metabolic demands of the tissues. The causes of heart failure are many, and some are consistent with R.F.'s history of angina pectoris, myocardial infarction, and longstanding hypertension with left ventricular hypertrophy. Although one can speculate that the recent change in propranolol with its adverse effect on inotropic function (beta blocker) may have compromised his left ventricular function, it is not likely without some evidence of his dependence on a sympathetic drive to maintain his cardiac function.

R.F. complained of weakness, cough, dyspnea on exertion (DOE), nausea, loss of appetite, and paroxysmal nocturnal dyspnea (PND). Clinically, symptoms have been divided into those reflecting failure of the right or of the left ventricles or both. In right ventricle failure, the venous blood pools in the intestine causing gastrointestinal (GI) complaints (e.g., nausea, loss of appetite, and bloating) and in the lower extremities causing pedal edema. When only the left ventricle fails, fluid accumulates in the lungs creating exertional shortness of breath and a non-productive cough, which sometimes is the initial complaint especially in the elderly. When R.F. engaged in the activities of daily living (ADL), his heart could not supply enough oxygen-rich blood and he became short of breath (SOB). During sleep, fluid collected and redistributed to his lungs, causing him to awaken short of breath (i.e., paroxysmal nocturnal dyspnea). He also reported that he felt some relief in the semi-inclined position with his head elevated (i.e., orthopnea). Many patients with left ventricular failure report sleeping on pillows (e.g., 2 or 3 pillow orthopnea) with a fan blowing in their face or next to an open window to help them breathe.

In R.F., exam findings consistent with left ventricular failure include S_3 gallop, bilateral diffuse moist crackles, wheeze, and an enlarged left ventricle evidenced by the PMI located at the level of the 6th intercostal space at the anterior axillary line, well outside its normal limits (i.e., 5th intercostal space, medial to midclavicular line). Left ventricular hypertrophy is noted on the ECG. Hypertension leads to left ventricular hypertrophy which leads to congestive heart failure. Exam findings consistent with right ventricular failure include positive hepatojugular reflux (which, combined with elevated liver enzymes, suggests hepatic congestion), hepatomegaly, jugular vein distention, and pitting pretibial edema to the knees. The Cheyne-Stokes pattern of breathing and peripheral cyanosis signify hypoxia (e.g., peripheral and central) and may or may not be present with congestive heart failure depending upon the severity of the failure.

R.F. had several physical findings suggesting CHF. His heart was tachycardic (i.e., 120 beats/min) which was in response to sympathetic stimulation to supply more tissue oxygen.

Cheyne-Stokes respiratory pattern may be found in CHF and other diseases or drug-induced respiratory depression. R.F. was breathing in a cyclic pattern of deep breathing followed by a period of apnea. As the heart enlarges, the apical impulse shifts to the left chest wall.

In the failing heart, rapid left ventricular filling accentuates the third heart sound. If the heartbeats are rapid, the sounds simulate a galloping horse. With less effective heart pumping, fluid accumulates in the lung bases (e.g., crackles) and sometimes wheezing may be heard. Engorgement of the liver is felt extending below the right costal margin. The neck jugular veins are distended (JVD). Firm hepatic palpation squeezes excess blood up the jugular vein, confirming hepatojugular reflux (HJR). Extracellular fluid is palpated in the ankles, extending up the legs. Poor blood oxygenation makes the skin appear bluish-purple (cyanosis). R.F. demonstrated signs and symptoms of both right and left ventricle failure.

Management. The key to management of CHF is to reduce the workload on the heart, specifically to reduce the preload and afterload. This is accomplished by reducing intravascular volume with diuretics and restriction of fluids and salt. Further reduction of afterload with vasodilation is employed in some cases. Work of the heart is improved by increasing oxygenation, increasing inotropic forces, and decreasing preload and afterload. There are many different ways to manage CHF with various drug combinations. Decreasing intravascular volume and improving the cardiac output (i.e., work of the heart) would result in fluid moving from the alveoli of the lungs (e.g., crackles), the liver (e.g., hepatomegaly), the soft tissues (e.g., pitting edema), the intravascular space (e.g., jugular distention, hepatojugular reflux) as diuresis occurs. With reversal of failure, the S_3 gallop should disappear. The left ventricular hypertrophy will not change. Tissue oxygenation should improve with reversal of findings related to hypoxia.

Early treatment for a failing heart includes rest, along with restricted intake of fluids and salt. Sometimes, simply limiting activity can provide relief. The patient should rest in bed with the head of the bed elevated at 30°. Reassuring the patient often is calming and provides some relief. Diuresis can reduce excessive vascular volume, and water and salt must be consumed in moderation. Minor sodium restriction (e.g., avoiding salty foods and not adding salt during or after cooking) frequently is helpful. Daily fluid intake and output should be recorded.

If necessary, a diuretic is added to excrete excess fluid and control daily fluid buildup. The patient should be weighed daily at first and then periodically to judge response. Until symptoms improve, the patient should lose about 1 kg daily.

Furosemide was started in R.F. because a prompt diuresis was desirable to give quick symptomatic relief. Furosemide, a loop diuretic, diminishes vascular volume which reduces peripheral and pulmonary edema. It also reduces preload by vasodilation.

Table 11.7

Heart Failure Management Principles

Reduce Workload on Heart

Acute:
1. Bed rest
2. Oxygen by mask or nasal cannula
3. Control hypertension
4. Minimize emotional stress

Long Term:
1. Decrease activity
2. Weight loss to ideal body weight
3. Control hypertension
4. Minimize emotional stress

Control Water/Fluid Retention

Acute:
1. Restrict fluid intake
2. Restrict salt intake
3. Remove fluid by diuresis
4. Bed rest to improve renal function

Long Term:
1. Controlled restriction of dietary sodium
2. Keep fluid off by use of diuretics (In hypertensive patients, this may be accomplished with use of ACE inhibitors only.)

Drug Therapy

Acute: Highly variable depending on compounding factors (i.e., hypertension, cardiac arrhythmias, asthma, myocardial infarction, hepatic and/or renal failure, drug allergy or history of adverse response, etc.)

Long Term:
1. Diuretics for control of sodium and water retention
2. Cardiac inotropic agents (digitalis, sympathomimetic drugs, amrinone, milrinone
3. Decrease workload on heart (vasodialtors)

With effective treatment, signs of venous excess (e.g., HJR, NVD) regress. Breathing becomes less labored and skin color normalizes. R.F.'s heartbeat slowed and the gallop rhythm disappeared. However, diuretics may have serious side effects. For postural hypertension, check for dizziness, weakness, and dropping blood pressure (e.g., greater than 15 mm Hg systolic) upon sitting up or standing. To detect irregular beats, count the pulse. Serum electrolytes, muscle cramps, and weakness are found with electrolyte wasting.

Some might elect to use an angiotensin-converting enzyme (ACE) inhibitor in the situation where there is moderate hypertension and a need to block the renin angiotensin cascade which will be triggered with improvement and resultant decreased renal perfusion.

Digoxin improves heart contractility and slows the rate. Both these actions work to increase cardiac output. Because of the need to achieve prompt relief, R.F. was given a loading dose followed by a daily replacement dose. Following the loading of digoxin, an ECG would reflect the effects of digoxin. Digoxin may be associated with non-specific ECG changes (e.g., ST segment depression, shorten QT interval). Its antiarrhythmic action is to slow conduction through the AV node. These properties correlate poorly with the serum concentration. For CHF, a serum concentration of 0.5 to 2.0 ng/mL has been accepted as the therapeutic target; however, a normal serum level may be therapeutic or toxic in a patient, depending upon electrolyte balance (especially potassium and magnesium) and hypoxia. In R.F., serum levels can serve as a guide to a subtherapeutic response or possible toxicity, but clinical judgment is the most essential guide to rational drug therapy.

Digoxin toxicities are multiple and appear insidiously or dramatically. Digoxin can cause all types of arrhythmias because it irritates the atria and ventricles, and blocks the SA/AV nodes. Any time a patient taking digoxin complains of a disturbing symptom, the drug should be considered as a possible iatrogenic agent. A complete cardiac examination (especially noting bradycardia, arrhythmias), an ECG, serum electrolytes and serum digoxin concentration should be evaluated and the digoxin should be withheld pending test results. A serum concentration of digoxin that is within the usual therapeutic range does not exclude digoxin-induced toxicity. Digoxin can also affect the central nervous system (e.g., irritability, confusion, lethargy, headache, yellow-green or halo vision) and the gastrointestinal tract (e.g., anorexia, nausea, vomiting, diarrhea).

In summary, the clinical evaluation of R.F. involves improvement of the signs and symptoms caused by the congestive heart failure. The patient should be less dyspneic and less cyanotic. As cardiac pumping action improves, abnormal lungs sounds (e.g., crackles and wheezes) should resolve. On chest x-ray, the cardiac silhouette should decrease, as will hilar vascular markings (see Figure 11.13b). R.F. should be able to sleep in a lying position without pillows. Due to the action of the diuretic, hepatojugular reflux and neck vein distention should disappear. The pulse should slow and be checked regularly for changes in rate and rhythm that might reflect digoxin toxicity. Also, with serial cardiac auscultation, the third heart sound (S_3) may eventually be inaudible. Over time the ECG should show digoxin effects and resolution of ventricular hypertrophy.

Therapeutic Drug Monitoring Examples

CONGESTIVE HEART FAILURE (CHRONIC)

The approach to therapuetic drug monitoring by clinicians varies depending upon many factors. Some of these include preferences among clinicians in a given community or region; concurrent medical problems which dictate that certain drugs be used or avoided; the patient's response to selected medication. The following outlines of therapeutic drug monitoring offer examples which may serve to stimulate discussion and further understanding of initiating and monitoring drug use. The drugs and dosages presented should not be applied to any clinical situation without proper medical supervision.

Drug Therapy

Furosemide 40 mg tablet 1 PO TID. Digoxin 0.25 mg tablet 1 PO QD. Captopril 12.5 mg tablet 1 PO TID. Potassium chloride 10 mEq SR capsule 1 PO BID.

Monitoring

Symptoms: Ask the patient to describe his ability to perform the activities of daily living (ADL). How far can the patient walk before feeling short of breath (SOB)? How many flights of stairs can the patient climb before becoming SOB? Is the patient SOB lying down or does he need to sit to breath comfortably? Does the patient sleep on more than one pillow? Does the patient awaken SOB? Ask about the following right-sided failure symptoms: abdominal pain, anorexia, nausea/vomiting, constipation. Has the patient noted shoes or clothes being tighter? Ask about the following left-sided failure symptoms: non-productive cough, orthopnea, dyspnea, or feeling heartbeats?

Signs: *Gen:* Describe signs of distress, body stature, and weight changes. Is the patient sitting or lying down? *VS:* Count the pulse rate (i.e., tachycardia versus bradycardia) and rhythm (i.e., regular or irregular?). Measure the blood pressure, noting pulsus alternans (see Chapter 10: Blood Vessels). *MSE:* Measure the patient's level of consciousness and

Therapeutic Drug Monitoring Examples

CONGESTIVE HEART FAILURE (CHRONIC)
(continued)

Monitoring

orientation. Describe the patient's appearance and behavior (e.g., manner of speech, body movements, and posture). *Skin:* Observe the skin and nail bed for cyanosis. *Chest/Lungs:* Inspect for Cheyne-Stokes respiratory pattern (see Chapter 9: Chest and Lungs). Percuss for any areas of dullness (e.g., pleural effusion in right hemithorax). Check for vocal and tactile fremitus. Listen for normal breath sounds (e.g., Are they faint/distant?). Describe the presence of crackles in the bases or wheezing on deep respiration. *Heart:* Look for chest heaves and pulsations. Find and measure the primary apical impulse (PMI) area and distance from the left sternal border (LSB). Listen in each valvular area for S_1 and S_2. Using the bell in the left lateral position, listen for the S_3 and S_4 sounds of heart failure. If tachycardia is present, is a summary gallop heard? *Abd:* Survey for signs of ascites (e.g., tight, shiny skin with radiating umbilical varicosities). Auscultate for bowel sounds. Percuss for shifting dullness and fluid wave. Palpate for hepatomegaly and splenomegaly. Check for HJR. (see Chapter 12: Abdomen). *PVS:* Inspect the right external jugular vein for fullness (NVD) and pulsatile movements. Measure the jugular vein height above the sternal angle. Feel for weak carotid pulsations. Listen to the carotid arteries for bruits and radiating heart murmurs. *Ext:* Check for pitting edema in the feet. Grade the degree of pitting and distribution (e.g., to the

Therapeutic Drug Monitoring Examples

CONGESTIVE HEART FAILURE (CHRONIC)
(continued)

Monitoring	knee). In the supine position, check for sacral edema. Note the presence of the severe form of edema known as anasarca.
Laboratory Tests	The clinician may elect to order all, none, or some of these laboratory studies depending upon history and physical findings, as well as other significant clinical indications. Electrocardiogram (ECG), chest x-ray, serum digoxin, serum creatinine, urine protein, white blood cell (WBC) count, serum electrolytes.
Adverse Drug Event Monitoring	**Furosemide:** Question about dizziness when getting out of bed or a chair. Ask if the patient has any problems with muscle weakness, fatigue, or cramps (i.e., signs of electrolyte loss, especially potassium). Is the patient unusually thirsty? Measure the supine and sitting or standing blood pressure to check for postural hypotension. Weigh the patient often (e.g., water retention secondary to worsening congestive heart failure leads to weight gain).

Digoxin: Ask about loss of appetite, nausea or vomiting, irregular heartbeats, or visual disturbances (e.g., blurring or halos around lights). Count the apical pulse. Is the pulse slow or fast? Is the pulse regular? New onset of irregular pulse may suggest digoxin toxicity.

Captopril: Ask about dizziness, lightheadedness, or fainting. Is the patient complaining of coughing or loss of taste? Ask if the patient has experienced fever,

Therapeutic Drug Monitoring Examples

CONGESTIVE HEART FAILURE (CHRONIC)
(continued)

Adverse Drug
Event Monitoring

sore throat, joint pain, or skin rash. Measure the blood pressure both supine and sitting or standing to check for postural hypotension.

Potassium Chloride: Check for symptoms/signs of hyperkalemia: irregular heartbeat, unusual tiredness, weakness or heaviness of legs, or arms; tingling feeling (paresthesia). Test the ankle DTR for areflexia (Chapter 14: Neurological System). Ask about GI complaints such as epigastric pain.

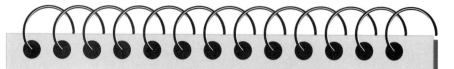

Therapeutic Drug Monitoring Examples

ANGINA PECTORIS

The approach to therapuetic drug monitoring by clinicians varies depending upon many factors. Some of these include preferences among clinicians in a given community or region; concurrent medical problems which dictate that certain drugs be used or avoided; the patient's response to selected medication. The following outlines of therapeutic drug monitoring offer examples which may serve to stimulate discussion and further understanding of initiating and monitoring drug use. The drugs and dosages presented should not be applied to any clinical situation without proper medical supervision.

Drug Therapy	Nitroglycerin (NTG) 0.4 mg tablet 1 SL Q 5 min PRN chest pain to 3 doses. Nifedipine 30 mg capsule 1 PO QID. Propranolol 20 mg tablet 1 PO TID. Nitroglycerin 10 mg transdermal patch apply one to chest Q a.m.; remove at HS.
Monitoring	**Symptoms:** Ask about attacks and the activity the patient was engaged in during the attack. Ask the patient to describe the pain, duration and its location, and whether it is felt as a radiating sensation. Is the pain relieved by rest and medicine? Does the pain occur at rest?
	Signs: *Gen:* Record body stature (e.g., overweight) and any finding of distress. *VS:* Measure the blood pressure for hypertension. *Skin:* Check the fingers for yellow tobacco stains. *Heart:* During an attack, listen for abnormal S_3 or S_4 sounds.
Laboratory Tests	The clinician may elect to order all, none, or some of these laboratory studies depending upon history and physical findings, as well as other specific clinical indications. ECG, exercise stress testing, ambulatory ECG, coronary arteriography.
Adverse Drug Event Monitoring	**Nitroglycerin (tablets and patches):** Question about unusual headaches, dizziness on standing, and skin irritation at

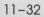

Therapeutic Drug Monitoring Examples

ANGINA PECTORIS
(continued)

Adverse Drug Event Monitoring

the patch site. Measure the blood pressure both sitting and standing.

Nifedipine: Question about feelings of lightheadedness when getting up suddenly from a supine or sitting position. Ask if the patient has had problems with headaches or swollen feet. Palpate the feet for edema. Measure the blood pressure.

Propranolol: Question about symptoms of depression, fatigue, sexual dysfunction, or numbness of the toes or fingers. Count the pulse for bradycardia or irregularity. Measure the blood pressure. Examine the legs and feet for cyanosis or edema.

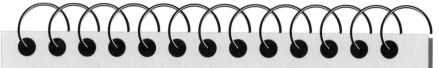

Therapeutic Drug Monitoring Examples

SUPRAVENTRICULAR TACHYCARDIA (RECURRENT)

The approach to therapeutic drug monitoring by clinicians varies depending upon many factors. Some of these include preferences among clinicians in a given community or region; concurrent medical problems which dictate that certain drugs be used or avoided; the patient's response to selected medication. The following outlines of therapeutic drug monitoring offer examples which may serve to stimulate discussion and further understanding of initiating and monitoring drug use. The drugs and dosages presented should not be applied to any clinical situation without proper medical supervision.

Drug Therapy	Verapamil 80 mg tablet 1 PO QID. Quinidine 200 mg tablet 1 PO TID.
Monitoring	**Symptoms:** Ask the patient about dizziness, lightheadedness, skipping or rapid heartbeats, episodic difficulty breathing, or fatigue.
	Signs: *Gen:* Check for signs of distress, and note the patient's weight. Note skin color. *MSE:* Evaluate the patient's orientation and level of consciousness. *VS:* Measure blood pressure, radial pulse rate and rhythm, and respiration. *Neck:* Palpate and listen to the carotid pulse for rate and rhythm, bruits, or murmur radiation. With the patient at a 30° incline, measure the jugular vein height above the sternal notch for jugular vein distention (JVD). *Chest/Lungs:* Listen to the lung bases for crackles. *Heart:* Auscultate the apical rate; note any difference between radial and apical pulse. Listen for normal and abnormal sounds (e.g., S_3, gallop, or murmur). *Ext:* Inspect and palpate the lower legs for pitting edema.
Laboratory Tests	The clinician may elect to order all, none, or some of these laboratory studies depending upon history and physical findings, as well as other significant

Therapeutic Drug Monitoring Examples

SUPRAVENTRICULAR TACHYCARDIA (RECURRENT)
(continued)

Laboratory Tests	clinical indications. ECG, serum quinidine concentration, serum electrolytes, complete blood count (CBC).
Adverse Drug Event Monitoring	**Verapamil:** Question about constipation, tiredness, nausea, headache, dizziness, feeling faint, or irregular heartbeats. Count the pulse for bradycardia or irregular rhythm.
	Quinidine: Ask about any problems with diarrhea, nausea/vomiting (N/V), unusual bruising (i.e., thrombocytopenia), headache, blurred vision. Ask if the patient has fainted or has nearly fainted. Check the pulse rate and rhythm.

Abdomen

*T*he abdominal cavity contains many organs that can be affected by various categories of drugs (e.g., antacids, antidiarrheals, anti-infectives, H_2-antagonists, diuretics, corticosteroids, cholinergics, laxatives, insulin, and oral hypoglycemic drugs). The physical assessment of organs within the abdominal cavity, therefore, should always be tempered by knowledge of the medications being taken by the patient.

ANATOMY AND PHYSIOLOGY

Abdominal Cavity

The abdominal cavity extends superiorly to the diaphragm, anteriorly and laterally to the abdominal wall, posteriorly to the spine and paraspinous muscles, and inferiorly to the pelvic brim. Located within this large body compartment are **hollow organs** (e.g., the stomach, small and large intestines, gallbladder, and urinary bladder) and **solid organs** (e.g., the liver, pancreas, spleen, kidneys, adrenal glands, ovaries, and uterus). (See Figure 12.1.) The wall of the abdominal cavity is lined by a membrane called the **parietal peritoneum**; the abdominal organs are covered by a continuation of the membrane called the **visceral peritoneum**. The membranous fold of parietal peritoneum that attaches or suspends an organ (e.g., small intestine) from the posterior wall of the abdominal cavity is called the **mesentery**. Mesenteries connect visceral and parietal peritoneum and carry blood vessels and nerves to and from the suspended organs. The **peritoneal space** refers to the area between the visceral and parietal peritoneum. The peritoneal space, like the pleural space and the pericardial space, contains a small amount of fluid to facilitate frictionless movement of one membranous covering over the other.

Stomach

The **stomach** is located within the epigastrium (i.e., the upper middle region of the abdomen) just under and below the xiphoid process and to the left and right of the medial aspects of the subcostal margins. The stomach consists of three anatomically and functionally distinct regions: the fundus, the body, and the antrum (see Figure 12.2). The **fundus** (or cardia) is the small region near the esophagus that contains mucus-secreting cells. The **body** constitutes 80% to 90% of the stomach and contains the parietal cells which secrete acid and intrinsic factor. The body of the stomach also

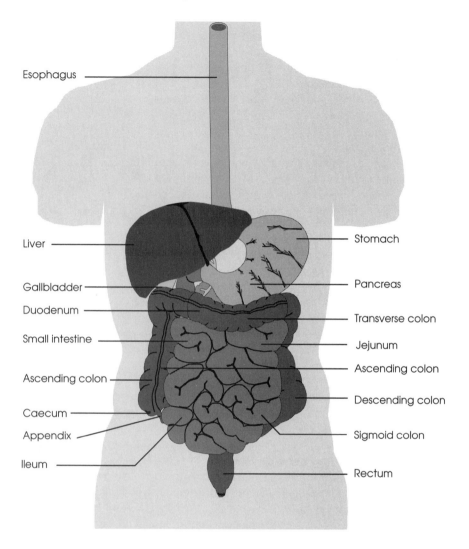

Fig. 12.1 The location of organs in the abdominal cavity.

contains chief cells which secrete pepsinogen. The **antrum** constitutes about 10% to 20% of the stomach and contains G cells that secrete the hormone, gastrin.

The stomach attaches to the lower esophageal sphincter at the diaphragm at about the level of thoracic vertebrae 10 and 11 and ends about one inch to the right of the first lumbar vertebra at the duodenum. The stomach mixes, stores, and partially digests food. While in the stomach, food is mixed with acid, mucus, and pepsin, and becomes a liquefied material known as **chyme**. When the smooth muscles of the stomach contract, the liquefied gastric contents squirt into the duodenum.

Small Intestine

The small intestine is divided histologically and physiologically into the **jejunum** and **ileum**. The small intestine, about 21 feet long and located in the mid-abdominal area, completes the digestive process that begins in the mouth and stomach (see Figure 12.3). Proteins, fats, and complex carbohydrates are broken down into absorbable units and digested primarily in the small intestine. These nutrients, along with vitamins, minerals, and water, cross

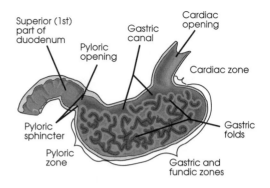

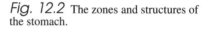

Fig. 12.2 The zones and structures of the stomach.

the mucosa and are absorbed from the small intestine into the lymph or blood. These functions of digestion and absorption depend upon digestive enzymes (e.g., aminopeptidase, lactase), hormones (e.g., gastrin), chemical mediators (e.g., acetylcholine), gastrointestinal mucosal cells, smooth muscle peristalsis, and intact neural mechanisms (e.g., vagal nerves increase intestinal motility and secretion; sympathetic nerves slow motility and secretion).

About 7 L of fluid enter the gastrointestinal (GI) system each day from secretions of the pancreas, bile, duodenum, and intestines, and about 2 L come from dietary ingestion. Most of the 9 L of fluid are reabsorbed into the circulation and only about 100 to 150 mL are excreted in the feces each day. An imbalance in these absorptive and secretory processes leads to water and electrolyte imbalance and gastrointestinal conditions such as diarrhea or constipation.

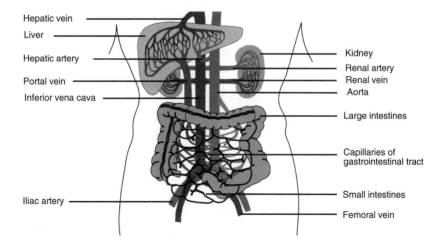

Fig 12.3 Circulatory system within the abdomen.

Large Intestines

The colon or large intestine continues from the ileum and is located 1 to 2 inches to the right of the fourth and fifth lumbar vertebrae. The colon begins as a small pouch called the **caecum** to which the appendix is attached and moves cephalad (i.e., upward toward the head) as the **ascending colon**. At the level of the right kidney, just beneath the liver (i.e.,

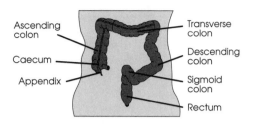

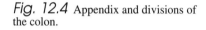

Fig. 12.4 Appendix and divisions of the colon.

hepatic flexure), the large intestine continues horizontally across the upper abdomen in front of the stomach as the **transverse colon**. At the spleen (i.e., splenic flexure), the large intestine turns toward the left pelvic brim as the **descending colon**. At the pelvic brim the colon is suspended by a mesentery and is called the **sigmoid colon**. At the level of the mid-sacrum, the colon loses its mesentery and becomes the rectum (see Figure 12.4). The colon functions as a storage and absorptive-secretory unit for the final stages of digestion. The upper two-thirds of the colon participate in the final stages of absorption and secretion; the lower one-third of the colon serves as the storage site for the feces. Normal bowel movements begin with the conscious sensing of filling and stretching of the rectum. External and internal anal sphincter muscles prevent incontinence and participate in the control of defecation.

Pancreas

The pancreas, an exocrine and endocrine gland, is located in the epigastric area on both sides of the midline. As an exocrine gland, the pancreas secretes digestive enzymes (e.g., amylase, trypsin, chymotrypsin, and lipase) into the jejunal part of the small intestine primarily to digest proteins and fats. The pancreas also secretes bicarbonate to neutralize the acidic chyme in the duodenum to a pH of approximately 6 to 7 which is optimal for activity of pancreatic digestive enzymes. As an endocrine gland, the pancreas participates in the synthesis, storage, and secretion of insulin and glucagon. Examples of pancreatic disorders include simple bicarbonate loss with diarrhea, diabetes mellitus, pancreatic cancer, and pancreatitis.

Gallbladder

The gallbladder is located beneath the liver in the right costal area. At periodic intervals, the gallbladder secretes bile salts into the common bile duct for delivery into the duodenum. The bile salts combine with lipids to form micelles (i.e., emulsified fat droplets) to facilitate fat absorption and digestion. The liver synthesizes about 1 L of bile salts each day for storage in the gallbladder. In response to a meal, the vagus nerve and the intestinal hormone, cholecystokinin, stimulate contraction of the gallbladder to release bile salts into the duodenum.

Liver

The liver is located below the right rib margin with the left lobe of the liver extending across the midline. In most adults, the liver consists of four lobes; however, various configurations are normally found in healthy persons. Blood flows through the liver at a rate of about 1.5 L/min at rest. The **portal veins** from the intestine and spleen drain their contents into the liver, while the **hepatic arteries** bring oxygenated blood to the liver from the lungs and heart. The **hepatic veins** drain blood from the liver into the inferior vena cava which, in turn, empties into the right atrium of the heart (see Figure 12.5).

The liver plays a significant role in the metabolism of carbohydrates, fats, and proteins. The carbohydrate, glucose, is stored in the liver as glycogen and released when needed by the body. Fats are oxidized and proteins are converted into glucose when needed by the body for energy. The liver also stores vitamins and iron, and synthesizes blood coagulation-lysis proteins and albumin. Nutrients and drugs that are orally ingested must pass through the liver before entering the systemic circulation, unlike nutrients and drugs that are parenterally administered.

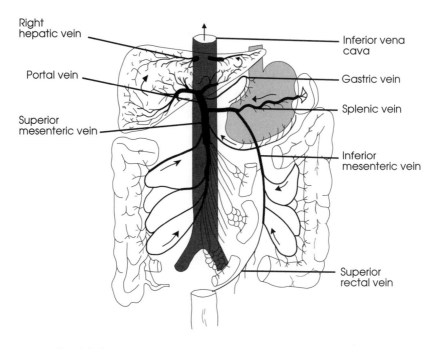

Fig. 12.5 Portal circulation.

The liver is the primary organ for detoxification of drugs and clearance of metabolic wastes such as nitrogen and senescent red blood cells (RBCs). Since the liver is the clearinghouse of drug metabolism, dosages of drugs may need to be adjusted in patients with liver dysfunction.

Kidneys, Ureters, and Bladder

The kidneys lie outside the abdominal cavity, behind a peritoneum and, therefore are said to be "retroperitoneal." Partially protected by the lower ribs, the kidneys are located on the back at the costovertebral angle (CVA), where the inferior margin of the 12th rib meets the vertebral column. Each kidney receives a blood supply from a renal artery (i.e., right or left; see Figure 12.3).

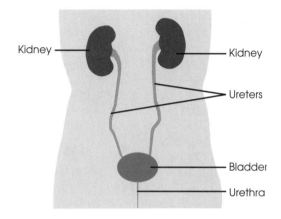

Fig. 12.6 Urinary tract consisting of kidneys, ureters, bladder, and urethra.

The kidneys play a vital role in the elimination of drugs and waste products, and in the maintenance of fluid and electrolyte balance. The kidneys filter about 100 mL/min of and selectively reabsorb certain nutrients, fluids, and electrolytes. The metabolic products that are not reabsorbed flow from the nephrons of the kidneys into the collecting ducts and concentrate as urine. Urine flows from the kidneys through the ureters for storage in the urinary bladder (see Figure 12.6). The adult bladder can generally hold about 400 to 500 mL of urine before initiating the "full bladder" signal. After voiding, a small residual volume (e.g., 50 to 100 mL) of urine may remain in the bladder.

Adrenal Glands

An adrenal (i.e., suprarenal) gland sits atop each kidney and receives blood from arteries that branch from the aorta (see Figure 12.7). The medulla of the adrenal gland secretes norepinephrine and epinephrine. The cortex of the adrenal gland secretes hydrocortisone and aldosterone into the blood stream.

Spleen

The spleen, located in the left upper quadrant of the abdomen, directly connects to the liver via the splanchnic vasculature (see Figure 12.8). The spleen stores several

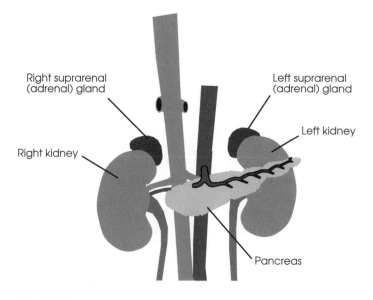

Right suprarenal (adrenal) gland

Left suprarenal (adrenal) gland

Left kidney

Right kidney

Pancreas

Fig. 12.7   Adrenal gland's relationship to kidney and pancreas.

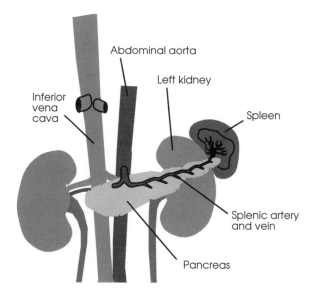

Abdominal aorta

Left kidney

Inferior vena cava

Spleen

Splenic artery and vein

Pancreas

Fig. 12.8   Spleen's relationship to pancreas, left kidney, and blood supply.

hundred milliliters of blood and functions as part of the reticuloendothelial system to filter blood and to make monocytes and lymphocytes. The spleen serves an important role in our immune defense, and splenectomized patients are highly susceptible to infection with microorganisms such as *Streptococcus pneumoniae*.

PHYSICAL ASSESSMENT

Conduct the examination of the abdomen in a well-lit, warm room, and be sure to provide the patient with adequate covering to prevent shivering and tensing of abdominal muscles. Place the patient in a relaxed, supine position on an examination table with his head resting on a pillow. Drape the patient with a sheet or blanket; cover the lower half of the body up to the symphysis pubis and expose the abdomen from the inferior costal margin to the pubis. In addition, cover the breasts of the female patient with a towel or pillow case.

If you are right-handed, start your examination of the patient's abdomen by standing on the patient's right side. Warm your hands by rubbing them together vigorously before touching the patient. Relax the patient's abdominal muscles by bending the patient's knees and placing the soles of the patient's feet flat on the bed. Place the patient's arms at her sides. If the abdominal muscles are still not supple, place a pillow under the knees to provide additional support and help relax the abdominal muscles.

Explain what you will do and enlist the patient's assistance as needed to keep the abdomen relaxed. Examine the abdomen slowly; avoid quick, unexpected movements and facial expressions. Remember the patient is studying your facial expressions and reading your body language. Identify locations of pain or tenderness by asking the patient to point to the area with one finger and note whether the location of the pain is generalized or localized to a specific spot. Because the patient with abdominal pain may have difficulty relaxing, areas of pain or tenderness should be examined last.

Abdominal Landmarks

The location of findings from the physical examination of the abdomen can best be described by dividing the abdomen into four quadrants with imaginary horizontal and vertical lines that intersect at a right angle through the umbilicus. The rib cage above and the inguinal ligaments below serve as the upper and lower boundaries to the four quadrants created by the intersecting imaginary horizontal and vertical lines. These quadrants help to pinpoint the location of organs within each quadrant (see Figure 12.9).

The upper right abdominal quadrant contains the right kidney, right adrenal gland, hepatic flexure of the colon, part of the pancreas, liver, gallbladder, distal stomach, and parts of the small intestine. The spleen, major parts of the stomach, the major part of the pancreas, splenic flexure of the colon, left kidney, left adrenal gland, and parts

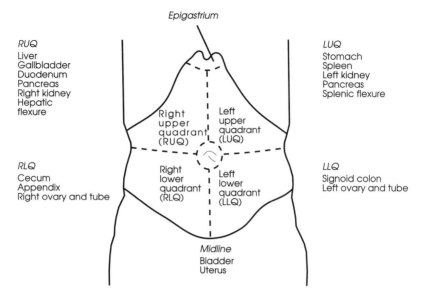

Fig. 12.9 Location of physical findings in the abdomen are described in terms of the four-quadrant scheme illustrated above.

of the small intestine are found in the upper left quadrant. Part of the small intestine and the sigmoid colon are placed in the lower left quadrant. Part of the small bowel, the cecum, and appendix are located in the lower right quadrant. The bladder, uterus (in a female patient), prostate (in a male patient), and the rectum are below (i.e., caudad) the pelvic inlet and pubic symphysis in the midline. The aorta is located just to the left of the vertebral column. The aorta bifurcates at about the level of the umbilicus to form the right and left iliac arteries that supply blood to the legs and the bladder and other pelvic organs.

Inspection

The examination of the abdomen generally begins with **inspection**, followed by **auscultation**, and then **percussion** and **palpation**. The inspection of the abdomen is conducted with the patient in the supine position and adequately draped by a sheet or a blanket. Expose the patient's abdomen and sit down on the patient's right side at about eye level with the patient's abdomen. Use oblique lighting to illuminate the patient's abdomen and gaze across the surface. Discipline yourself to carefully inspect the abdomen and avoid being overly eager to palpate and auscultate. Look at the patient's face for signs of distress such as fear or grimacing. Does the patient appear restless and agitated, or is the patient quietly resting? Is the abdomen relaxed or does it look tense? Does the patient have knees drawn to the chest?

Inspect the skin for color, scars, striae, rashes, dilated blood vessels, and lesions. A yellowish skin and sclera suggest abnormal accumulation of bile pigments. Jaundice can be detected in incandescent or natural lighting; however, florescent lighting will not reveal excessive bile pigment in the skin. Jaundice is also accompanied by such intense itching that telltale scratch marks often can be detected on the skin. If a scar is noted on the skin, record its location, configuration, and length. Striae or stretch marks on the abdominal skin surface often result from pregnancy, ascites, or rapid weight loss or gain. Striae look pink or blue if new and turn silvery if old. With Cushing's disease, striae are purplish. In addition, inspect the skin for ecchymoses, petechiae, and other evidence of bleeding. With acute abdominal bleeding, the skin often looks pale, cool, and moist.

Inspect the **umbilicus**, which normally is inverted and located half the distance between xiphoid and symphysis pubis in the midline. An everted umbilicus can be the result of a hernia, ascites, congenital defect, gross obesity, increased intra-abdominal pressure, or an intra-abdominal mass.

Next, look at the contour and symmetry of the abdomen, and also look for the presence of enlarged organs and masses. With your head at a level slightly higher than the patient's abdomen, gaze horizontally across the surface and look from the feet to the head. The horizontal abdominal contours are usually scaphoid, flat, or protuberant in appearance depending upon the body habitus. Is the abdomen symmetrical or do you see localized bulging? Generalized symmetrical distention can be suggestive of intestinal gas or fluid, or obesity. Distention of the abdomen below the level of the umbilicus can be the result of pregnancy, abnormal ovarian or uterine pathology, or a distended bladder. When the abdomen is distended above the umbilicus, consider the possibility of a pancreatic cyst or tumor, tumor of the bowel or liver, or intestinal dilation caused by obstruction or ileus. When the abdomen bulges asymmetrically, consider fecal impaction, hernia, bowel obstruction, aortic aneurysm, a singularly enlarged organ, or normal variant.

Ask the patient to take a deep breath and hold it while you look at the contour of the abdomen again. The deep inhalation causes the abdominal diaphragm to squeeze the abdominal contents and make more obvious previously unseen protrusions. An abdominal protrusion in the midline can be caused by **diastasis recti** which is the separation of the two abdominal rectus muscles from their normal juxtaposition.

Using tangential light, watch for **abdominal movement, gastrointestinal peristalsis**, and **pulsations** of the aorta. Looking from the patient's right side, evaluate the normal abdominal movement from respiration, especially in the male. This is more difficult to observe in women who breathe more quietly with less abdominal movement.

Note if the patient's breathing is shallow to guard against abdominal pain. Look for **intestinal peristalsis** as a rippling movement that is usually more noticeable in the scaphoid abdomen. **Aortic pulsations** are easily seen as rhythmic waves moving from the xiphoid to caudad (i.e., motion from the feet toward the head). Marked aortic pulsations can be caused by a large pulse pressure, a tortuous aorta, or an aortic aneurysm. You may be able to observe your own aortic pulsations the next time you lie in the bathtub: fill your navel with water, look toward your feet, and watch your water-filled navel bounce with each heartbeat.

The veins in the abdominal wall are usually difficult to see. If seen, this fine venous network could be normal or could reflect increased collateral circulation as seen with portal hypertension. Although the abdominal veins below the umbilicus normally fill toward the feet and those above the umbilicus fill toward the head, diseases can change this normal fill pattern. If the patient has engorged, palpable, abdominal veins, check the venous filling pattern by placing both index fingers touching one another on top of a dilated vein. Compress the vein with your fingers and separate your fingers in opposite directions to milk the venous blood; then release one finger and note the direction of venous refilling and refill time. The superficial abdominal veins appear to radiate from the umbilicus and refill in the normal upward pattern in patients with portal hypertension; however, the refill flow is reversed when the superior vena cava is obstructed (see Figure 12.10). When the inferior vena cava is obstructed, you can see abnormally distended upper abdominal veins that drain toward the head. With chronic liver disease and portal hypertension, you may occasionally see a venous pattern radiating from the navel called **caput medusae** (i.e., the veins have a snake-like configuration). If you see this venous pattern, inspect the chest, face, neck, and upper extremities for **spider nevi**, another sign of late-stage liver disease.

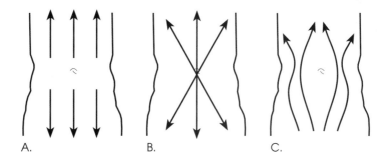

Fig. 12.10   Abdominal venous filling patterns. A shows a normal pattern; B, a pattern seen with portal hypertension; and C, a pattern resulting from obstruction of the inferior vena cava.

Auscultation

Auscultation of the abdomen evaluates bowel and vascular sounds. If you want to hear normal bowel sounds, do not palpate or percuss the abdomen until after completion of auscultation because manipulation of the abdomen can stimulate artificial peristaltic sounds. Gently place the warmed bell of the stethoscope on the abdomen and listen. Auscultate the abdomen in an orderly, clockwise sequence, beginning in the right upper quadrant, moving to the left upper, then left lower, and lastly the right lower quadrant. The intestine normally produces sounds heard as gurgles at an irregular frequency of five to thirty-five times per minute. Listen in each abdominal quadrant until bowel sounds are heard, or for at least three minutes if no bowel sounds are heard. The absence of bowel sounds, or the presence of extremely weak and infrequent sounds suggest possible bowel obstruction or ileus. The presence of increased frequency of bowel sounds with a high-pitched, rushing, tinkling quality might represent early intestinal obstruction or diarrhea (gastroenteritis). The tinkling sounds are made by air and water under higher than normal bowel pressure squeezing through a narrow opening. Sometimes, the familiar prolonged growling sounds known as **borborygmi** can be heard. These loud, prolonged gurgles of hyperperistalsis are heard after a meal as a growling noise or may be present with some diseases. Take time to listen with your stethoscope to your normal bowel sounds.

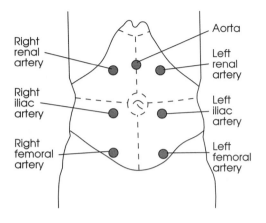

Fig. 12.11 Sites for auscultation of abdominal bruits.

If the patient has arterial vascular disease, auscultate over the areas of the aorta and the renal, iliac, and femoral arteries. It is especially important to evaluate patients with arteriosclerotic-associated diseases (e.g., hypertension, peripheral vascular disease, coronary artery disease) for the presence of **abdominal bruits** (see Figure 12.11). Using the bell of the stethoscope, listen for the high-pitched systolic sounds of a bruit caused by the turbulence of blood flowing through a constricted, dilated, or tortuous artery. These abdominal bruits or murmurs may be heard in an aortic aneurysm and over liver cancer. In addition, a bruit may be heard over a narrowed renal artery as a soft, medium, or low-pitched systolic sound, commonly associated with renovascular hypertension. These renal murmurs are best heard just above and slightly to the left of the navel. Auscultation of the abdomen also might detect the sound of a **venous hum** heard over the upper abdomen, especially around the liver and associated with hepatic cirrhosis or hepatoma.

A peritoneal **friction rub** may be heard over a cancerous liver, a splenic infarction, or an inflamed gallbladder. The sound of a friction rub is soft in quality and is created by the rubbing of an irritated surface of an organ (e.g., liver, spleen, gallbladder) against the parietal peritoneum of the abdominal wall. Friction rubs are best heard upon deep inspiration.

Percussion and Palpation

Percussion and palpation of the abdomen assist in estimating the size of organs, and in identifying the presence and localization of tenderness, air, fluid, or masses in the abdomen.

Begin by percussing in the four quadrants to assess the distribution of normal **tympany** and **dullness**. Percuss the quadrants in the same clockwise sequence used during auscultation. Ordinarily, tympany is heard over the hollow viscera such as the stomach, air-filled bowel, and bladder. Percussion over solid viscera (e.g., the liver, spleen, kidneys, pancreas, uterus, ovaries, and stool-filled bowel) usually generates dull sounds. Solid viscera also can be distinguished from hollow viscera by palpation (i.e., solid viscera are palpable but hollow, tympanitic viscera are usually not palpable unless an associated mass is felt).

Light Palpation. Following general percussion, lightly palpate the entire abdomen in a systematic fashion. **Light palpation**, in contrast to **deep palpation** provides a general sense of regions of resistance, superficial masses, and tenderness. This is the time to study the patient's face for grimacing or flinching in reported areas of tenderness. Note whether the patient's body language agrees with a reported tender region.

To palpate abdominal structures, rest your right hand parallel to the ribs in the upper left quadrant. Gently press your fingers in a rolling motion to a shallow depth in the abdomen. The skill of palpation using light pressure can be learned by palpating a partially inflated blood pressure cuff to raise the sphygmomanometer gauge about 20 mm Hg above zero. Move your fingers as if you are waving good-bye or kneading bread dough. Once you have learned this technique, palpate your way around the abdomen sequentially in each quadrant. Unless the abdominal muscles are tense, the abdominal surface should feel supple and resilient. If any superficial masses, fluid, gas, or edema are felt, explore the area later with deep palpation. If any point of tenderness is encountered, consider whether the cause is attributable to localized inflammation of abdominal muscles, an inflamed organ, or peritonitis.

If the abdomen is tender, try to elicit **rebound tenderness** (i.e., Blumberg's sign) by applying slow and firm pressure over the abdomen and then suddenly withdrawing the pressure. A positive test generates pain in the rebounding tissue at the point of reported tenderness. For known areas of tenderness, apply pressure to an area distant from the tender spot to detect **referred pain**. For example, when the patient reports tenderness in the left upper quadrant, press slowly and deeply into the left lower quadrant and quickly release the pressure. A positive referred pain test in the above example is the finding of pain in the upper left quadrant at the point of tenderness. Additionally, a complaint of sharp or stabbing pain might indicate peritoneal irritation. For example, pressure applied in the left upper quadrant and suddenly released may cause pain in an area over the right lower quadrant in a patient with appendicitis. An alternative method for assessing referred pain in the ambulatory patient with appendicitis is the use of **Markle's test** (i.e., the heel-drop jarring test). The patient participates in the Markle's test by rising on tiptoes, then suddenly dropping to the heels of the feet resulting in pain in the area of an irritated appendix. This maneuver can also elicit pelvic pain in a patient with acute pelvic inflammatory disease (PID). These tests are positive in several other abdominal inflammatory diseases including intra-abdominal abscess, pelvic inflammation, and acute diverticulitis.

If abdominal wall muscle resistance to palpation is encountered, try to determine if it is voluntary or involuntary. To differentiate the etiology of muscle resistance, flex the patient's knees (about 90°), place a pillow under the patient's head, and ask the patient to breathe slowly through an open mouth. These maneuvers will help relax the abdominal wall muscles. Feel the abdomen on each expiration; identify the point of least resistance. Involuntary rigidity or local **guarding** is associated with muscle spasm caused by peritoneal inflammation (e.g., peritonitis, appendicitis). These involuntary muscle spasms cannot be relaxed by voluntary efforts. Voluntary guarding of the abdominal muscles is generally associated with fear or nervousness and is not necessarily associated with an intra-abdominal pathology. Usually, voluntary guarding can be overcome by reassurance and by conversing with the patient.

When the patient reports a tender spot on the abdomen, explore for **cutaneous hyperesthesia** (i.e., hypersensitive skin pain perception). Hyperesthesia is associated with zones of parietal peritoneal irritation and, in the setting of acute appendicitis, may signal impending perforation. To test for cutaneous hyperesthesia, gently stroke the skin with a pin or lift the skin away from the underlying muscle. Watch the patient's face for signs of pain. Be careful not to pinch the skin painfully.

Deep Palpation. Following light palpation, explore the abdomen with deeper palpation. Using your finger pads, feel within the abdominal quadrants for any masses, unusual tenderness, or pulsations. Deep palpation can be accomplished by either **single-handed palpation** or **bimanual palpation**. Most often simply pressing more firmly with one hand is adequate for deep palpation; however, the bimanual method of placing one hand on top of the other sometimes is necessary. With the bimanual method, the hand on top exerts the pressure while the finger pads of the underlying hand concentrate on tactile sensations.

The choice of using one or two hands for deep palpation is less important than the movement of the hand that is deeply palpating. The fingers of the palpating hand should slide with the underlying abdominal wall over the organ or mass being studied (i.e., do not simply slide your fingers over the skin). Move your fingers in a back and forth motion in the horizontal plane. Deep palpable pressure is equal to 40 to 60 mm Hg; practice with a partially inflated blood pressure cuff. If a mass is detected, map its borders and note these characteristics: **location, consistency, shape, tenderness, mobility**, and **pulsation**. Additionally, determine if the mass is in the abdominal wall or within the abdominal cavity. An intra-abdominal mass becomes more difficult to palpate when the patient tenses the abdominal muscles by lifting her head while supine. An abdominal wall mass, in contrast, is still easily palpated in this situation. Sometimes, tender areas are noticed only with deep palpation. Deep palpation of some abdominal areas (e.g., the aorta, cecum, sigmoid colon, and the epigastrium just below the xiphoid process) will normally elicit complaints of tenderness by the patient.

Palpation and Percussion of Specific Organs

Along with providing a general evaluation of the abdomen, palpation and percussion can be used to examine specific organs.

Liver. Liver size varies with age, gender, height, disease process, and body build, and can be estimated by percussion. Ask the patient to take a deep breath and to hold it in before initiating percussion. Begin in the right midclavicular line at nipple level and percuss from normal lung resonance downward to liver dullness: mark the spot with a washable ink pen. Starting at the point of tympany below the navel in the right midclavicular line, percuss upward to liver dullness; mark the spot. These points along the right midclavicular line are the upper and lower limits of the percussed liver, or the "liver span." In the right midclavicular line of the adult, the usual liver span is 6 to 12 cm. A smaller liver span may represent atrophy (e.g., alcoholic liver cirrhosis), whereas a larger liver span may indicate hepatomegaly (e.g., acute hepatitis). If percussion is repeated at the midsternal line, the liver span usually is about 4 to 8 cm. The size of the liver span is extremely variable and these estimates of liver span size should only be used as a guide.

A normal lower liver border generally does not extend more than 1 to 3 cm below the right costal margin at the midclavicular line. However, this measurement must be correlated with a measurement of liver span. If the patient has a lung disease such as emphysema, lung expansion and flattening of the right diaphragm push the normal liver out from under the ribs. In this situation, the lower liver edge is greater than 1 to 3 cm below the right subcostal margin at the midclavicular line; however, the liver span is still within normal limits.

To palpate the liver, place your left hand under the lower right part of the patient's back and lift. Lay your right hand on the lower abdomen at the umbilicus in the right midclavicular line with the fingers pointing toward the ribs. Deeply palpate with the fingertips while asking the patient to inhale and hold a deep breath. Moving the hand at 1 to 2 cm intervals along the right midclavicular line, tell the patient, "Each time I move my hand, take a deep breath and hold it." Try to feel the liver as it moves down to touch your fingertips with each deep inspiration. Keep repeating your directions to the patient as your hand moves at 2 cm intervals. Ordinarily, the liver is not palpable. When palpable, a normal liver feels firm, nontender, and has a smooth edge and surface.

If intra-abdominal fluid (e.g., ascites) is suspected, special procedures must be utilized to detect it. The first is by checking for a **fluid wave**. With the patient lying flat on his back, have an assistant press the ulnar edge of his right hand vertically in the abdominal midline; this prevents a false positive test. Place your left hand against the patient's right flank. Next, sharply tap the patient's left flank with your right hand. In the presence of a large amount of ascites, a wave passes through the intra-abdominal fluid from the left flank to the right flank. This movement of fluid is felt as a sharp impulse or tap on your left hand. This finding identifies a significant amount of fluid in the peritoneal space. However, you should be aware of the possibility of false positive findings with this test.

To practice experiencing the tactile sensation of a fluid wave, partially fill a balloon with water and lay it on a table. Position your hands as above. Now, slosh the water with your right hand so that it ripples in a wave to the other palpating hand.

Another method for assessing ascites is to test for **shifting dullness**. Percuss from the umbilicus to the left flank, noting the change from tympany to dullness. Be sure to mark the spot of dullness. Then roll the patient to her left side and percuss from the umbilicus to the flank to identify a change from tympany to dullness. If ascites is present, the point of dullness or "fluid level" shifts to the umbilicus or it would be above the first mark. This change of dullness is called "shifting dullness." These signs (i.e., shifting dullness and fluid wave) seldom detect less than 500 mL of fluid in the abdomen.

Spleen. After completing the assessment of the liver, identify the splenic area in the left, lateral, lower, anterior rib cage. From the left anterior axillary line below the left subcostal margin, and moving to the posterior axillary line, percuss from bowel tympany to splenic dullness. If enlarged, the splenic edge is noted by a change from resonance or tympany to dullness. While standing to the right of the patient, reach across with your left hand and lift the posterior ribs to raise the spleen. Now, palpate with your right hand in the same manner used to palpate the liver, with the patient taking a deep breath to bring the spleen closer to your fingertips.

Unless it is enlarged or the abdomen is thin, the spleen is difficult to detect in an adult. If the spleen is felt, it is probably enlarged (i.e., splenomegaly). As a more sensitive check for splenomegaly, roll the patient *toward* his right side (i.e., 45°, not 90° off the table). Place your left hand under the patient's lower left ribs on his flank/back. Place your right hand low on the anterior abdomen along the anterior axillary line. Instruct the patient to "Inhale deeply through your open mouth then exhale each time I move my hand." You may have to coach the patient by breathing along or repeating your instructions. If the spleen is enlarged, you will feel it sliding beneath your fingers.

Kidneys. To examine the left kidney, place the patient in a supine position, then slide your left hand behind the patient's back while supporting the patient's left lower rib. Ask the patient to take deep breaths. Try to feel the lower lying, left kidney move beneath your fingers. You must use deep palpation. Unless the patient is very thin or the kidneys are swollen, normal kidneys cannot be palpated. However, if the kidney has been detected by palpation, it should be smooth, firm, and nontender. To examine the right kidney, place your left hand under the right side and lift. Feel deeply with your right hand as described. Occasionally a patient complains of kidney tenderness or experiences kidney pain.

If the kidney is tender or if symptoms are suggestive of inflammation, have the patient sit, and stand behind the patient. If the patient cannot stand or sit, roll the patient onto one side and then the other. Lay your hand on the patient's back over the healthy kidney at the costovertebral angle (CVA), make a fist, then strike a brisk blow to the CVA with the fist's ulnar surface. Normally, the patient perceives a thud or dull sensation, but no pain. Now, check the involved kidney. If the patient complains of sharp pain, this is CVA tenderness and it suggests kidney inflammatory disease, especially pyelonephritis.

PHARMACOTHERAPEUTIC CASE ILLUSTRATION

History

S.F., a 67-year-old female, complained of "stomach aches, vomiting, and diarrhea."
She stated, "It started last night and I've had to go every hour." S.F. has symptoms of
myalgia, lethargy, and anorexia. She lives in a nursing home.

Her past medical history included chronic atrial fibrillation (AF), chronic constipation,
hypertension, abdominal aortic aneurysm, history of (H/O) gastrointestinal (GI)
bleeding secondary to duodenal ulcer, and osteoarthritis.

Her family history (FH) showed her father died of myocardial infarction (MI) at about
age 66; her mother died of CVA at age 87; and her brother died of lung cancer at age
54. Her social history (SH) showed that she is a nonsmoker and does not drink
alcohol.

She is taking the following drugs: digoxin 0.125 mg PO Q a.m.; hydrochlorothiazide
25 mg PO QD; verapamil SR 240 mg PO Q a.m.; sorbitol 70% 30 mL with cascara
5 mL PO QD PRN constipation; docusate 200 mg PO Q HS; cimetidine 300 mg PO Q
HS; magnesium/aluminum hydroxide suspension 30 mL PO 1 hr PC and HS; tap
water enema PRN; aspirin 80 mg PO QD; and acetaminophen 325 mg tablets 2 PO Q
4 hr PRN pain.

S.F. has no known drug allergies. Her review of systems (ROS) was not contributory
except as outlined in the history of present illness.

Physical Examination

S.F. appeared to be a 67-year-old cachectic, chronically ill female in moderate
distress.

Her vital signs (VS) were as follows: temperature 98° F; respiratory rate (RR) 18/min;
pulse (PR) 78 beats/min (supine), 102 beats/min (sitting) irregular; blood pressure
(BP) 135/68 mm Hg (supine), 115/54 mm Hg (sitting); weight 115 lb (recent loss of 4
lb). Her mouth was dry and she had poor skin turgor. Her abdomen was scaphoid, with
no scars, striae, dilated veins, or masses. Hyperactive bowel sounds with borborygmi
were present in all quadrants. She had an aortic bruit at the umbilicus. Her abdomen
was soft with generalized abdominal tenderness and no rebound tenderness. Her
bladder was not tender. Liver dullness and span were normal. She displayed no sign of
costovertebral angle (CVA) tenderness. Her kidneys and spleen were not palpable.
There was no fecal impaction.

Laboratory

The urinalysis with microscopic examination, complete blood cell count (CBC), and serum chemistries were not significantly different from previous examinations except the serum potassium was 3.2 mEq/L, HCO_3 19 mEq/L, albumin 3 gm/dL, and urine specific gravity 1.028. Stool hemoccult test was negative. Serum digoxin concentration was 1.0 ng/mL.

Diagnosis and Management

S.F. was diagnosed with acute viral gastroenteritis. She was ordered Gatorade, a Bratty diet as tolerated, promethazine 25 mg PO/IM Q 4 to 6 hr PRN nausea, and kaolin/pectin suspension 30 mL PO after each loose bowel movement. She was told to stop using laxatives. She was prescribed potassium chloride 40 mEq PO BID for 2 days, then 30 mEq PO every morning and repeat laboratory tests in 4 days.

Discussion

Disease. Acute viral gastroenteritis is caused by various viral agents. A common cause among adults is the Norwalk agent. This organism can cause a single case, but often causes outbreaks in communal situations. The infection is spread from patient to patient or caregiver to patient, and by food-borne or water-borne contamination. Once started, the outbreak spreads rapidly through the population. S.F. lived in a nursing home which put her at risk. Nursing home patients are frequent victims of a community epidemic because the virus is carried by a caregiver.

Following a 24- to 48-hour incubation period, the patient is inflicted with "flu-like" complaints (e.g., malaise, myalgia, anorexia), nausea, vomiting, watery diarrhea, and abdominal cramping. Usually, the illness remits in 24 to 48 hours without sequelae; however, severe fluid and electrolyte losses or aggravation of a pre-existing disease could complicate the recovery in some patients (e.g., sick elderly patients or infants).

S.F.'s abdominal findings support a generalized intestinal disease. The key signs are tenderness with a soft abdomen and hyperactive bowel sounds. These findings point to an acute, inflammatory bowel disease. The absence of rebound tenderness indicates no peritoneal involvement; no organomegaly eliminates some visceral diseases. The absence of CVA tenderness points away from a urinary tract infection (UTI) as the cause. Interestingly, fecal impaction in the elderly may present as an acute febrile diarrhea and should be digitally checked.

Management. The first step is to assess the severity of fluid and electrolyte losses. Generally, thirst is a good indicator of volume loss, but it is not a reliable sign in the elderly. On physical examination check for signs of dehydration. S.F. had dry mucus membranes in her mouth; however, mouth breathing can cause a false positive finding. It is necessary to look under the patient's tongue for dryness which better correlates with volume loss. Because of skin changes associated with normal aging, measuring the skin turgor has limited value in elderly persons. S.F. lost less than 5% percent of her body weight. Acute weight change is a useful index of body volume loss. A 10% loss is rated as a severe volume loss, 5% is moderate, and less than 5% is considered a mild volume deficit. S.F. did experience orthostatic hypotension which increased her pulse rate and caused a drop in her systolic blood pressure, both signs of volume depletion. Examining the jugular veins can be helpful in assessing volume depletion; they are flat in severe volume loss. Urine output should be carefully checked for oliguria. Satisfactory volume replacement is shown by adequate urine output, restored body weight, return of normal pulse and jugular vein pressure, wet oral membranes, and good skin turgor.

Drug-induced diarrhea is a common cause of acute diarrheal episodes in the chronically ill patient. S.F. was prescribed several agents associated with diarrhea: digoxin, sorbitol with cascara, an antacid, cimetidine, and docusate. Laxative abuse, especially in the elderly, occurs because patients mistakenly believe that a daily bowel movement is needed for good health. S.F.'s laxatives were held until the diarrheal episode cleared.

Fluid and electrolyte losses were managed with Gatorade; never use plain water. Water with electrolytes and glucose is needed to replenish losses. Glucose promotes the active small intestine reabsorption of sodium and water. The absorptive cells are damaged by the virus and need time to recover. A temporary lactose intolerance is expected and dairy products will aggravate the diarrhea for 7 to 10 days. Oral rehydration should be liberal. A simple way to judge adequate rehydration is that the patient drinks until she urinates often (i.e., assumes normal renal function). The key to dietary management is small, frequent feedings. A Bratty diet consists of bananas (B), rice (R), apples (A), toast (T), tea (T), and yellow vegetables (Y).

Diarrhea is a normal body response to rid itself of a noxious substance. Remember, the goal is to slow the diarrhea sufficiently to permit the administration of oral fluids for volume repletion. Aggressive management with antiperistaltic agents (e.g., loperamide) may lead to complications (e.g., toxic megacolon). If an invasive pathogen is the cause, systemic symptoms can be worsened by antiperistaltic agents. A kaolin-pectin mixture, an adsorbent agent with minimal risk to the patient, was prescribed. The greatest risk of such a medication would be to give it to a patient with a bowel obstruction or to iatrogenically create a bezoar.

Therapeutic Drug Monitoring Examples

GASTROESOPHAGEAL REFLUX DISEASE (GRD)

The approach to therapuetic drug monitoring by clinicians varies depending upon many factors. Some of these include preferences among clinicians in a given community or region; concurrent medical problems which dictate that certain drugs be used or avoided; the patient's response to selected medication. The following outlines of therapeutic drug monitoring offer examples which may serve to stimulate discussion and further understanding of initiating and monitoring drug use. The drugs and dosages presented should not be applied to any clinical situation without proper medical supervision.

Drug Therapy	Metoclopramide 10 mg tablet 1 PO 30 min AC and HS. Gaviscon liquid 30 mL PO 30 min PC and HS with ½ glass of water. Omeprazole 20 mg capsule 1 PO QD.
Monitoring	**Symptoms:** Ask the patient to describe the pain and any associated activities such as sleeping, bending, or squatting. Does the patient smoke or drink alcohol? If the patient answers "yes" ask about the quantities consumed. Ask the patient how often heartburn occurs. Does the patient have any complaints of dysphagia (i.e., difficulty swallowing) or odynophagia (i.e., pain on swallowing)? Are there any foods associated with worsening or easing of the heartburn?
	Signs: *Gen:* Do the patient's clothes fit comfortably around the waist? Measure the weight for obesity. Look for signs for distress and/or discomfort. *VS:* Check blood pressure, pulse, respiration, and temperature. *Abd:* Inspect for scars, symmetry, and mass. Listen for normal bowel sounds. Palpate for epigastric tenderness.
Laboratory Tests	The clinician may elect to order all, none, or some of these laboratory studies depending upon history and physical findings, as well as other specific clinical

Therapeutic Drug Monitoring Examples

GASTROESOPHAGEAL REFLUX DISEASE (GRD)
(continued)

Laboratory Tests	indications. Barium swallow, esophagogastroduodenoscopy (EGD).
Adverse Drug Event Monitoring	**Metoclopramide:** Assess the patient's level of consciousness by looking for signs of drowsiness, confusion, or restlessness. Ask about feelings of tiredness or weakness. Evaluate bowel functions (e.g., diarrhea or constipation). Examine the patient for the following signs of extrapyramidal side effects: shuffling gait, shaking hands, bradykinesia, or stiffness. Watch for signs of tardive dyskinesia which presents as abnormal orofacial movements.
	Gaviscon: Ask about any changes in bowel function (e.g., constipation or diarrhea).
	Omeprazole: Does the patient describe problems with headache, diarrhea, abdominal pain, nausea/vomiting, or dizziness? Monitor for possible drug interactions.

Therapeutic Drug Monitoring Examples

DUODENAL ULCER

The approach to therapeutic drug monitoring by clinicians varies depending upon many factors. Some of these include preferences among clinicians in a given community or region; concurrent medical problems which dictate that certain drugs be used or avoided; the patient's response to selected medication. The following outlines of therapeutic drug monitoring offer examples which may serve to stimulate discussion and further understanding of initiating and monitoring drug use. The drugs and dosages presented should not be applied to any clinical situation without proper medical supervision.

Drug Therapy	Cimetidine 800 mg tablet 1 PO Q HS. Sucralfate 1 gm tablet 1 PO 30 min AC and HS.
Monitoring	**Symptoms:** Evaluate the patient's response to drug therapy by asking for a description of epigastric pain (e.g., "hunger-like," "burning," "gnawing"). Has the pain awakened the patient? Are there any associated factors that make it worse or better? Is the pain worse at a particular time of the day (e.g., at night versus mid-morning)? What is the frequency and duration of the pain? Has the patient vomited any "coffee grounds" vomitus? Does the patient have any complaints of epigastric cramping, regurgitation, excessive belching, bloating, or distention.
	Signs: *Gen:* Study the patient for signs of distress. *Abd:* Inspect for scars, pulsations, or masses. Auscultate all quadrants for bowel sounds. Palpate for epigastric tenderness (e.g., the 3 cm area just below the xiphoid process).
Laboratory Tests	The clinician may elect to order all, none, or some of these laboratory studies depending upon history and physical findings, as well as other specific clinical indications. Complete blood count (CBC),

Therapeutic Drug Monitoring Examples

DUODENAL ULCER
(continued)

Laboratory Tests	hemoccult stools, serum creatinine, endoscopy, barium swallow.
Adverse Drug Event Monitoring	**Cimetidine:** Check the patient's mental status for signs of confusion such as disorientation, agitation, delirium, hallucinations, or anxiety (see Chapter 3: Mental Status Examination). Monitor for potential drug interactions.
	Sucralfate: Has constipation been a new problem for the patient? If yes, palpate the abdomen for fecal mass.

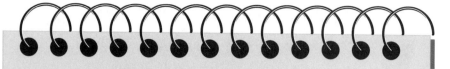

Therapeutic Drug Monitoring Examples

NON-INSULIN DEPENDENT DIABETES MELLITUS (TYPE II)

The approach to therapeutic drug monitoring by clinicians varies depending upon many factors. Some of these include preferences among clinicians in a given community or region; concurrent medical problems which dictate that certain drugs be used or avoided; the patient's response to selected medication. The following outlines of therapeutic drug monitoring offer examples which may serve to stimulate discussion and further understanding of initiating and monitoring drug use. The drugs and dosages presented should not be applied to any clinical situation without proper medical supervision.

Drug Therapy   Glyburide 10 mg tablet 1 PO Q a.m.

Monitoring

Symptoms: Ask questions to determine if the patient is experiencing polyuria, polyphagia, polydipsia, tingling/numbness of the extremities, impotence or decreased libido, weakness, weight changes, and blurred vision. Does the patient have any foot infections or lesions? How are the bowel functions (e.g., chronically constipated or diarrhea)? Are there any complaints of peripheral vascular disease (e.g., intermittent claudication)? Has the patient experienced any cardiac chest pain (i.e., chest pain with exertion)? Does the patient have any symptoms suggesting transient ischemic attacks (TIAs) (i.e., brief neurological deficits)? Does the patient feel bloated, experience early satiety or nausea (e.g., gastroparesis)?

Signs: *Gen:* Measure the patient's weight and note any loss or gain of weight. *MSE:* Check the patient's orientation and alertness. Is the patient's speech coherent and logical? Describe the patient's physical appearance, behavior, and attention (see Chapter 3: Mental Status Examination). *VS:* Measure the patient's pulse, respiration, temperature, and blood pressure (both sitting and standing for

Therapeutic Drug Monitoring Examples

NON-INSULIN DEPENDENT DIABETES MELLITUS (TYPE II)
(continued)

Monitoring

postural changes). *Skin:* Carefully examine the patient's skin for dryness and poorly healing lesions. Look for signs of dehydration (e.g., turgor/mobility). *Eyes:* Using a Snellen chart and newspaper, assess the patient's visual acuity (see Chapter 5: Eye). Check extraocular muscle movements (e.g., cranial mononeuropathy). With tangential lighting, inspect the corneas and lens for opacities. Check the intraocular pressure (IOP). Examine the retina for diabetic damage (e.g., neovascularization, microaneurysm, various hemorrhages, hypertensive vessel changes; see Chapter 5: Eye). *CVS:* Examine for signs of coronary artery disease (CAD), high blood pressure (HBP), and congestive heart failure (CHF) (see Chapter 11: Heart). Listen for normal and abnormal heart sounds. Is an S_3 or S_4 heard? *Abd:* Auscultate the aorta, renal, iliac, and femoral arteries for bruit sounds. *Ext:* Inspect the legs, noting any signs of peripheral vascular disease (PVD) (see Chapter 12: Blood Vessels). Carefully inspect and palpate the feet for ingrown toenails or infection. Look at the plantar surfaces for neurotrophic ulcers or callus formations. Palpate the popliteal, dorsalis pedis, and posterior tibial pulses. Note any edema. *Neuro:* Tell the patient to walk normally, then heel-to-toe across the room; note coordination and balance. Check for Romberg's sign (see Chapter 14: Nervous

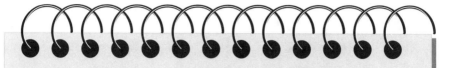

Therapeutic Drug Monitoring Examples

NON-INSULIN DEPENDENT DIABETES MELLITUS (TYPE II)
(continued)

Monitoring	System). Assess strength by grip and shallow knee bend. Screen for sensory defects with pin prick or vibration (e.g., peripheral polyneuropathy). Measure deep tendon reflexes (DTRs), especially for absence of ankle or knee jerks.
Laboratory Tests	The clinician may elect to order all, none, or some of these laboratory studies depending upon history and physical findings, as well as other specific clinical indications. Fasting blood glucose, glycosylated hemoglobin, urinalysis with microscopic exam, serum blood urea nitrogen (BUN)/creatinine.
Adverse Drug Event Monitoring	**Glyburide:** To detect hypoglycemia, observe for sweating, palpitation, tremor, nervousness, night sweats, weakness, and tachycardia (i.e., sympathetic symptoms). Check for central nervous system (CNS) symptoms, including headache, diplopia, nightmares, confusion, and motor incoordination.

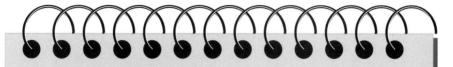

Therapeutic Drug Monitoring Examples

ALCOHOLIC LIVER DISEASE

The approach to therapuetic drug monitoring by clinicians varies depending upon many factors. Some of these include preferences among clinicians in a given community or region; concurrent medical problems which dictate that certain drugs be used or avoided; the patient's response to selected medication. The following outlines of therapeutic drug monitoring offer examples which may serve to stimulate discussion and further understanding of initiating and monitoring drug use. The drugs and dosages presented should not be applied to any clinical situation without proper medical supervision.

Drug Therapy | Spironolactone 25 mg tablet 2 PO QID. Lactulose syrup 30 mL PO TID.

Monitoring | **Symptoms:** Ask about the patient's appetite, weight loss, fatigue, or weakness. Has the patient noticed any dark/black stool or yellowish foamy urine? Does the patient bruise easily?

Signs: *Gen:* Describe the patient's body habitus. Weigh the patient. Smell the patient's breath for an ammonia-like or alcohol odor. *MSE:* Is the patient alert, and oriented to person, place, and time? Is the patient irritable, forgetful, or neglecting personal hygiene? Has the patient undergone any change in usual personality? *VS:* Check the patient's blood pressure, pulse, respiration, and temperature. Is the pulse bounding? Is the pulse pressure wide? *Skin:* Look attentively at the patient's skin. Do you find petechiae or ecchymoses? Examine the fingernails for clubbing or cyanosis. *HEENT:* Inspect the sclera for icterus (jaundice). Examine around the eyelids for xanthomas. Check for rhinophyma, and facial and chest telangiectasia. Also, inspect for palmar erythema. *Abd:* Inspect for scars, pulsations, or mass. Note the symmetry of the abdomen. Is it protuberant? When the patient is supine,

Therapeutic Drug Monitoring Examples

ALCOHOLIC LIVER DISEASE
(continued)

Monitoring	do the flanks bulge? Survey for signs of ascites [i.e., tight, shiny with radiating umbilical varicosities (caput medusae)]. If the patient has ascites, measure the girth at the umbilicus. Look at the upper chest for spider nevi. Percuss for shifting dullness and fluid wave. Palpate for hepatomegaly and splenomegaly. Check for hepatojugular reflux. *Ext:* Check for pitting edema in the feet. Rate its quality (i.e., 1+, 2+, 3+, or 4+) and distribution (e.g., to the knee). *MUS:* Survey the arms and legs for muscle wasting. Check muscle strength (see Chapter 13: Musculoskeletal System) by hand grip. *Neuro:* Test the patient's deep tendon reflexes (DTRs) for hyperreflexia. Extend the patient's arm and dorsiflex the hand (i.e., asterixis or "bye-bye" sign). Ask the patient to write his signature each day for comparison.
Laboratory Tests	The clinician may elect to order all, none, or some of these laboratory studies depending upon history and physical findings, as well as other specific clinical indications. Liver enzymes (AST, ALT), serum electrolytes, urinalysis for bilirubin, serum albumin/globulins, clotting tests (PT/aPTT), serum bilirubin.
Adverse Drug Event Monitoring	**Spironolactone:** Ask about dizziness and thirst. Check for signs of excessive electrolyte loss. Watch serum electrolytes, especially for hyperkalemia (e.g., slow heartbeat, confusion, severe muscle weakness.) Measure the blood pressure with the patient both sitting and standing. Weigh the patient.

Therapeutic Drug Monitoring Examples

ALCOHOLIC LIVER DISEASE
(continued)

Adverse Drug
Event Monitoring

Lactulose: Ask about diarrhea. Watch for signs/symptoms of excessive water/electrolyte loss in stools.

Therapeutic Drug Monitoring Examples

DIARRHEA (ACUTE, BACTERIAL)

The approach to therapeutic drug monitoring by clinicians varies depending upon many factors. Some of these include preferences among clinicians in a given community or region; concurrent medical problems which dictate that certain drugs be used or avoided; the patient's response to selected medication. The following outlines of therapeutic drug monitoring offer examples which may serve to stimulate discussion and further understanding of initiating and monitoring drug use. The drugs and dosages presented should not be applied to any clinical situation without proper medical supervision.

Drug Therapy

Bismuth subsalicylate suspension 30 mL for each loose stool, to 8 doses daily. Trimethoprim-sulfamethoxazole (TMP/SMX) 2 tablets PO BID.

Monitoring

Symptoms: Determine the onset, duration, and number of bowel movements per day. Ask if the diarrhea is associated with other symptoms such as fever, vomiting, or abdominal pain. Has the patient noticed any blood in the stool? What food has the person eaten in the last 24 hours? Have other family members or close friends experienced the same problem? Ask about feelings of thirst and hunger.

Signs: *Gen:* Observe the patient's general state of health; look for signs of distress or discomfort. Weigh the patient. Note posture, motor activity, and demeanor. *VS:* Is the patient's temperature elevated? Is the patient experiencing tachycardia? Is the pulse weak/thready (see Chapter 10: Blood Vessels)? Is the blood pressure low? Does the blood pressure drop, heart rate go up, and the patient become dizzy when standing? Note the respiratory rate. *MSE:* Note the patient's level of consciousness and alertness. *Skin:* Check turgor and mobility for dehydration. Feel the skin temperature and texture. Note if it is warm and dry. *Eyes:* Look for "sunken"

Therapeutic Drug Monitoring Examples

DIARRHEA (ACUTE, BACTERIAL)
(continued)

Monitoring	appearance. Are tears present? Palpate the eyeballs for softness. *Mouth:* Inspect the mucus membrane surface. Is it moist or dry? Does the saliva seem "stringy"? *CVS:* Inspect the precordial areas for pulsations or heaves. Feel for the primary apical impulse (PMI). Auscultate for normal and abnormal heart sounds. Is the apical rate tachycardiac? Feel the carotid pulse. Is it bounding, or weak? *Abd:* Carefully evaluate the shape of the patient's abdomen. Is it bloated? Can you see hyperperistalsis waves? Auscultate for hyperactive bowel sounds in all quadrants. Percuss for generalized tympanitic sound. When palpating, describe any tenderness. Is tenderness generalized or localized?
Laboratory Tests	The clinician may elect to order all, none, or some of these laboratory studies depending upon history and physical findings, as well as other specific clinical indications. Complete blood count (CBC) with differential, urinalysis with microscopic exam, serum chemistries, serum electrolytes, stool for ova/parasites.
Adverse Drug Event Monitoring	**Bismuth Subsalicylate Suspension:** Question about tinnitus, especially if concurrently taking aspirin. Avoid warfarin; it interferes with coagulation. Watch for signs/symptoms of bleeding. **Trimethoprim-Sulfamethoxazole (TMP/SMX):** Interview for new onset skin rash, sore throat, fever, or unusual bruising or bleeding. Does the patient have

Therapeutic Drug Monitoring Examples

DIARRHEA (ACUTE, BACTERIAL)
(CONTINUED)

Adverse Drug Event Monitoring	any new complaints of nausea, vomiting, or anorexia since starting antibiotic therapy. Check CBC for thrombocytopenia, especially if in an elderly patient who is also taking a thiazide diuretic.

Musculoskeletal System

*T*he musculoskeletal system (MSS) provides the means of locomotion and support for the human body. The bony component of the MSS also is the site of hematopoietic functions. This chapter, however, will focus on locomotion-related disorders and their treatment. Millions of patients suffer with rheumatic diseases and many drugs are used to treat these disorders. To clinically evaluate drug efficacy and toxicity, a clinician should be familiar with the physical examination of the musculoskeletal system.

ANATOMY AND PHYSIOLOGY

The bony skeleton, muscles, blood vessels, and nerves that comprise the musculoskeletal system must work in harmony to carry out the tasks of locomotion and support for the body. Disease involving any one or more of these components can result in malfunction.

The primary function of the skeleton is to permit purposeful motion. Human bones connect with one another in a variety of ways. However, there are three basic types of joints: movable joints (i.e., diarthroses), partially movable joints (i.e., amphiarthroses), and immovable joints (i.e., synarthroses). (See Figure 13.1.) The design of a joint depends upon its function. In clinical practice, one most frequently evaluates diarthrodial joints. Unlike the other two types of joints, diarthrodial joints contain synovial membranes and synovial fluid and, therefore, are also called **synovial joints**. Rheumatic diseases most often affect these joints. Because of the prevalence of rheumatic disease and its association with synovial joints, this chapter focuses on the movable joints, their structures, and examination.

Skeletal Structures

Movable joints are composed of two adjacent bones connected by muscles, ligaments, cartilage, and tendons. Each of these components must function normally for the joint to move freely and carry on locomotion. Based upon the type of joint function, other

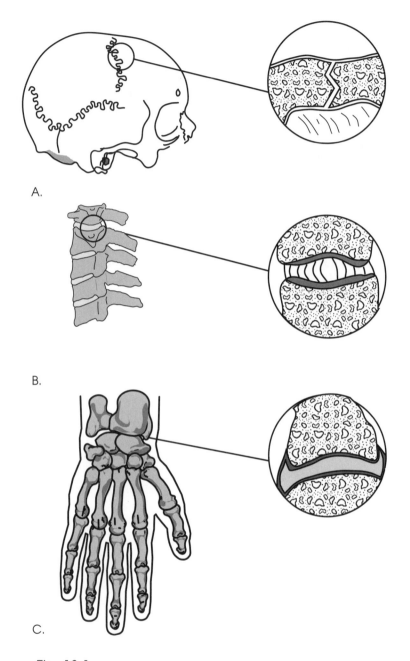

Fig. 13.1 The three basic types of skeletal joints: A. synarthroses; B. amphiarthroses; and C. diathroses.

structures associated with movable articulations may be found, such as bursae and articular disks. Diarthrodial joints are well-lubricated to allow various movements such as **flexion** (i.e., bending), **extension** (i.e., straightening), **adduction** (i.e., movement toward the midline), and **abduction** (i.e., movement away from the midline).

Ligaments are composed of collagenous fibers that connect bones to other bones, and serve to strengthen and stabilize joints. Ligaments anchor and align the joint surfaces. For example, when the medial collateral ligaments are torn or stretched, the knee alignment is weakened and its range of motion is limited.

Cartilaginous plates reduce bone friction by covering the articular surface of bones. A fibrous capsule stretches across the joint and surrounds it. A synovial membrane (i.e., synovium) covers the inner surface of the joint capsule to form the lining of the synovial cavity. The synovium covers all intracapsular structures except articular cartilage. The synovium is richly fed by microvascular vessels and secretes a clear, egg white-like fluid known as synovial fluid, which lubricates the joint surface. **Bursae** are closed synovial sacs that form at points of friction, usually near bony prominences close to joints, and facilitate ease of joint movement. A bursa may be located between muscle layers, between bone and muscle, or around ligaments or tendons.

Skeletal muscles are held together by non-contractile connective tissue, including fasciae, tendons, aponeuroses, and ligaments. Fasciae are composed primarily of fibrous connective tissues and spread like sheets over muscles to reduce friction and allow for ease of movement. Tendons and aponeuroses connect muscles to bones.

Skeletal muscles are essential for stability and locomotion. They attach across each joint and hold the joint surface in apposition for proper alignment and stability. Over 600 individually identifiable muscles comprise about 40 percent of body weight. Muscles vary in size from very small (e.g., the stapedius muscle of the middle ear) to very large (e.g., the gastrocnemius muscle of the calf). Skeletal muscles are richly supplied with blood, receiving about 4 to 7 mL/min/100 gm of muscle at rest, and 50 to 75 mL/min/100 gm during extreme exercise.

The nervous system is very important to skeletal muscle function. A detailed discussion of the relationship between muscles and the nervous system is presented in Chapter 14: Nervous System. Nerves transmit electrical impulses to motor end plates causing contraction. Voluntary contractions send the joint through its range of motion while preventing extremes of flexion or extension. Any interruption of nerve function leads to muscular paralysis and subsequent atrophy.

Voluntary movement is controlled by the contraction and relaxation of skeletal muscles. Muscles are arranged in groups across joints and work by synchronous contraction and relaxation. The contracting muscle exerts a force on the bone and pulls the bone at the joint in the direction of contraction. Simultaneously, an opposing muscle group relaxes to permit the movement. For example, in order for the biceps muscle of the arm to flex the elbow, the triceps muscle (used for extension of the elbow) must relax.

Joint Movement

Joint movements are described as **gliding, angular (i.e., flexion, extension, adduction, and abduction), circumduction**, and **rotation**. The normal range of motion of various joints is described in Table 13.1. A joint may be designed to move in only one way, or it may move in more than one way. For example, the knee can only execute angular movements which is one reason it is prone to injury. In contrast, the shoulder is quite versatile and performs circumduction, angular, and rotation movements.

In clinical practice, injury and disease are more frequently encountered involving certain joints. These joints are located in the hand, elbow, shoulder, foot, knee, hip, and spine. This chapter will focus on the examination of these diarthrotic joints.

Upper Extremity Joints

The identifying landmarks of the hand are the phalangeal joints, the connecting dorsal and ventral tendons, the ulnar bony prominence, and the radial and ulnar bones (see Figure 13.2). Viewed posteriorly (i.e., the extensor surface), the landmarks of the elbow include the medial and lateral epicondyles of the humerus and the olecranon process of the ulna (see Figure 13.3). The bursa in the elbow joint may be clinically visible if it is enlarged. The ulnar nerve lies between the medial epicondyle of the humerus and the ulnar olecranon process.

The shoulder joint is a ball and socket articulation whose bony structures are the clavicle, the scapula, and the humerus. Other important palpable points in the shoulder are the acromion and coracoid processes of the scapula. The greater and lesser tubercles are located on the humeral head (see Figure 13.4). The bursa resting on top of the humeral head is a common site of bursitis.

Lower Extremity Joints

The ankle and foot meet at a hinge type joint whose landmarks include the medial malleolus (tibia), lateral malleolus (fibula), Achilles tendon, talus, and calcaneus (see Figure 13.5). The landmarks of the knee include the tibial tuberosity, the medial and lateral condyle of the tibia, the patella, the medial and lateral epicondyle of the femur, proximal head of the fibula, and the patellar ligaments (see Figure 13.6).

The identifying features of the hip joint are the pelvic iliac crest, anterior superior iliac spine, and the greater trochanter of the femur; all other bony structures are clinically, for the most part, not easily distinguishable (see Figure 13.7). A posterior view of the back allows one to identify the spinous processes (especially cervical vertebra 7 and thoracic vertebra 1), the scapulae, and the iliac crests. Viewed from the side, the vertebral column has four normal curves: the cervical (concave), thoracic (convex), lumbar (concave), and sacral (convex) (see Figure 13.8).

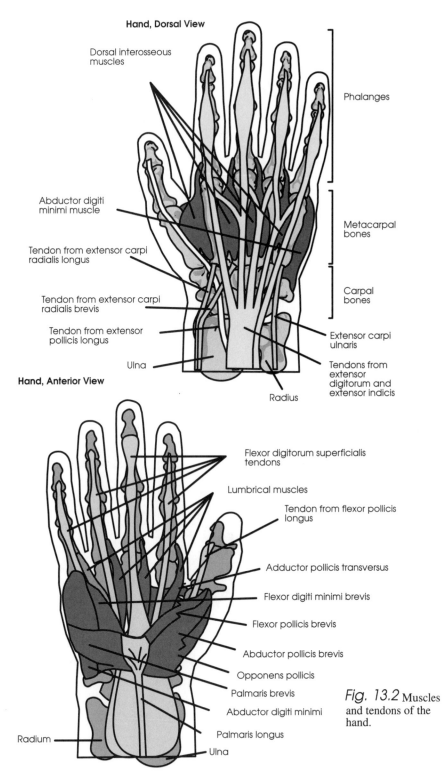

Hand, Dorsal View

Dorsal interosseous muscles

Phalanges

Abductor digiti minimi muscle

Metacarpal bones

Tendon from extensor carpi radialis longus

Tendon from extensor carpi radialis brevis

Carpal bones

Tendon from extensor pollicis longus

Extensor carpi ulnaris

Ulna

Tendons from extensor digitorum and extensor indicis

Hand, Anterior View

Radius

Flexor digitorum superficialis tendons

Lumbrical muscles

Tendon from flexor pollicis longus

Adductor pollicis transversus

Flexor digiti minimi brevis

Flexor pollicis brevis

Abductor pollicis brevis

Opponens pollicis

Palmaris brevis

Abductor digiti minimi

Radium

Palmaris longus

Ulna

Fig. 13.2 Muscles and tendons of the hand.

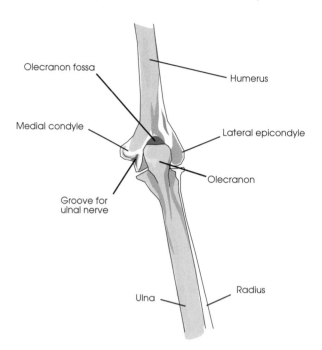

Fig. 13.3 Right elbow, posterior view.

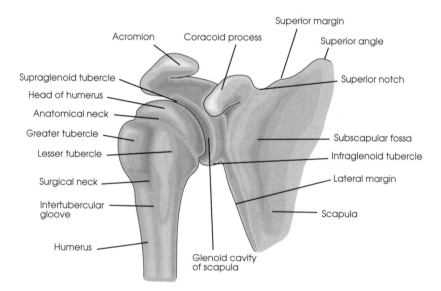

Fig. 13.4 Shoulder, anterior view.

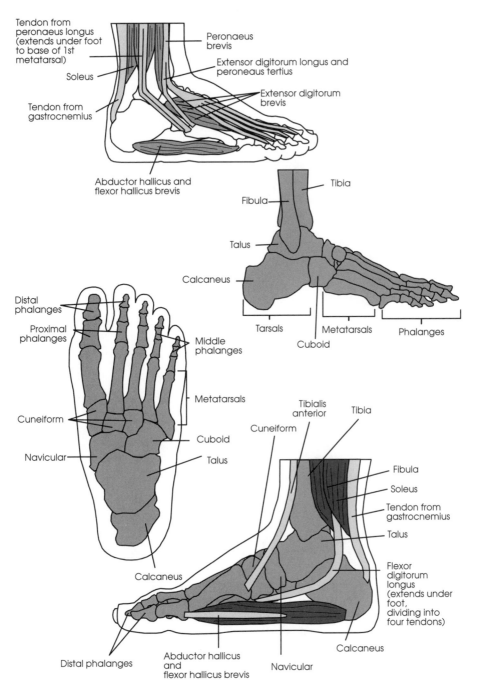

Tendon from peronaeus longus (extends under foot to base of 1st metatarsal)

Soleus

Tendon from gastrocnemius

Peronaeus brevis

Extensor digitorum longus and peroneaus tertius

Extensor digitorum brevis

Abductor hallicus and flexor hallicus brevis

Tibia

Fibula

Talus

Calcaneus

Tarsals

Cuboid

Metatarsals

Phalanges

Distal phalanges

Proximal phalanges

Middle phalanges

Cuneiform

Cuboid

Navicular

Talus

Metatarsals

Calcaneus

Tibialis anterior

Cuneiform

Tibia

Fibula

Soleus

Tendon from gastrocnemius

Talus

Flexor digitorum longus (extends under foot, dividing into four tendons)

Calcaneus

Distal phalanges

Abductor hallicus and flexor hallicus brevis

Navicular

Fig. 13.5 The ankle and foot.

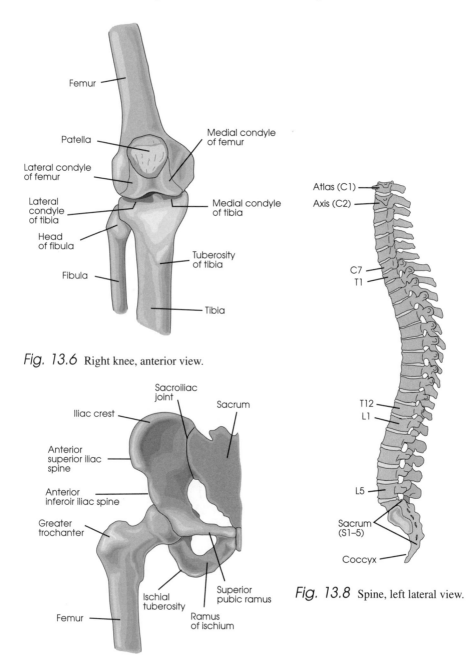

Fig. 13.6 Right knee, anterior view.

Fig. 13.7 Hip, anterior view.

Fig. 13.8 Spine, left lateral view.

PHYSICAL ASSESSMENT

A thorough examination of the musculoskeletal system must include evaluation of both structure and function of skeletal muscles and joints. Examine the patient in an area with good lighting and a comfortable room temperature. Usually, the patient is draped in a short, sleeveless gown. As with other organ system assessments, begin with a general evaluation by observing body movements and positions such as leaning over, sitting, standing, posture, and gait. These types of general observations are valuable as they relate directly to the activities of daily living (ADL) assessment. If the patient has difficulty with ADL, then a more detailed evaluation is warranted.

Posture and Gait

Normal **posture** places the head over the center of gravity with four separate curvatures of the spine: the cervical concavity, the dorsal (i.e., thorax) convexity, the lumbar concavity, and the sacral convexity. Abnormal postures and deformities are described in Table 13.2. **Gait** is the description of the way a person walks. Individuals tend to have distinct and characteristic walks (e.g., the characteristic walk of actor John Wayne). Certain diseases are also associated with specific gait patterns (see Table 13.3). For example, a patient with Parkinson's disease usually walks with a distinctive shuffling gait. After observing the patient's gait, examine specific muscles or joints by inspection and palpation, and evaluate range of motion, deformity, muscle strength, surrounding soft tissue abnormalities, crepitus, and symmetry.

Range of Motion

Range of motion is evaluated by asking the patient to move the joint in specific directions (see Table 13.1), measuring the angle of joint movement with a goniometer, and then comparing the measurement obtained with expected norms for that joint. For example, the fully extended elbow is defined to be at zero degrees. The range of full extension of the elbow to full flexion is normally 160°. "Normal" range of motion varies depending upon age and gender. During clinical evaluation, compare the range of motion between similar joints of the same individual. Joint deformities commonly result from bony enlargements or remodeling of the joint. Selected deformities of the spine, shoulder, elbow, hand, foot, knee, and hip are described in Table 13.2.

Muscle Strength

Muscle strength is tested by asking the patient to push or pull against an applied force or resistance. For example, quadriceps muscle strength can be tested by having the

Normal Range of Motion

Table 13.1

Articulation	Joint Position	Degree
Upper Body Joints		
Hand and wrist		
Wrist	Adduction (ulnal flexion)	55
	Abduction (radial flexion)	20
	Extension	70
	Flexion	90
	Supination	90
	Pronation	90
Distal interphalangeal joint (DIP)	Extension	0
	Flexion	80
Proximal interphalangeal joint (PIP)	Extension	0
	Flexion	120
Metacarpal phalangeal joint (MP)	Hyperextension	30
	Flexion	90
Elbow	Extension	0
	Flexion	160
Shoulder	Forward flexion	180
	Backward extension	50
	Abduction	180
	Adduction	50
	External rotation	90
	Internal rotation	90
Lower Body Joints		
Ankle/Foot	Dorsiflexion	20
	Plantar flexion	45
	Inversion	30
	Eversion	20
Hip and Knee		
Knee	Hyperextension	15
	Flexion	130
Hip with knee straight	Forward flexion	90
	Backward extension	15
Hip with knee flexed	Forward flexion	120
	Backward extension	30
	Adduction	30
	Abduction	45
	Internal rotation	40
	External rotation	45
Spine and Neck		
Spine	Right lateral flexion	35
	Left lateral flexion	35
	Right rotation (shoulder forward)	30
	Left rotation (shoulder forward)	30
	Forward flexion	80
	Backward extension	30
Neck	Right lateral flexion	40
	Left lateral flexion	40
	Right rotation (chin to right)	70
	Left rotation (chin to left)	70
	Forward flexion	45
	Backward extension	55

[a]To evaluate articular function, one must be familiar with these movements and their normal range of motion.

Table 13.2

Postures and Deformities

Ankylosing Spondylitis	A seronegative spondyloarthropathy producing stiffness and pain as a result of inflammation of the sacroiliac, intervertebral, and costovertebral joints which may lead to complete rigidity in the spine.
Baker's Cyst (Popliteal Cyst)	A swelling behind the knee caused by the leakage of synovial fluid into the gastrocnemius bursa causing a bulge in the popliteal fossa of the knee joint.
Bouchard's Nodes	Small, hard nodules in the proximal interphalangeal joints of the fingers usually associated with osteoarthritis.
Boutonniere Deformity	Deformity of the finger with flexion of the proximal interphalangeal joint and hyperextension of the distal joint. It is seen in chronic arthritis.
Dupuytren's Contracture	Shortening, thickening, and fibrosis of the palmar fascia, producing a flexion deformity of a finger.
Ganglion Cyst	A cyst within the tendon sheath. It is also termed a subchondral cyst.
Hallux Valgus	Angulation of the great toe from the midline; the great toe may overlap or underlap the adjacent toe.
Hammer Toe	The proximal portion of the toe is extended, and distal and second portions are flexed, causing a claw-like appearance.
Heberden's Nodes	Small, hard nodules, associated with osteoarthritis, that usually form at the distal interphalangeal articulations of the fingers.
Kyphosis	Abnormal increased convexity in the curvature of the thoracic spine when viewed from the side. It is commonly termed humpback.
Lordosis	Anterior concavity in the lumbar and cervical spine as viewed from the side. It is also termed swayback, hollow back, and saddle back.
Scoliosis	Abnormal lateral deviation in the spine.
Swan Neck Deformity	Deformity of the finger in which the proximal interphalangeal joint is flexed. The deformity is found in advanced chronic arthritis.
Ulnar Deviation	Lateral deviation of the hand associated with chronic arthritis. It occurs when the proximal phalanx dislocates from the metacarpal heads.

Gaits

Table 13.3

Festinating Gait	A gait that includes short, hurried steps. One of the gaits associated with Parkinson's disease.
Spastic Hemiparesis	The paralytic foot is held in plantar flexion, and is either dragged or swung in a semicicular (outward to inward) movement when walking. The affected arm is positioned fixed across the body and slightly flexed at the elbow and wrist. Stroke victims may exhibit spastic hemiparesis.
Steppage Gait	The knees are bent, legs are lifted higher than normal, and ankle flexed in the plantar position. The person appears to be walking up steps. Steppage gait is associated with foot drop secondary to lower motor nerve disease, such as neuropathy of diabetes mellitus.
Ataxic Gait	There are two types: sensory and cerebellar. In both types, the gait is staggering, unsteady, and wide-based. The patient's eyes are watching the ground with each step. In cerebellar ataxia, balance is difficult with either the eyes open or closed. Sensory ataxia is seen with some of the polyneuropathies. Drug-related cerebellar toxicity (e.g., alcohol, phenytoin) is associated with cerebellar ataxia.
Parkinsonian Gait	The head is displaced forward, trunk stooped forward, with arms and legs flexed. The center of gravity is more forward. The patient slides or shuffles his feet across the floor with very little arm swing. Initiating and stopping walking are difficult. In fact, once walking, the patient has difficulty stopping and another person may have to help the patient stop.
Senile Gait	With normal aging, the gait becomes wide-based, slow, deliberate, and forward displaced. The hips and knees are slightly flexed.

patient extend a 90° flexed knee by pushing (extending the knee) against your hand placed at the ankle. Compare each muscle to its contralateral twin. Muscle strength is rated on a five point scale, with five representing normal muscle strength and zero the absence of any muscle activity (see Table 13.4).

Joint Findings

Using inspection and palpation, evaluate each joint for range of motion, muscle strength, and abnormal findings. The following abnormal findings should prompt a closer examination of the joint: signs of **soft tissue injury** (e.g., redness, tenderness, heat, swelling, or muscle atrophy); **bone deformities** (e.g., nodules, dislocation, or contracture); **range of motion abnormalities** (e.g., limitation or instability); **joint distribution pattern** (e.g., single or multiple joint injury, symmetrical or

Muscle Strength Rating Scale

Table 13.4

Grade	Amplitude
0	No evidence of muscle contraction
1	Slight muscle contraction without joint motion
2	Muscle and joint movement without gravity
3	Slight muscle and joint movement with gravity
4	Muscle and joint movement with gravity and some resistance
5	Muscle and joint movement against gravity and full resistance (This is normal muscle and nerve function)

asymmetrical pattern); **pain** (e.g., with and without movement); **crepitus** (i.e., a crackling sensation heard or felt when the joint moves); and **muscle strength**.

Examining Specific Joints

Temporomandibular Joint (TMJ). Locate the temporomandibular joint (TMJ) just anterior to the tragus of each ear. Using your fingertips, palpate the TMJ as the patient gently opens and closes her mouth. The degeneration of this joint can cause headaches and can be felt as crepitus.

Spine. With the patient in a seated or standing position, inspect the neck and cervical spine for its normal concave curvature; look for deformities. Ask whether the patient has experienced any sore or painful areas in the neck. Palpate the bony and soft tissue of the neck for tenderness and evaluate the neck for range of motion limitations. First, gently flex the patient's head forward until the chin touches the chest; then, extend the patient's head backward until the chin is pointing toward the ceiling. Return the patient's head to the neutral anatomic position. Turn the patient's head from side to side toward each shoulder, then laterally flex the head in an effort to touch each ear to the corresponding shoulder.

While observing from the side, assess the curvature of the spine. The normal curvature of the spine can be described as being cervical concave, thoracic convex, or lumbar concave. Next, stand behind the patient and observe whether the spinous processes form a straight vertical line from the base of the skull to the tip of coccyx. Run your index finger up and down the spine (i.e., spinous processes) to check its midline position. Also, note whether the shoulders are of equal height.

Step away from the patient and observe the patient from the side. Evaluate the range of motion of the spine by asking the patient to bend forward and touch his toes. When the patient is bent over at a 90° angle observe the scapulae. They should be symmetric in their positioning. If not, suspect abnormal curvature of the spine. Then ask the patient to lean (i.e., hyperextend) backward while holding his knees straight with both hands on his hips. To test lateral range of motion of the spine, ask the patient to bend from side to side (i.e., lateral extension) as far as possible. Stand near the patient and be ready to prevent a fall if the patient bends over too far. With his hands on his hips, have the patient rotate or twist from side to side (i.e., rotate the right shoulder forward and the left one backward and visa versa). The patient should be able to move freely without pain or limitation. Finally, palpate down the spinous processes for areas of tenderness. Also palpate the paravertebral muscles to identify areas of tenderness or spasm.

Shoulders. While standing in front of the seated patient, look down the patient's shoulders and inspect and palpate each shoulder for deformities, inflammation, joint swelling, and muscle wasting. Next, palpate the sternoclavicular joint, acromio-clavicular joint, biceps groove, and glenohumeral joint for crepitus. Use your stethoscope to listen for fine crepitus.

Test shoulder range of motion by asking the patient to undertake the following movements:

- **forward flexion:** raise the arms forward and overhead;

- **backward extension:** hyperextend the arms backward;

- **abduction:** lift the arms laterally until they are parallel to floor;

- **elevation:** lift the arms from an abducted position to a vertical position overhead;

- **adduction:** bring both arms across the front of the body or from a fully abducted position down to the side of the body or neutral position;

- **internal rotation:** with elbows bent, place both arms behind the lower back;

- **external rotation:** with elbows bent, place both arms behind the upper part of the head.

Elbows. Support the patient's arm in a slightly bent position, and observe for nodules, swelling, or inflammation about the elbow. Then palpate the elbows for tenderness, crepitus, or swelling. Check the elbow's range of motion by instructing the patient to extend and flex the joint, then with the wrist in a neutral position direct the patient to turn her palms downward (i.e., pronation) and then upward (i.e., supination).

Hands and Wrists. Inspect the hands and wrists for normal symmetry and range of motion. Ask the patient to extend and spread apart all fingers, and then make a tight fist. Next, have the patient flex, extend, abduct (e.g., radial deviation), and adduct (e.g., ulnar deviation) each wrist. Carefully palpate each joint in the hands and wrists.

Some abnormal findings might include deformities, swelling, inflammation, nodules, or muscle atrophy. Measure the circumference of swollen or inflamed joints with a cloth metric tape or ring size loops.

Hips and Knees. With the patient in a supine position, inspect the hips and knees for normal symmetry and alignment. The angle of alignment between the femur and tibia should be less than 15°. Look for atrophy of the quadriceps, contractures, and deformities. Feel each joint for tenderness, swelling, nodules, and crepitus.

Palpate the tibiofemoral joint and popliteal space for deformity, tenderness, and crepitus. Test knee range of motion by flexing, then hyperextending the knee. To check hip motion, raise the patient's straight leg (i.e., hip flexion); flex the hip with the knee flexed; with the knee flexed at 90°, rotate the leg inward and then outward (i.e., internal and external rotation, respectively); and, with legs straightened, adduct then abduct each leg.

Feet and Ankles. Inspect the feet and ankles for deformities, calluses, nodules, bunions, or swelling. The toes are common sites for deformities such as hallux valgus, claw toes, and hammer toes (see Table 13.2). Palpate the feet and ankles for nodules, tenderness, and edema. Test ankle range of motion by gripping the lower leg just above the ankle while inverting and everting the ankle joint by the heel. Ankle range of motion also can be evaluated by instructing the patient to dorsiflex and plantar flex the ankle. Complete the examination of the feet and ankles by asking the patient to curl, then straighten his toes.

PHARMACOTHERAPEUTIC CASE ILLUSTRATION

History

W.K., a 68-year-old male, complained of pain in his hands. Upon questioning he stated, "Doc, my fingers hurt when I move them." Further questioning revealed that both hands had been stiff, especially after he had not moved them for an extended period of time (e.g., overnight). He further stated that he had this problem "off and on" for several years and had taken various self treatments for the problem. For the past several days, pain had been particularly severe.

His medical history revealed the following problems: kidney stones; diverticulosis; resection squamous cell cancer of right ear helix; hypertension; gastrectomy with Billroth II repair; angina pectoris; chronic constipation; gastrointestinal (GI) bleeding; chronic itching; and bilateral cataracts.

His current medications were: hydrochlorothiazide 25 mg tablet 1 PO QD; acetaminophen 325 mg tablet 2 tablets Q 4 hr PRN pain; trimeprazine (Temaril)

2.5 mg tablet 1 Q 4 hr PRN itching; sucralfate (Carafate) 1 gm tablet 1 tablet 30 min AC and HS; aluminum/magnesium suspension 30 mL 1 hr PC and HS; kaolin/pectin suspension 30 mL PO after each loose stool PRN; sorbitol 70% 15 mL PO Q HS PRN constipation; docusate 100 mg capsule 2 capsules Q HS; and vitamin B12 injection 200 µg IM every month.

Physical Examination

W.K. was a 5 ft 8 in, 150 lb 68-year-old male in mild distress. He had the following vital signs (VS): blood pressure (BP) 100/70 mm Hg; pulse 81 beats/min, regular; temperature 97.1° F, oral; respiratory rate (RR) 18/min regular.

Gross screening showed normal gait and posture for his age and general health. Inspection and palpation of both hands demonstrated warm, swollen proximal inter-phalangeal (PIP) and metacarpophalangeal (MP) joints; mild ulnar deviation; mild muscle wasting; and the presence of nodules. No Heberden's nodes, Bouchard's nodes, swan neck deformity, joint crepitus, or Boutonniere deformity were observed. Range of motion was reduced in the PIP, MCP, and distal interphalangeal (DIP) joints in both hands.

Laboratory

The erythrocyte sedimentation rate (ESR), rheumatoid factor (RF), and uric acid serum concentrations were analyzed and an x-ray of W.K.'s hands was obtained.

Diagnosis and Management

W.K.'s problem was tentatively diagnosed as acute rheumatoid arthritis flare-up. He was prescribed ibuprofen 400 mg tablet 1 QID for 15 days and physical therapy once the acute changes begin to subside. W.K. was instructed to return in two weeks for re-evaluation and discussion of laboratory test results.

Upon revisit, W.K. did not complain of hand pain. He stated that his ability to perform activities of daily living (ADLs) had improved. He demonstrated this by showing that he could now tie his shoes. Improvement was also noted in increased range of motion and decreased ring size measurements. Physical findings were the same, except acute inflammatory joints were not evident. Laboratory results showed an ESR of 52 mm/hr (normal: <15 mm/hr), serum uric acid 7 mg/dL (normal: 4.0 to 8.0 mg/dL), and positive serum RF; x-ray findings were consistent with rheumatoid arthritis. The patient was advised of the chronic progressive nature of the disorder. A conservative treatment plan of physical therapy and ibuprofen would be used until otherwise indicated.

Discussion

Disease. Pain is a frequent complaint associated with musculoskeletal disease. Pain may be described as sharp, dull, or aching in nature. The interview of the patient should determine if the pain began suddenly or slowly, and if an acute traumatic event can be identified. Ask if the pain involves one joint (i.e., monoarticular) or more than one joint (i.e., polyarticular), and whether joint involvement is symmetrical (e.g., both knees involved) or asymmetrical (e.g., one knee involved). W.K. was not in severe pain; but complained, "Doc, my fingers hurt when I move them, especially in the morning." The involvement was bilateral, polyarticular, and symmetrical; the time course was insidious and progressive, with remissions and exacerbations. After prolonged inactivity, joint movement stiffened and contracted, but "loosened-up" with movement. This history is consistent with the diagnosis of rheumatoid arthritis (RA).

Physical findings were characteristic of an acute flare-up. Proximal interphalangeal (PIP) and metacarpophalangeal (MP) joints were swollen, painfully tender, and warm to palpation, indicating acute inflammation. Usually, distal interphalangeal (DIP) joints are spared. As the disease progresses, soft tissue laxity leads to other hand deformities such as ulnar deviation. In advanced stages of the disease, muscle wasting and subluxation of the MP joints occurs. Also, PIP hyperextension accompanied by DIP flexion forms the familiar swan-neck deformity. Another physical change is the Boutonniere deformity in which PIP flexion is combined with DIP extension. The examiner did not find physical deformities associated with degenerative joint disease (i.e., Heberden's or Bouchard's nodes were not noted). Although a nonspecific finding, the range of motion was decreased in the affected joints.

Management. W.K. was initially treated with ibuprofen, a nonsteroidal anti-inflammatory drug (NSAID). The specific NSAID with which to begin therapy is arbitrary in terms of efficacy. The choice is based upon safety, cost, and compliance. With a history of gastrointestinal (GI) bleeding, aspirin was not an initial choice. Although ibuprofen is also associated with gastric irritation, it has a good safety and efficacy profile and is relatively inexpensive. The relief of pain was achieved within a few hours and the inflammatory response was under control within a few days as evidenced by reduced joint swelling and redness. The long-term physical findings such as ulnar deviation are unpredictable; chronic damage may be slowed with continued therapy or it may rapidly progress regardless of therapy. The clinician should observe the patient's ability to perform activities of daily living (e.g., dressing and eating). Joint size was evaluated by ring size measurement and was found to be smaller after therapy. This was related to decreased inflammation swelling of the soft tissue of the joint.

Physical therapy was also prescribed for W.K. Physical and occupational therapy are important in rehabilitation care and help to maximize functions, as well as slow the progression of the disease. Drugs such as NSAID allow the patient to be pain-free and, therefore, more functional. Drugs and rehabilitation services are necessary for the total care plan and, if used properly, maximize musculoskeletal function and minimize the need for rheumatoid arthritis medications.

Therapeutic Drug Monitoring Examples

RHEUMATOID ARTHRITIS (RA)

The approach to therapuetic drug monitoring by clinicians varies depending upon many factors. Some of these include preferences among clinicians in a given community or region; concurrent medical problems which dictate that certain drugs be used or avoided; the patient's response to selected medication. The following outlines of therapeutic drug monitoring offer examples which may serve to stimulate discussion and further understanding of initiating and monitoring drug use. The drugs and dosages presented should not be applied to any clinical situation without proper medical supervision.

Drug Therapy — Piroxicam (Feldene) 20 mg capsule 1 PO QD.

Monitoring — **Symptoms:** Ask how long the patient has experienced symptoms such as feelings of malaise, fatigue, and joint pain. What joints are involved? Is the joint pattern symmetrical and bilateral? Does the patient complain of stiffness from prolonged inactivity such as sleep or sitting? After inactivity, how long is it before the joints "loosen up?" Ask the patient to describe any limits to activities of daily living (ADLs), such as walking, standing, opening doors, opening containers, or writing. Is the patient experiencing low-grade fevers or anorexia with weight loss? Question about depressive symptoms (e.g., mood, affect). Ask if the treatment has helped. If yes, ask the patient to describe what has changed.

Signs: *Gen:* Watch how the patient moves. Note the patient's posture and gait. Check for signs of recent weight loss (e.g., loose fitting clothes). Ask the patient to walk, stand, and to undertake a delicate manipulation (e.g., tying shoe laces). Note the degree of difficulty and pain the patient experiences during these movements. Note whether the patient appears depressed. *VS:* Check for a low-grade fever. *MUS:* For

Therapeutic Drug Monitoring Examples

RHEUMATOID ARTHRITIS (RA)
(continued)

Monitoring	each affected joint, determine the range of motion (ROM), muscle strength, soft tissue changes, crepitus, and deformities. Give extra attention to pathognomonic findings such as ulnar deviation, swan neck deformity, Boutonniere deformity, or rheumatoid nodules. Look for bilateral symmetry. Palpate each joint for swelling (e.g., boggy synovium), tenderness, and inflammation. Look for signs of muscle wasting (e.g., atrophy of thenar eminence; quadriceps hollowness) and subluxation. Ask the patient if joint pain is continuously present or only experienced with movement. Using a metric tape, measure and compare symmetrical joint circumferences.
Laboratory Tests	The clinician may elect to order all, none, or some of these laboratory studies depending upon history and physical findings, as well as other specific clinical indications. Complete blood count (CBC), rheumatoid factor (RF), erythrocyte sedimentation rate (ESR), serum creatinine, serum electrolytes.
Adverse Drug Event Monitoring	**Piroxicam:** Ask about any gastrointestinal (GI) problems such as epigastric distress or nausea. Examine for signs of peripheral edema and congestive heart failure (CHF).

Therapeutic Drug Monitoring Examples

OSTEOARTHRITIS (DEGENERATIVE JOINT DISEASE)

The approach to therapeutic drug monitoring by clinicians varies depending upon many factors. Some of these include preferences among clinicians in a given community or region; concurrent medical problems which dictate that certain drugs be used or avoided; the patient's response to selected medication. The following outlines of therapeutic drug monitoring offer examples which may serve to stimulate discussion and further understanding of initiating and monitoring drug use. The drugs and dosages presented should not be applied to any clinical situation without proper medical supervision.

Drug Therapy

Diclofenac sodium 50 mg tablet 1 PO TID.

Monitoring

Symptoms: Measure treatment response with questions such as "Are the symptoms limited to just your joints or are general symptoms troubling you?" "Does the pain happen only with movement of involved joints or is pain present at rest?" "Is joint stiffness present?" Get an accurate description of the joints afflicted. Determine if the pattern is monoarticular or polyarticular, bilateral or symmetrical. Ask if the patient's medication has changed any of the symptoms. Ask if the patient's treatment has improved the ability to perform activities of daily living?

Signs: *MUS:* Study the patient's gait and posture. Look for a limp (e.g., a sign of a diseased hip). Does the patient have trouble rising from a chair? Carefully inspect each diseased joint for soft tissue swelling and inflammation. Meticulously inspect the hands for Heberden and Bouchard nodes, and lateral DIP joint deviation. Examine the knee joints for localized tenderness, passive movement pain, crepitus, and muscle atrophy. Compare bilateral muscle strength. Test the range of motion, comparing it

Therapeutic Drug Monitoring Examples

OSTEOARTHRITIS (DEGENERATIVE JOINT DISEASE)
(continued)

Monitoring	bilaterally. Does the patient experience pain in the joint with passive ROM? Palpate inflamed joints for tenderness and warmth. Feel for crepitus in afflicted joints. When bending forward to touch her toes, is the patient's spinal ROM decreased with associated pain and tenderness in the lumbar region?
Laboratory Tests	The clinician may elect to order all, none, or some of these laboratory studies depending upon history and physical findings, as well as other specific clinical indications. Liver function tests (LFTs), especially ALT and AST; serum creatinine; serum electrolytes (especially potassium); complete blood count (CBC).
Adverse Drug Event Monitoring	**Diclofenac Sodium:** Question the patient for the most common complaints: abdominal pain, headache, fluid retention, and dizziness. Ask about and examine for the following signs and symptoms of hepatotoxicity: fatigue, nausea, anorexia, jaundice, right upper quadrant tenderness, or "flu-like" symptoms.

Therapeutic Drug Monitoring Examples

ACUTE GOUTY ARTHRITIS

The approach to therapuetic drug monitoring by clinicians varies depending upon many factors. Some of these include preferences among clinicians in a given community or region; concurrent medical problems which dictate that certain drugs be used or avoided; the patient's response to selected medication. The following outlines of therapeutic drug monitoring offer examples which may serve to stimulate discussion and further understanding of initiating and monitoring drug use. The drugs and dosages presented should not be applied to any clinical situation without proper medical supervision.

Drug Therapy	Indomethacin 50 mg capsule 1 PO TID.
Monitoring	**Symptoms:** Ask the patient to describe the pain, its onset, duration, and precipitating cause (e.g., trauma, heavy ethanol use, low dose aspirin, proximal loop diuretic). Describe the number of joints affected. Note whether it is monoarticular. Ask the patient to describe the number and frequency of previous attacks. Ask if the drug treatment has relieved the pain.
	Signs: *Gen:* Is the patient obese? *Skin:* Look for tophi (i.e., gouty deposits) in the joints, olecranon bursa, infrapatellar and Achilles tendons, and extensor surface of the forearms. *MUS:* Examine the painful joint for warmth, redness, and tenderness. Inspect uninvolved joints for chronic arthritis-like changes.
Laboratory Tests	The clinician may elect to order all, none, or some of these laboratory studies depending upon history and physical findings, as well as other specific clinical indications. Serum uric acid, 24-hour urine uric acid (sometimes), serum creatinine/blood urea nitrogen (BUN), LFTs, CBC.
Adverse Drug Event Monitoring	**Indomethacin:** Check for central nervous system (CNS) effects such as fatigue, mild

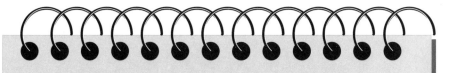

Therapeutic Drug Monitoring Examples

ACUTE GOUTY ARTHRITIS
(continued)

Adverse Drug Event Monitoring	confusion, vertigo, and headache. Assess GI side effects for nausea, dyspepsia, diarrhea, or epigastric pain. Does the patient have a history of aspirin-sensitive bronchospasm, nasal polyps associated with angioedema, or recent peptic ulcer?

Nervous System

*T*he nervous system functions to receive, interpret, and respond to stimuli and can be affected by the actions of many drugs.

ANATOMY AND PHYSIOLOGY

The neuron is the basic unit of the nervous system. Structurally, it is composed of a nerve cell body, nerve fiber (i.e., axon), and a dendrite. **Efferent** nerve fibers (i.e., axons) connect to other nerve cell bodies, muscles, glands, or sensory organs and conduct nerve impulses from the central nervous system (CNS) to the periphery. **Afferent** nerve fibers conduct nerve impulses from the periphery (e.g., sensory nerves of the fingertips) to the CNS (e.g., sensory nerves of the cerebral cortex). Efferent nerve fibers conduct nerve impulses from the CNS (e.g., motor area of the cerebellar cortex) to the periphery (e.g., biceps muscle of the arm causing the elbow to flex). After recognition of afferent impulses, a response is sent from the CNS by efferent neurons to effectors such as skeletal muscles, involuntary muscles, and glands.

Central and Peripheral Nervous Systems

The nervous system is composed of the central nervous system and the peripheral nervous system (see Figures 14.1 and 14.2). The components of the central nervous system are the brain, the brain stem, and the spinal cord. The spinal cord is attached to the brain through the brain stem and consists of 31 pairs of spinal nerves (i.e., 8 cervical, 12 thoracic, 5 lumbar, 5 sacral, and 1 coccygeal nerve pair). Each paired spinal nerve has dorsal and ventral roots carrying hundreds of individual nerve fibers to and from the spinal cord. These nerve roots are located in rows along the spine. Though the spinal cord ends at the first lumbar vertebra, the spinal nerves continue to exit at their respective vertebral level (e.g., L2, L3, L4). Thus, in the more distal spinal cord, the spinal nerve level in the cord is higher than the vertebral level at which the spinal nerve exits to the rest of the body (see Figure 14.3).

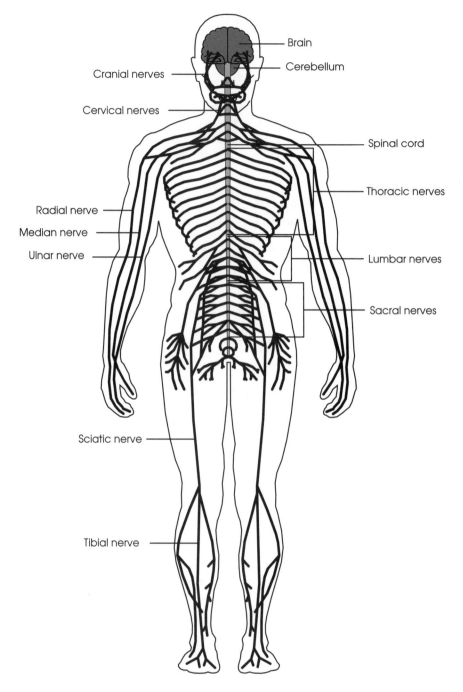

Fig. 14.1 The peripheral nervous system.

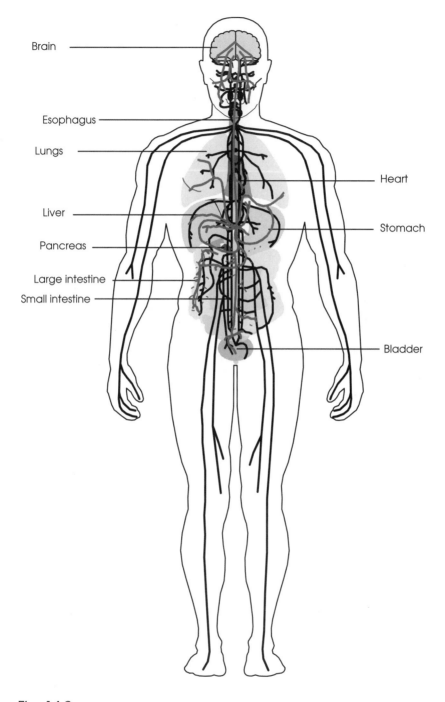

Fig. 14.2 The sympathetic and parasympathetic nervous systems.

The brain weighs approximately 1300 to 1400 gm in the young adult and is divided into three regions: the **cerebrum**, the **cerebellum**, and the **brain stem**. The cerebrum is separated into two hemispheres: the right and the left. Each cerebral hemisphere has four lobes: the frontal lobe, the parietal lobe, the temporal lobe, and the occipital lobe (see Figure 14.4).

The **frontal lobe** controls voluntary skeletal movements and some personality characteristics. The **parietal lobes** control complex functions such as speech, reasoning, and sensation. The **temporal lobes** are associated with the senses of hearing, taste, and smell. The **occipital lobes** are associated with vision. The **cerebellum** attaches to the brain stem and is divided into right and left cerebellar hemispheres. It functions primarily to coordinate balance. The **brain stem** consists of the medulla, pons, midbrain, and diencephalon. Certain "vital" centers (e.g., the centers that control respiration and body temperature) are located in the brain stem. Outside the central nervous system, the peripheral nervous system is divided into nerves associated with the motor pathways, the basic reflex arcs, and the sensory pathways.

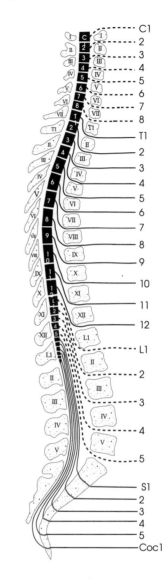

Fig. 14.3 Points at which spinal nerve segments exit the vertebral column.

Motor Pathways

Voluntary movements originate in the motor cortex of the frontal lobe. The left motor strip (i.e., cortex) controls the right side of the body while the right motor strip controls the left side of the body. Each motor strip corresponds to specific muscle functions. For instance, the left motor strip controls the larynx, tongue, right side of the face, thorax, abdomen, and the right thigh, calf, foot, hand, and arm. Thus, injury to the left motor

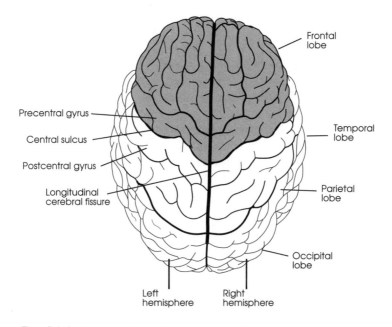

Fig. 14.4 The superior surface of the brain illustrating the location of the four lobes of each hemisphere (right and left).

cortex could result in an inability to voluntarily move the right arm. The efferent pathway from the motor cortex to the skeletal muscles consists of **pyramidal** (i.e., upper motor neurons) and **peripheral** nerve fibers (i.e., lower motor neurons). The upper motor neuron fibers descend from the cerebral cortex to the spinal cord in bundles known as tracts. These nerve tracts are named by compound words which contain the name of their place of origin followed by the name of their termination. In the case of the cortex motor fibers going to the spinal cord, the tract is called the **corticospinal tract**. Most motor neurons follow the corticospinal tract and cross over to the opposite side of the body in a part of the brain stem called the **pyramid** (e.g., the right cortex controls function of the left arm). Some motor nerve fibers, however, diverge from the corticospinal tract in the midbrain to form the **corticobulbar tract**. The motor neurons in the corticobulbar tract terminate in the brain stem on the cranial nerve nuclei (e.g., the trigeminal, hypoglossal, glossopharyngeal, vagus, facial, oculomotor, trochlear, abducent, and accessory nerves). Both corticospinal and corticobulbar neurons are often called upper motor neurons.

Lesions in the upper and lower neurons often cause distinctive symptoms. For example, a lesion that damages the pyramidal tract prevents voluntary motor impulses from reaching the spinal motor horn cells below the lesion site. Such an upper motor neuron lesion would still leave the reflex arch intact. Normally, the motor cortex sends impulses to reduce muscle tone; however, this dampening action is lost when a lesion in the upper motor neuron develops. Over several days to a few weeks following such injury [e.g., a cerebrovascular accident (CVA) or stroke], the stretch reflexes of the intact reflex arch become hyperactive. Hyperactive stretch reflexes increase muscle tonus resulting in stiff, firm muscles (i.e., spasticity) and resistance to passive movements of the limb. In the absence of motor cortex signals to reduce muscle tone, the tendon reflexes in the affected limbs become hyperactive with clonus (i.e., rhythmic jerks). If passive exercises are not performed, the flexor muscles, being stronger than extensor muscles, contract and prevent the joint from being extended. The joint becomes rigid and "fixed" in a flexed or "drawn-up" position.

Lower motor neuron damage usually retards function in more discrete muscle groups while upper motor damage results in more generalized disorders. In contrast to lower motor neuron disease, disruption to the pyramidal (i.e., the upper motor neuron) tract affects whole body muscle groups (e.g., the leg). For example, cervical level disease destroys motor function in both the leg and arm on the same (i.e., ipsilateral) side as the lesion. If the lesion is above the crossover of the tract, then the loss of motor function occurs in the limbs on the opposite (i.e., contralateral) side.

Destruction of the lower motor neurons abolishes both voluntary and reflex responses, causing normal muscle tonus to disappear. In the early stages of lower motor neuronal damage, the muscles fasciculate, the limb becomes flaccid, and tendon reflexes become absent. Within a few weeks the muscles atrophy and may ultimately disappear.

Sensory Pathways

The sensory nerves receive a variety of stimuli and organize the sensations for recognition and reaction in the cerebral cortex. Stimulation of peripheral sensory receptors generates afferent impulses that are carried by various nerve tracts through the spinal cord to the midbrain where the impulses are reorganized and transferred to the cerebral sensory cortex. Since lesions at different places in sensory pathways produce varying kinds of sensory loss, testing with various stimuli can help to localize pathologic lesions. Some of the sensations that can be tested include proprioception (i.e., sense of position), pain, temperature, light touch, and vibration. These various stimuli are carried to the cerebrum by different pathways or tracts within the spinal cord and brain. Three nerve tracts of clinical importance are the posterior column, the lateral spinothalamic, and anterior spinothalamic tracts (see Figures 14.5 and 14.6).

In the **posterior column tract**, nerve impulses associated with **proprioception, light touch**, and **vibration** are carried to the medulla where the nerve fibers cross over and convey these sensations to other contralateral higher nerve centers (i.e., the cerebrum, the cerebellum, and certain nuclei). Upon reaching the thalamus, the posterior column tract is on the opposite side from its entry into the spinal cord.

Pain and **temperature** sensations are carried by the **lateral spinothalamic tract** from peripheral receptors in the skin, mucous membranes, muscles, and viscera into the spinal cord (see Figure 14.7). The impulses then cross over to the opposite side, and continue through the lateral spinothalamic tract to synapses in the thalamus. At the thalamic level, crude perceptions of pain and temperature occur. However, only in the sensory cortex is fine sensory discrimination possible. The **anterior spinothalamic**

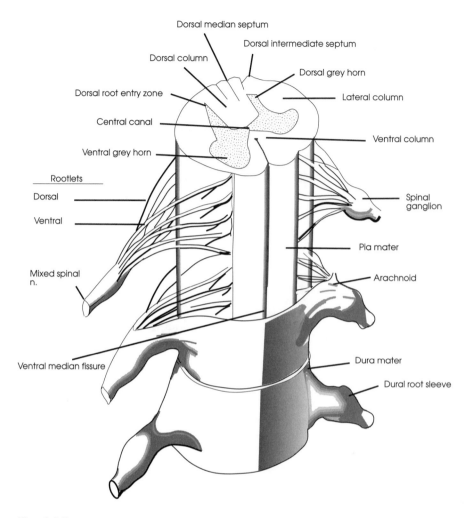

Fig. 14.5 General structure of the spinal cord, nerve roots, and meninges.

tract organizes **crude touch** sensations. Nerve fibers in this tract cross over to the opposite side in the spinal column and ascend to the thalamus. In the thalamus, the fibers reorganize before terminating in the sensory cortex. By examining any deficits in the patient's perception of these various sensations, the clinician can begin to localize possible sites of lesions. For example, the loss of crude touch sensations points toward damage to the anterior spinothalamic tract.

Reflex Arch

The skeletal muscles continuously maintain tension known as tonus through what is termed a **reflex arc**. When a person passively stretches a muscle, a small amount of

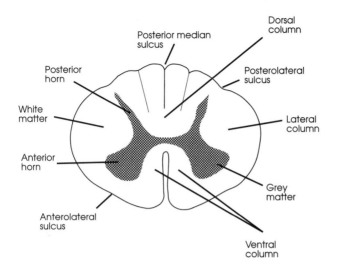

Fig. 14.6   Transverse section of the spinal cord. Ventral column carrying anterior spinothalmic tracts (crude touch); lateral column carrying lateral spinothalmic tracts (pain and temperature); and posterior column carrying nerve fibers associated with proprioception, light touch, and vibratory sense.

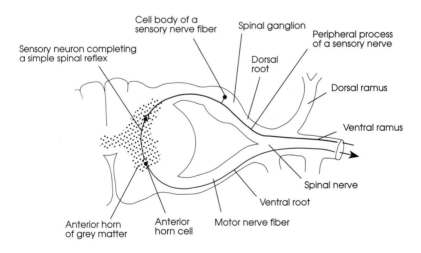

Fig. 14.7   Relationship of spinal nerves to spinal cord. Afferent doral spinal nerve fibers enter into cord terminating in gray matter or traveling various tracts to the brain. Efferent ventral spinal nerve fibers exiting the cord going to peripheral structures.

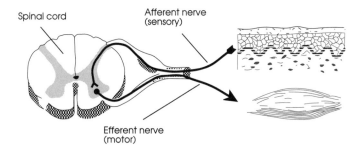

Spinal cord

Afferent nerve
(sensory)

Efferent nerve
(motor)

Fig. 14.8 Reflex arc: Babinski sign—scratching bottom of foot with blunt object creates afferent sensory input resulting in efferant motor output, flexion of the toes. Deep tendon reflex—striking patellar tendon with reflex hammer excites stretch receptors which carry afferent impulse to the spinal cord gray matter and creates lower motor neuron response through efferent nerve resulting in muscle contraction and knee jerk.

resistance is normally felt. When a muscle stretches, nerve impulses travel through afferent fibers to the spinal cord. Afferent (i.e., sensory) nerve fibers enter the spinal cord through the posterior (i.e., dorsal) root where they synapse on the motor neuron (i.e., the anterior horn cell). The impulses stimulate the motor neuron and exit the spinal cord through the efferent (i.e., motor) nerve fibers through the anterior (i.e., ventral) root to the muscle. The muscle contracts, thus completing what is known as the reflex arc (see Figure 14.8). Note that the reflex arc involves only the lower motor neurons and not the upper motor neurons. When a reflex hammer is used to test the reflex arc by stretching a muscle's tendon, the muscle contraction is called a deep tendon reflex (DTR). Specific spinal nerves are tested by striking specific muscle-tendon-nerve combinations. For example, the C5-C6 spinal nerve innervates the biceps. If you tap the biceps tendon at the elbow with a reflex hammer and the biceps muscle contracts, this indicates that the C5-C6 reflex arc is intact and functioning. An abnormality in the reflex arc helps to localize lesions. Table 14.1 presents a more complete listing of spinal segment levels and their associated deep tendon reflexes.

Dermatomes

Skin pain is transmitted by sensory fibers entering the spinal cord through the dorsal nerve roots. The band of skin innervated by the sensory nerve root of a single spinal segment is called a **dermatome** (see Figure 14.9). Through the use of a stimulus such as pin prick, an understanding of dermatome patterns can help determine the level or location of spinal nerve injury. The absence of sensation over a certain dermatome indicates that efferent sensation is not reaching the brain (e.g., the nerve has been cut or is compressed by a tumor). Sensory dermatomes are also used to determine the level of anesthesia when an epidural is given for labor and delivery or for a C-section

Spinal Nerve Segment Distribution and Reflexes

Table 14.1

Spinal Nerve Segment Level	Reflex
Deep Tendon Reflexes	
Cervical 5 and 6	Biceps
Cervical 5 and 6	Brachioradialis
Cervical 6, 7, and 8	Triceps
Lumbar 2, 3, and 4	Knee (patellar)
Lumbar 5	Ankle (Achilles)
Sacral 1 and 2	Ankle (Achilles)
Superficial Reflexes	
Thoracic 8, 9, and 10	Upper abdomen (above umbilicus)
Thoracic 11 and 12	Lower abdomen (below umbilicus)
Lumbar 4 and 5	Plantar (Babinski sign)
Sacral 1 and 2	Plantar (Babinski sign)

delivery. If sensation cannot be felt below the umbilicus, the anesthesia is effective from thoracic level 10 (i.e., the dermatome at level of umbilicus) on down (e.g., T10, T11, T12, L1).

Cranial Nerves

The names and functions of the 12 pairs of cranial nerves are outlined in Table 14.2; the superficial points of origin for the cranial nerves are illustrated in Figure 14.10. The **olfactory** nerves (CN1) have receptors in the nasal mucosa and their afferent impulses go directly to the cerebral cortex. In response to light, impulses conduct through the **optic** nerves (CN2) to the occipital cortex. Located in front of the pituitary gland, the afferent nerve fibers from the nasal side of the eye cross in the optic chiasm before synapsing in the thalamus, then travel to the occipital cortex. Different fields of vision can be lost depending upon the location of an injury on the nerve. For instance, damage in the optic chiasm causes the loss of the temporal field of vision in both eyes.

The **oculomotor** nerves (CN3) innervate all but two of the eye muscles. Oculomotor paresis (i.e., weakness) or paralysis will display such physical examination findings as external strabismus (i.e., outward eye turning), ptosis (i.e., upper lid drooping), and mydriasis (i.e., enlarged pupil). The **trochlear** nerves (CN4) control the superior oblique muscle of the eye. Damage to these nerves impairs downward and outward eye movement. The **abducens** nerves (CN6) control lateral eye movements (i.e., the lateral rectus muscle). Diplopia (i.e., double vision) is a complaint expressed by patients with paresis of the abducens nerve (see Chapter 5: Eye).

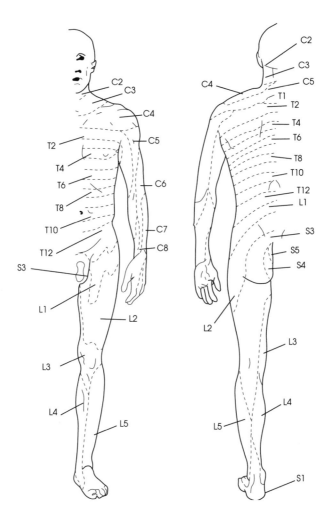

Fig. 14.9 Anterior and posterior views of dermatome distribution patterns.

The **trigeminal** nerves (CN5) have motor (i.e., efferent) and sensory (i.e., afferent) branches. Damage to the motor component can result in atrophy and weakness of the jaw muscles. Trigeminal lesions produce loss of pain and temperature perception on the same side of the face with a peripheral nerve lesion, but on the opposite side of the body if the lesion occurs in the medulla or lower pons. Trigeminal neuralgia (i.e., tic douloureux) is an extremely painful sensory branch nerve disorder. The **facial** nerves (CN7) have a motor component which controls facial expressions and closes the eyelids. Disorders of the facial nerves cause unilateral smiling, as well as a flattening of the nasal labial fold and the inability to wrinkle the forehead. Because the eyelid does not close properly, the involved eye suffers chronic irritation and dryness. Bell's palsy is usually a temporary facial muscle paralysis due to involvement of the facial nerve.

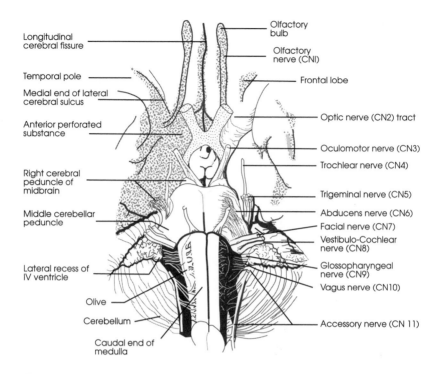

Fig. 14.10 The inferior surface of the brain showing the superficial origins of the 12 cranial nerves.

The **auditory** nerves (CN8) have two branches: the acoustic and vestibular. The acoustic nerve originates in the hair cells of the cochlea, enters the brain stem, and terminates in the temporal lobe of the cerebrum. Hearing loss and tinnitus are common complaints of acoustic dysfunction, excessive cerumen, or middle ear disease. The vestibular branch begins in the inner ear's three semicircular canals, reaches the medulla, and terminates on the cerebellum. Two vestibulospinal tracts descend the spine to maintain muscle strength against gravity and upright posture. The vestibular fibers are interconnected to eye motor functions that control eye position and enable the eyes to remain stationary on objects when the head turns. Stimulation of the vestibular apparatus produces subjective sensations of body motion. The patient may have a feeling of objects moving about (i.e., vertigo). If these sensations recur as attacks of vertigo, tinnitus, and nausea, then Meniere's syndrome may be the problem. Motion sickness is vertigo associated with air, auto, or sea travel (see Chapter 6: Ear).

The **glossopharyngeal** (CN9) and **vagal** (CN10) nerves originate in the medulla. The glossopharyngeal nerves control motor functions of the pharyngeal structures and receive sensory input from the ear canal, tympanic membrane, and posterior portion of the tongue. The vagus nerves overlap these areas. Vagal branches serve

Table 14.2

Cranial Nerves

Cranial Nerve	Number	Function
Olfactory	1	Smell: The nerve transmits impulses to the brain from the nasal receptors
Optic	2	Vision
Oculomotor	3	Pupillary constriction, elevation of the upper eyelid, eye movement
Trochlear	4	Downward and inward movements of the eye
Trigeminal	5	*Motor branch:* temporal and masseter muscle clenching of the jaw
		Sensory branch: facial sensations of touch and pain
Abducens	6	Lateral eye movement
Facial	7	*Motor branch:* forehead movement, muscles of facial expression
		Sensory branch: taste sensations (anterior tongue)
Acoustic	8	Hearing and balance
Glossopharyngeal	9	*Motor branch:* movement of pharyngeal structures
		Sensory branch: sensations of the ear canal, eardrum, and taste (posterior portion of the tongue)
Vagus	10	*Motor branch:* movement of the palate, pharynx, and larynx
		Sensory branch: sensations of the pharynx and larynx
Spinal Accessory	11	Movements of the shoulders and neck muscles
Hypoglossal	12	Movements of the tongue

[a] A useful mnemonic utilizes the first character from each word in the following sentence to identify the cranial nerves in order of ascendancy. "**On** old **O**lympus **t**owering **t**ops **a** **F**inn and **G**erman **v**iewed **s**ome **h**ops."

the external auditory canal, pharynx, soft palate, larynx, vocal cords, and cardiac muscle. Damage to cranial nerves 9 and 10 can affect swallowing (e.g., dysphagia), speaking (e.g., hoarseness, dysphonia, or dysarthria), tasting, coughing, or gagging.

The **spinal accessory** nerves (CN11) innervate the trapezius muscles and sternocleidomastoid muscles. Spinal accessory nerve damage presents as shoulder and neck muscle weakness. The **hypoglossal** nerves (CN12) innervate the muscles of the tongue. Speech impairment, tongue atrophy, tongue fasciculations, and deviation from the midline on tongue protrusion are signs of hypoglossal nerve damage.

PHYSICAL ASSESSMENT

Neurologic evaluation is extremely variable. This chapter reviews basic screening procedures for examining cranial nerve functions, motor functions, sensory functions, and deep tendon reflexes. If a patient has a chronic sensory deficit, chronic pain, or other neurologic complaints, more extensive examination techniques need to be explored and are beyond the scope of this chapter.

As discussed in earlier chapters, the neurologic assessment should be integrated throughout the entire physical examination. For example, most cranial nerves are evaluated while examining the head and neck (see Chapter 7: Head, Neck, and Face); motor and sensory functions are part of the musculoskeletal examination (see Chapter 12: Musculoskeletal System), while reflex testing stands alone. After the physical data have been collected, the information is organized in the neurologic write-up section of a complete exam. In a patient complaining of a specific neurologic problem, one performs specific evaluations that further define the problem.

Cranial Nerves

Begin the neurologic examination by assessing the 12 cranial nerves (see Table 14.2). Test the olfactory nerve (CN1) by asking the patient to close both eyes, occlude one nostril, and smell and identify a mildly aromatic substance such as alcohol or soap. Repeat the procedure with the other nostril. Next, evaluate the optic nerve by asking the patient to read the smallest print on a hand-held eye card or newspaper. Then use an ophthalmoscope to complete the eye exam (see Chapter 5: Eye). Check pupil reaction to light, accommodation, and the six fields of gaze to evaluate the second, third, fourth, and sixth (CN2, 3, 4, and 6) cranial nerves.

Examine fifth cranial nerve (CN5, i.e., trigeminal) motor functions by asking the patient to clench her teeth and then relax as you palpate the temporal and masseter muscles. Trigeminal nerve function can be tested by alternately stimulating the nerve with the dull and sharp ends of a safety pin along the nerve route. During normal conversation, evaluate the function of the facial nerve (CN7) by looking for any signs of facial asymmetry, loss of nasal labial folds, or abnormal facial movements. Auditory (CN8), glossopharyngeal (CN9), and vagus (CN10) nerve testing have been described in Chapters 6: Ear and 7: Head, Neck and Face. Evaluate the spinal accessory nerve (CN11) by instructing the patient to shrug her shoulders against your hands while observing strength and contraction of the trapezius muscles. Finally, assess hypoglossal (CN12) nerve functions by asking the patient to stick out her tongue. With normal nerve function, the tongue remains in the midline with minimal tremor.

Balance and Gait

Next, assess cerebellar and basal ganglia function by carefully inspecting the coordination and smoothness of the patient's gait and hand movements. To test cerebellar function, ask the patient to walk across the room, then return. The normal gait is relaxed, with the arms swinging smoothly, and balance maintained. Ask the patient to walk a straight line in a "heel-to-toe" fashion. This may be difficult for the aged; you should walk alongside the patient to guard against falling. Muscle weakness may impair a patient's ability to perform this test. However, if the patient has difficulty maintaining balance, evaluate cerebellar function further with the Romberg test. Balance is maintained by vision, vestibular sense, and proprioception. To complete the Romberg test, ask the patient to stand with both feet together and arms at the side. Note the patient's ability to maintain balance. Then, instruct the patient to maintain his position with both eyes closed. Be careful to stand close to the patient to prevent a falling injury. Normally, minimal swaying is seen. Loss of the ability to maintain balance is a positive Romberg sign usually associated with proprioception or vestibular malfunction. These tests reflect whole body coordination skills. If the patient has difficulty with coordination or if specific nerve deficits are identified, arm and leg coordination should then be tested.

Test arm coordination by having the patient hold his arms outstretched laterally with eyes closed. Then have the patient rapidly and alternately touch an index finger to the nose. An alternate method to test cerebellar function is to have the supine patient slowly move a heel along the shin from the knee to ankle and return to the knee. The patient performs the test smoothly without awkwardness when cerebellar function is normal.

Muscle Testing

To evaluate the motor system, inspect muscle groups for atrophy and asymmetry. If a muscle is not used, secondary to efferent nerve supply damage, atrophy or muscle wasting is seen. Always compare corresponding muscle groups in a symmetrical fashion.

Measure muscle tone by passive range of motion testing. Ask the patient to relax the muscle being evaluated while you move the limb freely in various directions. Normally, muscles maintain slight tension. Abnormal flaccidity, pain, rigidity, spasticity, or cogwheeling should be documented if noted.

Changes or differences in muscle strength may reflect underlying neurologic problems. The basic techniques for evaluating these changes involve asking the patient to make movements against the resistance of your hand or moving a limb against gravity. As in other physical examination procedures, it is important to bilaterally compare muscle groups in reference to the patient's age, gender, and physical condition. Table 14.3 provides a five-point rating scale for muscle strength.

Muscle Strength Rating Scale

Table 14.3

Grade	Interpretation
0	No evidence of muscle contraction.
1	Slight muscle contraction without joint motion.
2	Muscle and joint movement without gravity.
3	Slight muscle and joint movement with gravity.
4	Muscle and join movement with gravity and some resistance.
5	Muscle and joint movement against gravity and full resistance.

Upper Extremity Strength

To evaluate upper extremity strength, ask the patient to close both eyes and to extend both arms with the palms open upward. The patient should be able to hold this position without difficulty for 20 to 30 seconds. If the patient's arms drift downward, a mild hemiparesis may be present. Test the patient's hand grip strength by crossing your index and middle finger and asking the patient to squeeze your fingers with his hand while you try to remove your fingers from the patient's grip. This exercise tests the strength of the patient's forearm muscle group. You should have difficulty removing your fingers from the hand of a patient with normal grip strength. In contrast, patients with nerve or muscle disorders have difficulty restricting the withdrawal of your fingers from their hands. Now ask the patient to abduct (i.e., spread) his fingers against your resistance; weakness suggests possible ulnar nerve damage.

To evaluate proximal arm motor strength, have the patient flex the elbow at his side with the hand at the shoulder. To check the biceps (i.e., elbow flexion), place your left hand on the patient's right elbow to steady it while grasping the patient's left hand with your right hand and pull the hand toward you against the patient's resistance. Check the left arm in a similar manner. To evaluate the triceps muscle (i.e., elbow extension), again steady the patient's elbow, but have the patient push his hand toward you away from his shoulder against resistance of your hand. Do this for both the right and left arms. Instruct the patient to extend and flex at the elbow against your hand to test upper arm strength.

Lower Extremity Strength

To evaluate lower extremity motor function, place the patient in a supine position on an examining table or bed. With your hand on the patient's knee, have the patient flex at the hip. To test abduction at the hip, place your hands on the outside of the patient's knee and ask the patient to spread her legs against your hands; reverse the procedures and place your hands on the inside of the knees to test hip adduction. Then, flex one of the patient's knees and place your left hand on the patient's knee and your right hand behind the patient's ankle. Now instruct the patient to resist as you try to straighten (i.e., extend) the flexed knee; again, reverse the procedure with instructions to resist your flexing of the knee. Repeat these techniques on the other leg. Test dorsiflexion and plantar flexion by asking the patient to pull (i.e., dorsiflex) and push (i.e., plantarflex) against your hand placed on the patient's distal foot.

The phrase, "More marked in the distal than in the proximal joints," is frequently encountered in descriptions of weakness or abnormality. A joint is "distal" with respect to another joint in the same limb if it is further away from the body trunk. A joint is said to be "proximal" with respect to another joint if it is closer to the body trunk. For example, the ankle is "distal" with respect to the knee. If a weakness is greater in the distal joints, it is likely to be caused by a neurological problem. Whereas with proximal joint weakness, the problem is probably due to muscular weakness rather than nerve damage.

Sensory Testing

Accurate sensory testing requires the cooperation of a patient who is mentally alert, comfortable, and not impaired by analgesics or other central nervous system depressants. As in all situations, carefully explain the testing procedures to the patient. In a patient without suspected neurological deficit, screening procedures such as comparison of light touch in the arms and legs, or testing pain and vibration perception in the hands and feet usually are adequate. If sensory deficits are suspected, more focused testing is needed for the detection of specific neurological deficits.

When assessing sensory function always remember the following guidelines:

- Compare symmetrical areas of the body.

- Compare distal and proximal areas in the arms and legs when testing pain and touch.

- When examining vibration and position perception, test the knuckles of the fingers and toes.

- Vary the testing rhythm so that the patient does not anticipate the stimuli.

Findings of muscular atrophy, numbness, weakness, excessive pain, or abnormal reflexes indicate a need for more extensive testing.

Pain, Proprioception, Touch, and Vibration

Throughout the sensory test examination, the patient's eyes should be closed. First, test **superficial pain sensations** by applying random pressure to the patient's skin with both the sharp and dull ends of a safety pin. Press the safety pin lightly into the skin and ask the patient to identify the sensations as being "sharp" or "dull." Always test the hands, feet, and cheeks bilaterally by using two pins simultaneously for evaluation of superficial pain sensations.

With the patient's eyes closed, bend the big toe of each foot upward and downward to test for position sense (i.e., **proprioception testing**) by asking the patient to identify the position of the toe. Randomly repeat the procedure. Be sure to grasp the big toe on the sides to prevent giving the patient position clues. The neurological impairment associated with pernicious anemia or the peripheral neuropathy of isoniazid affects posterior column pathways and impairs position sense. The upper extremities are only tested for proprioception if the lower extremities are abnormal or if specific upper body neurologic symptoms are present (e.g., numbness or paresthesia).

Vibratory sense is evaluated by briskly tapping the handle of a 128 cycles per second (cps) tuning fork and firmly applying it to the bony prominence of the wrist and ankle. Ask the patient to indicate when the vibration of the tuning fork is felt. Differentiate the patient's ability to distinguish vibration sensation from pressure sensation by stopping the vibrations of the tuning fork and asking the patient whether the sensation is different. Aged patients normally have reduced vibratory perception which begins distal, and, over time, moves proximal.

If pain and proprioception are normal, testing **tactile sense** or the ability to discern light touch is not necessary. To test light touch, use a fine cotton wisp and ask the patient to indicate when the sensation of touch is felt. Touch the hands, feet, and face in a symmetrically random fashion.

By conducting these testing procedures in an orderly fashion, you can identify sensory deficits and infer the possible location of lesions or pathologic processes (e.g., peripheral neuropathy of diabetes). If these tests are abnormal, then test for the ability to discern temperature and distinguish forms by placing objects in the patient's hands (i.e., stereognosis).

Reflex Testing: Deep Tendon Reflexes (DTRs)

Tests for deep tendon reflexes actually evaluate reflexes in which muscles are suddenly stretched by the tap of a reflex rubber hammer. Swing the rubber hammer freely between the thumb and index finger to deliver a brisk but reproducible, constant force to each target tendon. Observe the muscle group being tested and note its contraction and relaxation response. When the tendon is suddenly stretched, the attached muscle group normally responds by contracting. Table 14.1 lists the distribution of spinal nerves with their corresponding reflex testing sites. The interpretation of reflex responses is subjectively graded using a five point scale (see Table 14.4 and Figure 14.11). A normal person has symmetrically equal reflexes. The presence of asymmetry should be considered abnormal until demonstrated otherwise.

In the upper extremity, test the deep tendon reflexes of the biceps, triceps, and brachioradialis. Use the sharp end of the reflex hammer on the bicep and tricep tendons; however, use the dull hammer end on the brachioradialis. In the biceps test, the patient's arm is flexed at the elbow with the palm down. Hold the patient's arm at the elbow with your thumb pressing lightly against the biceps tendon in the antecubital fossa. Deliver a brisk tap to the tendon. If the reflex functions normally, the biceps muscle contracts, causing a slight flexion of the forearm. To test the triceps tendon response, flex the patient's

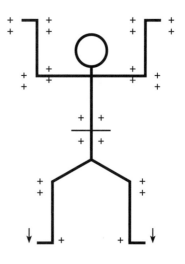

Fig. 14.11 An example of a stick figure used for deep tendon reflex (DTR) recording. The following grading scale is used to record DTR responses: 0 = no response; + = diminished response; ++ = normal response; +++ = increased response; ++++ = hyperactive response with or without clonus.

elbow, support the patient's arm at the wrist, and strike the triceps tendon. Normally, the triceps muscle contracts and the forearm extends. Next, with the patient's arm resting on her leg (if sitting) or across her abdomen (if supine), tap the brachioradialis tendon one inch above the wrist. You should see a normal flexion and supination of the forearm and maybe slight finger and hand flexion.

Table 14.4

Deep Tendon Reflex Grading Scale

Grade		Interpretation
0	0	No response[a]
1	+	Slight response
2	++	Normal
3	+++	Increased response
4	++++	Hyperactive with or without clonus[b]

[a] Sensory loss and absent or diminished reflexes associated with lower motor neuron damage or spinal segment damage. May also be seen with other medical conditions such as hypothyroidism and spinal cord injury.

[b] Associated with upper motor nerve damage (i.e., stroke). May also be seen with other medical conditions such as hyperthyroidism and pre-eclampsia of pregnancy.

In the lower extremity, test the deep tendon reflexes of the knee (i.e., patellar reflex) and ankle (i.e., Achilles reflex). First, with the patient's knees flexed by sitting on the bedside or supported by the examiner, briskly tap the patella tendon below the knee and watch for the normal contraction of the thigh quadriceps muscles and extension of the lower leg. The ankle or Achilles tendon reflex involves contraction of the calf muscle. While slightly pushing against the foot plantar surface over the metatarsal heads, tap the Achilles tendon just above the heel, level with the ankle. The calf muscle should contract, causing the foot to plantar flex.

Reflex Testing: Superficial Reflexes

Superficial reflexes are elicited by briskly stroking the skin with the blunt end of the reflex hammer. The deep tendon reflexes are important because they do not involve the brain, but are dependent upon the integrity of the reflex arc and spinal cord of the particular spinal nerve. In contrast, superficial reflexes test the higher motor centers in the brain as well as the reflex arc and spinal cord.

Examine the superficial reflexes in the abdomen and foot with symmetrical testing to reference and compare responses. Using the dull end of the reflex hammer or tongue blade, lightly stroke toward the patient's umbilicus in all four abdominal quadrants. The normal response is contraction of the abdominal muscles and deviation of the umbilicus toward the stimulus. In an obese patient, stretch the skin near the umbilicus away from the umbilicus on the side opposite to the side being stimulated. To test the foot or plantar response (i.e., Babinski reflex), use a blunt object to stroke the lateral and metatarsal surface in a smooth inverted L-shaped motion across the bottom of the foot. Normally, the toes plantar flex. Big toe dorsiflexion and fanning of the other toes is an abnormal response and is termed a positive Babinski sign which is associated with upper motor neuron dysfunction (e.g., stroke).

PHARMACOTHERAPEUTIC CASE ILLUSTRATION

History

A.T., a 64-year-old male was evaluated in the clinic because of frequent falls. His wife stated that he fell yesterday and that a neighbor had to help get him up. A.T. was in his usual state of health until ten years ago when he began to display symptoms of lethargy and weakness. His family physician diagnosed him as having Parkinson's disease. At that time, A.T. was able to feed himself, but unable to shave and dress himself. As the disease progressed, he developed resting tremor and slow awkwardness of movement. Presently, his parkinsonism has progressed and he needs assistance with dressing, standing, and other activities of daily living (ADL). Although the course of his disease has been marked with symptoms worsening and then improving, his condition has gradually worsened. In the past several months, he developed dysphagia which required hospitalization. At that time, endoscopic examination of the esophagus and stomach revealed gastritis along with impaired motility of the esophagus which was presumed secondary to his parkinsonism.

Past medical history (PMH) revealed hydrocele repair, mumps, and pneumonia. Social history (SH) indicated no tobacco or alcohol use. He has an 8th grade education. His father died at age 70 of myocardial infarction (MI), and his mother is alive at age 81. He has four sisters and two brothers living with no known medical problems.

Review of systems (ROS) was significant as follows: Mouth: History of difficulty swallowing. Cardiovascular: An episode of heart failure. Gastrointestinal (GI): Blood in stool. Neuropsychiatric: One episode of hallucinatory reaction to Mellaril; some difficulty with memory of recent events; history of depression associated with parkinsonism.

Current medications were amitriptyline (Elavil) 50 mg tablet HS, alprazolam (Xanax) 1 mg tablet TID, and a multivitamin capsule every day. He had no known drug or food allergies.

Physical Examination

Physical findings revealed a 64-year-old male, well-developed and well-nourished (WDWN) with expressionless face, poverty of movements, and walking with a stooped shuffling gait. His heart had a regular rhythm without murmur or extra heart sounds. His lungs were clear to auscultation and percussion. His abdomen had normal bowel sounds and no masses or enlarged organs. There was some moderate tenderness to deep palpation of the epigastrium and right upper quadrant. Rectal stool was heme positive for occult blood and he had external hemorrhoids. Sensory exam was intact to light touch, pin prick, vibration, and proprioception. Muscle strength was 4/5 bilaterally in all extremities. He had generalized fasciculations in the upper extremities and fine hand tremor at rest that disappeared with directed movement. Cogwheeling movements were present with passive flexion and extension of elbows and wrists. DTRs were 2/4 bilaterally in biceps, triceps, and patella. Achilles reflex was 1/4 bilaterally. Plantar reflex was negative for Babinski response. Cranial nerves 2 through 12 were grossly intact.

Laboratory

The following diagnostic tests were ordered and had no significant abnormal findings: chest x-ray, electrocardiogram (ECG), urinalysis (UA) with microscopic exam, SMA-18, and complete blood cell count (CBC).

Diagnosis and Management

A.T. was continued on his current medications and started on carbidopa/levodopa 10/100 tablet BID. Initially, the patient responded to the drug satisfactorily. However,

15 months later, the carbidopa/levodopa dose had to be steadily increased to control symptoms until abnormal involuntary movements (AIM) became a problem. Because of worsening dysphagia, bromocriptine (Parlodel) was added at 1.25 mg TID.

Discussion

Disease. Parkinsonism is a progressive, degenerative disorder of the motor system. This disease is a syndrome comprising rigidity, postural instability, gait disturbance, resting tremor, and bradykinesia. The classic triad of signs (i.e., rigidity, resting tremor, and bradykinesia) may be present to varying degrees. Some patients are predominantly bradykinetic while others have mostly tremor. The most disabling symptom is bradykinesia. These patients also suffer orthostatic hypotension, dystonia, ophthalmoplegia, and affective disorders. Disabling dementia is frequently diagnosed in these patients. A.T. initially complained of "lethargy and weakness" which are early symptoms of parkinsonism. As the disease progressed, he developed the more familiar resting tremor and bradykinesia.

Management. Newly diagnosed patients with only mild disability and no current drug therapy should have the nature of the illness explained to them. A.T. came to the clinic complaining of worsening disability. The activities of daily living (ADL) are the primary indicators of disability. Routine daily functions include feeding, dressing, grooming, bathing, walking, and bowel and bladder care. The decision to begin drug treatment depends upon the degree to which these functions are disrupted. For example, if the patient's work is disrupted, drug therapy might be started earlier than in a retired person. Before prescribing drugs, one must provide adequate physical therapy, occupational therapy, and psychological counseling to the patient and family.

Once the decision to use drugs is made, which one to prescribe must be determined. The choice is controversial. Some clinicians prefer amantadine (Symmetrel) and anticholinergic agents, while others prefer carbidopa/levodopa or bromocriptine. Identifying the predominant symptoms is helpful when making this decision. If the patient predominantly suffers from tremor, then an anticholinergic such as trihexyphenidyl (Artane) or benztropine (Cogentin) could be prescribed since tremor is believed to be secondary to acetylcholine stimulation. Carbidopa/levodopa or bromocriptine are very effective in rigid or bradykinetic states.

In this particular case, A.T. was employed until he was forced to retire. During the following eight years he has had adequate daily function. His tremor is worsened with onset of anxiety and disappears as his anxiety is relieved by psychotherapy or medication. For example, talking to the patient increased resting tremor and bodily movement which disappeared if he was not disturbed. A.T. was prescribed alprazolam (Xanax) for anxiety.

The presence of dysphagia raised concern. Decreased esophageal motility may result in aspiration of saliva and/or gastric contents into the lung. This is a leading cause of morbidity and mortality in the parkinsonian patient. A.T. had a history of pneumonia from aspiration. He must be fed very carefully with a pureed diet. Zealous feeding by family or nursing personnel increases the risk of aspiration pneumonia and possible death. Because of dysphagia, A.T. was started on carbidopa/levodopa 10/100 tablets BID.

Carbidopa/levodopa was the most useful drug adjuvant. However, its effectiveness diminished within three to five years with abnormal involuntary movements (AIM) increasing. Initially, you begin with a low dose and titrate to desired response or toxicity. The primary means of assessing efficacy is to determine the drug's effect on activities of daily living. The initial toxicities of this therapy are hypotension, gastrointestinal (GI) distress, and abnormal involuntary movements (AIM). AIM consists of dyskinesias of the neck, face, mouth, tongue, arms, or legs which are seen with too high of a dose. Over several years, the ability to perform activities of daily living worsens, requiring increasing dosage adjustments. As the disease progresses, frequent small doses will be needed to maintain some degree of activities of daily living. This loss of efficacy is known as "wearing off."

The "on-off" phenomenon is another problem associated with fluctuation in mobility. The patient alternates between periods of hyperkinesia, normal function, and hypokinesia. Involuntary movements, seen with the hyperkinetic state, include lip smacking, grimacing, motor restlessness, and neck twisting. The patient may revert to normal functions and then become hypokinetic. Hypokinesia is described as "freezing" posture which lasts for minutes to hours. A.T.'s carbidopa/levodopa dosage titration was limited by the onset of AIM. However, dysphagia worsened and bromocriptine was added to carbidopa/levodopa.

Dopamine agonists have several attractive advantages, including direct stimulation of dopamine receptors, longer duration of action, and possible D2 receptor selectivity. Bromocriptine has been used as monotherapy, combination therapy in advanced disease, and in mild disease. A.T. had advanced disease with carbidopa/levodopa toxicities. The addition of bromocriptine might lead to disease control and improvement in ADL. The most common, dose-related adverse effects are hallucinations, confusion, hypotension, and nausea. The initial dose of bromocriptine is 1.25 mg tablet BID and increased at 1.25 mg every three days. The total daily range is 20 to 40 mg. When adding bromocriptine, the carbidopa/levodopa dose may need to be reduced.

To assess treatment response, measure improvement in the patient's ability to function in his surroundings. For example, evaluate the patient's ability to feed, dress, shave, walk, groom, and transfer from bed to wheelchair.

Therapeutic Drug Monitoring Examples

PARKINSONISM

The approach to therapeutic drug monitoring by clinicians varies depending upon many factors. Some of these include preferences among clinicians in a given community or region; concurrent medical problems which dictate that certain drugs be used or avoided; the patient's response to selected medication. The following outlines of therapeutic drug monitoring offer examples which may serve to stimulate discussion and further understanding of initiating and monitoring drug use. The drugs and dosages presented should not be applied to any clinical situation without proper medical supervision.

Drug Therapy	Carbidopa/levodopa 25/250 mg tablet 1 PO TID.
Monitoring	**Symptoms:** Probe for a description of ADL functions: feeding, dressing, grooming, and walking. Then check more difficult motor functions such as driving and writing. Determine the patient's perception of his disability. Does the patient have dysphagia? Is falling a problem? Under treatment, have the symptoms progressed, stayed the same, or improved?
	Signs: *Gen:* Describe the patient's functional status. Look for the classic resting tremor. Is it bilateral? Or is bradykinesia dominant? *VS:* Check the blood pressure (BP) both supine and standing, pulse, respiration, and temperature. Did the BP decrease upon standing (see Chapter 10: Blood Vessels)? *MSE:* Is the patient's speech monotone and low in volume? Note orientation, memory, judgment, abstract reasoning, thought content/processing, and language skills (see Chapter 3: Mental Status Examination). Is the patient's handwriting small (i.e., micrographia) and tremulous? Is dementia present? Observe for signs of depression. *Skin:* Does the skin feel greasy? Examine the face and hair for

Therapeutic Drug Monitoring Examples

PARKINSONISM
(continued)

Monitoring	signs of seborrheic dermatitis (e.g., dandruff). *HEENT:* Characterize the facial expression ("mask face"). Is the patient drooling? Ask the patient to stick out her tongue. Do you see tremor or fasciculation? *Neuro:* Ask the patient to walk. Is bradykinesia present? Does the patient pass from a walking pace to running? Look for the classic parkinsonian gait and posture. Check balance with the Romberg test. Test the arms for rigidity (i.e., "cogwheel movement") and grip strength. Assess sensory function by pin prick and light touch. Investigate DTR response.
Laboratory Tests	None.
Adverse Drug Event Monitoring	**Levodopa/Carbidopa:** Ask the patient about feeling nauseated or vomiting. Look for the following abnormal involuntary movements (AIM): dyskinesias, myoclonus, choreiform, and dystonia. Question about "wearing off" effects. Ask about the "on-off" phenomenon. Determine any problem with **new onset** nightmares, anxiety, irritability, depression, delirium, and other psychiatric symptoms. Carefully measure the blood pressure for a 20 to 30 mm Hg drop. Count the pulse rate and judge the rhythm to determine if it is rapid or irregular.

Therapeutic Drug Monitoring Examples

TONIC-CLONIC SEIZURE

The approach to therapuetic drug monitoring by clinicians varies depending upon many factors. Some of these include preferences among clinicians in a given community or region; concurrent medical problems which dictate that certain drugs be used or avoided; the patient's response to selected medication. The following outlines of therapeutic drug monitoring offer examples which may serve to stimulate discussion and further understanding of initiating and monitoring drug use. The drugs and dosages presented should not be applied to any clinical situation without proper medical supervision.

Drug Therapy	Phenytoin 100 mg capsule 3 PO Q HS.
Monitoring	**Symptoms:** Ask the patient or witness to describe what happened before, during, and after the attack. Did the patient have an aura, abruptly lose consciousness, fall to the floor, stiffen out, stop breathing and become cyanotic, bite his tongue, and become incontinent of urine and bowel? During the seizure did the patient have alternating rhythmic jerking of total body and flaccidity? How long did the attack last? After the attack, did consciousness gradually return with a confusional state, lethargy, or postictal sleep? How often do the seizure attacks happen? On the present treatment, has the frequency of attacks decreased?
	Signs: No specific physical findings are associated with the disorder between seizure attacks.
Laboratory Tests	The clinician may elect to order all, none, or some of these laboratory studies depending upon history and physical findings, as well as other specific clinical indications. Complete blood count (CBC), serum phenytoin concentration, liver function tests (LFTs).

Therapeutic Drug Monitoring Examples

TONIC-CLONIC SEIZURE
(continued)

Adverse Drug Event Monitoring	**Phenytoin:** Listen for slurred speech. Has the patient experienced vertigo or diplopia? Note any report of symptoms of blood dyscrasia such as sore throat, fever, easy bruising, epistaxis, or petechiae. Listen for symptoms of hepatotoxicity (e.g., anorexia, abdominal discomfort, jaundice, enlarged liver, or dark urine). Examine the skin for a morbilliform rash. Conduct a mental status exam; listening for symptoms of poor memory, inattentiveness, lethargy, or slow learning. Evaluate the eyes for nystagmus (see Chapter 5: Eye). Examine the gums for hyperplasia. Have the patient walk across the room; watch for ataxia. If ataxia is seen, test for the Romberg sign.

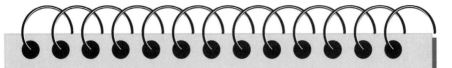

Therapeutic Drug Monitoring Examples

TRANSIENT ISCHEMIC ATTACKS (TIAS)

The approach to therapeutic drug monitoring by clinicians varies depending upon many factors. Some of these include preferences among clinicians in a given community or region; concurrent medical problems which dictate that certain drugs be used or avoided; the patient's response to selected medication. The following outlines of therapeutic drug monitoring offer examples which may serve to stimulate discussion and further understanding of initiating and monitoring drug use. The drugs and dosages presented should not be applied to any clinical situation without proper medical supervision.

Drug Therapy | Aspirin 325 mg tablet 2 PO BID.

Monitoring | **Symptoms:** How often do the attacks happen? How long do they last (e.g., minutes versus hours)? How severe are the attacks; does the patient have to stop any activity during an episode? Inquire about neurological symptoms. Inquire about symptoms such as a sensation of swelling or numbness of the hand, arm, or side of the face; loss of strength in one arm, hand, or leg; seeing double or half of an object, or loss of vision in one eye; dizziness; difficulty speaking or reading; ataxia; loss of consciousness. Since starting aspirin, have the attacks changed? If so, describe how.

Signs: *Gen:* Record the patient's age, gender, and race. Note the weight; is the patient overweight? *VS:* Analyze the radial pulse for arrhythmias, especially atrial fibrillation. Check blood pressure (BP) for orthostatic blood pressure changes and hypertension. *MSE:* Observe the patient's appearance, behavior, level of consciousness, orientation, memory, judgment, abstract reasoning, thinking, and language. *HEENT:* Auscultate the carotid arteries for bruits. *CVS:* Listen to the heart rate and rhythm. Is atrial fibrillation present. Do you hear a murmur;

Therapeutic Drug Monitoring Examples

TRANSIENT ISCHEMIC ATTACKS (TIAS)
(continued)

	if so, characterize it (see Chapter 11: Heart). *Abd:* Examine the abdominal arteries for vascular sounds (i.e., bruits). *Neuro:* Check the motor system by asking the patient to walk across the room, turn around, and come back. Then have the patient walk heel-to-toe. Determine the strength of the upper body by hand grip and the lower body with shallow knee bends. Move to sensory testing with pin prick and light touch in the hands, feet, and face. Lastly, measure DTRs.
Laboratory Tests	The clinician may elect to order all, none, or some of these laboratory studies depending upon history and physical findings, as well as other specific clinical indications. CBC, serum glucose, prothrombin time and partial prothrombin time (PT/PTT), electrocardiogram (ECG), serum electrolytes, serum lipid profile, stool occult blood.
Adverse Drug Event Monitoring	**Aspirin:** Inquire about GI complaints.

Reproductive System: Breast

A ccounting for 29% percent of malignancies in women, breast cancer is the most common female malignancy. A woman has a 1 in 8 to 1 in 12 chance of developing breast cancer during her life. In 1990, 150,000 new cases were diagnosed. Approximately 40,000 women died of breast cancer that same year. Fortunately, breast examination and mammography screening will discover up to 89% percent of breast cancers, many early enough to effect a cure.

ANATOMY AND PHYSIOLOGY

Breast Development

Under the hypothalamic pituitary stimulation of gonadotropin releasing hormone (GnRH), follicle stimulating hormones (FSH) and luteinizing hormones (LH) are released from the anterior pituitary and begin to stimulate the prepubertal ovary to produce estrogen. The first pubertal change resulting from estrogen stimulation is **thelarche** (i.e., breast bud formation) which occurs in girls 10.5 to 11 years of age on average and may occur as early as 9 years of age. Sometimes, to the young girl's concern and her parents' consternation, this breast bud development may initially be unilateral. At about the same time that breast bud development begins, the growth spurt starts. Before the growth spurt reaches its peak, but after the breast buds begin to develop, pubic hair growth is first noted. **Adrenarche** (i.e., pubic hair growth) is first noted on the average between ages 11 to 12 years. The onset of thelarche, adrenarche, and the maximum growth spurt are followed by **menarche**, signaled by the young woman's first menstrual period. Ovulation may occur before the first menstrual period. In the United States the average age of menarche is 13.5 years.

In order to characterize normal pubertal development and to identify abnormal growth patterns, Tanner has assigned stages to the development of public hair and the breast. In summary, these stages are outlined in Table 15.1 and Figure 15.1.

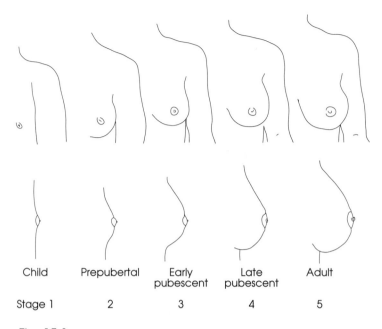

Child	Prepubertal	Early pubescent	Late pubescent	Adult
Stage 1	2	3	4	5

Fig. 15.1   Tanner classification of breast development.

Cyclic Breast Changes

With the onset of menarche, the breasts begin to undergo cyclic changes. Under estrogen stimulation during the first half of the menstrual cycle (i.e., the follicular or proliferative phase), the mammary gland ducts increase in number. During the second half of the cycle (i.e., the luteal or secretory phase), increased progesterone levels increase the mammary gland's secretory capacity with dilation of the ducts and differentiation of the alveolar cells into secretory cells. For many women, this results in a sense of increased "fullness" and, sometimes, heaviness of the breasts beginning a varying number of days before the onset of menstruation. The breast is preparing to nurture the newborn should pregnancy ensue. These premenstrual breast symptoms are produced by an increase in blood flow, vascular engorgement, and water retention. At the onset of menstruation, the alveoli and ducts become smaller, secondary to a regression of cellular activity.

Mammary Glands

The mammary glands, along with their surrounding supportive and adipose tissue, are located on the anterior chest wall, resting atop the pectoralis major and pectoralis minor muscles and the deep fascia surrounding these muscles. These muscles, in turn, rest on the ribs and connecting intercostal muscles of the thoracic cage. Superiorly, the breast begins at about the level of the second rib or second intercostal space and extends inferiorly to the level of the sixth intercostal space or rib at the midclavicular line. Medially, breast tissue usually begins at the lateral margin of the sternum and extends laterally to the anterior axillary line. The exception to this is in the area of the axilla itself, where breast tissue may extend into the axilla. When most women are in the supine position, the nipple is located at the midclavicular line at the level of the fourth intercostal space. However, the exact configuration of anatomical landmarks varies widely, depending upon the amount of breast tissue and the age of the patient (see Figures 15.2 and 15.3).

The breast is a modified sebaceous gland located within the superficial fascia of the anterior chest wall between the skin overlying the breast and the underlying deep fascia of the pectoralis muscle. Under proper stimulation, the mammary glands are capable of producing and secreting breast milk. The mammary gland is composed of 12 to 20 triangular lobes of glandular tissue; each lobe has its own central duct, collecting ducts, and secretory cells arranged as alveoli. Each lobe with its alveoli and collecting ducts empties into a single **lactiferous duct** and these 12 to 20 individual lactiferous ducts open through the skin at the nipple. On average, each breast weighs 200 to 300 gm and is composed primarily of fatty tissue with glandular tissue interspersed. Importantly, fibrous septa (i.e., Cooper's ligaments) separate the glandular lobes as the septa pass from the overlying skin of the breast

Tanner Developmental Stages

Table 15.1

Tanner Breast Development Stages

Stage B1	preadolescent; elevation of the nipple only
Stage B2	breast bud stage; elevation of the breast and nipple as a small mound; enlargement of the areolar diameter
Stage B3	further enlargement of the breast and areola with no separation of the contours
Stage B4	further enlargement with projection of the areola and nipple to form a secondary mound above the level of the breast
Stage B5	mature stage; projection of the nipple only, resulting from recession of the areola to the general contour of the breast

Tanner Pubic Hair Development Stages

Stage PH1	no pubic hair
Stage PH2	sparse growth of long, straight, only slightly curled hair along the labia
Stage PH3	thicker, coarser, and more curled hair extending sparsely over the junction of the pubis, mons pubis
Stage PH4	hair is adult in type and spreads over the mons pubis but not to the medial surface of the thighs
Stage PH5	hair is spread further laterally to the medial surface of the thighs and forms an inverse triangle

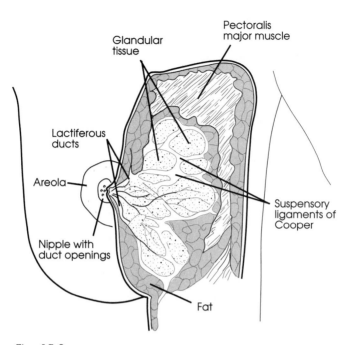

Fig. 15.2   Anterior view of the left breast showing the primary underlying structures.

to the deep fascia of the pectoralis muscles beneath; this relationship will take on added importance when breast exam for breast cancer is discussed.

The blood and lymphatic supply to the breast comes from many sources. These sources include the subclavian system above and behind each clavicle, the axilla, the intercostal lymphatic and vascular system, and paths to and from arteries and lymphatics deep to the chest wall within the thorax (see Figure 15.4). Though necessary for the physiologic function of the breast (i.e., production of breast milk and suckling), this rich blood supply and extensive lymphatic drainage also facilitate the multiple ways in which breast cancer can spread or metastasize.

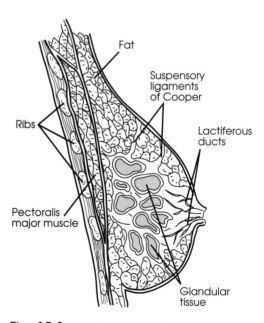

Fig. 15.3   Lateral, cross-section view of the breast

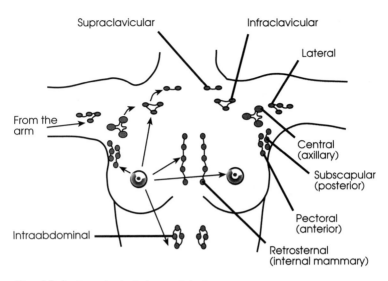

Fig. 15.4 Lymphatic drainage of the breasts.

Extra nipples (e.g., polythelia) and true accessory mammary glands (i.e., polymastia) may be located anywhere along "milk lines" which extend from the axilla to the groin (see Figure 15.5). The hyperpigmented areola with its central nipple contains the openings of the 12 to 20 collecting or lactiferous ducts. With pregnancy, the skin of the areola darkens and raised areas appear in a circular fashion on the areola around the nipple. These are **glands of Morgagni** which have hypertrophied and are an early sign of pregnancy. The nipple though most commonly everted, may be inverted. The inverted nipple may create some difficulty with attempts at breast feeding which can often be overcome using various breast feeding techniques and/or aids.

As discussed above, normal cyclic physiologic changes result from estrogen and progesterone stimulation during the menstrual cycle. In the absence of this stimulation (e.g., postmenopause state without estrogen replacement), the glandular

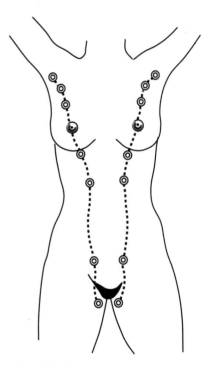

Fig. 15.5 Extra nipples and accessory mammary glands may arise anywhere along the "milk lines," embryonic ridges that extend from the axilla to the groin.

tissue of the breast will decrease in volume. This lost glandular tissue may be replaced by adipose tissue to varying degrees, depending upon the individual's nutritional status.

Since much of the breast is composed of adipose tissue, changes in weight can alter breast size and contour. With increasing age there is a "loosening" or loss in the strength of connective tissue throughout the body. This change also affects the connective tissue septa of the breast and may be reflected in a "sagging" of the breasts.

With pregnancy there is continuous stimulation of the glandular tissues of the breast in preparation for lactation following delivery. After delivery and with stimulation of the nipple through suckling or manipulation (e.g., the use of a breast pump), nerve endings in the nipple carry sensory impulses to the brain. Stimulation of certain centers in the brain results in the release of oxytocin from the posterior pituitary into the circulatory system. The oxytocin stimulates muscle fibers around the mammary gland alveoli and milk is expressed from the breast. The prolactin which has been circulating at high levels in the blood and preparing the glands to produce milk continues to be present, but at lower levels. During the first two to three days of suckling, the lactiferous glands are beginning the process of "milk let-down" so that breast milk will be available to the baby. During this time, colostrum, a yellow, alkaline liquid is secreted from the breast with suckling. Though not as nutritionally balanced as breast milk, colostrum contains many ingredients to support the baby's well being. For example, colostrum has greater anti-infective capabilities than the transitional milk or mature milk that follows. This provides protections for the newborn against its first exposure to many different types of infection. During breast feeding, it is important to empty one breast completely before changing to the other breast because the "hind milk," (i.e., the last milk to be suckled from the breast) is high in lipids and protein and is thus nutritionally the richest milk. Human milk is considered to be nutritionally complete except for fluoride and possibly vitamin D, which can be obtained by exposing the child to sunlight for brief periods of time during the day. When stimulation through suckling or the use of a breast pump ceases, breast milk production ceases. The opposite is also true. As long as the breast is stimulated to produce breast milk, it will be produced. This can continue for years.

PHYSICAL ASSESSMENT

Self-examination of the breasts and periodic breast exams by a physician are key to early detection of breast cancer. To help locate any suspicious findings detected during the exam, each breast is divided into quadrants by drawing imaginary vertical and horizontal lines through the nipple. This divides the breast into four parts: a lower outer quadrant, a lower inner quadrant, an upper inner quadrant, and an upper outer quadrant (see Figure 15.6). Generally, a greater proportion of the mammary gland tissue is found in the upper outer quadrant. Extending off the upper outer quadrant into the axilla is often a tail of mammary gland tissue (i.e., the axillary **tail of Spence**). The axilla is an area too frequently overlooked during the breast exam. This area is important to check not only for the possibility of enlarged lymph nodes but also to examine whatever breast tissue might be found there.

Inspection of the Breasts

Inspection and palpation are the two physical examination techniques used to assess the breast. Inspect the breast with the patient both sitting and lying supine. While sitting, the patient should lean forward causing the breast to become more pendulous and allowing the connective tissue septa of the breast to provide more support to the breast tissue. Ask the patient to place her hands on her hips and lean forward slightly. Stand in front of the patient and, with good indirect lighting to highlight abnormal skin shadows, carefully inspect the skin and areola of each breast. Examine the skin for:

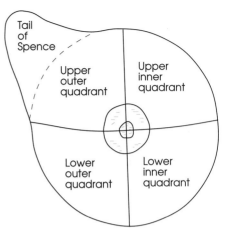

Fig. 15.6 Divisions of the breast used to describe the locations of physical findings.

- Abnormal discoloration or pigmentation (e.g., melanoma can occur on any body surface).

- Distortion or abnormal retraction of a nipple.

- A nodular fullness or tumor beneath the skin that might cause the skin to be raised and create a faint shadow.

- An orange peel appearance (i.e., Peu d'orange) to the skin associated with lymph edema from lymphatics being blocked more proximally by a tumor, preventing drainage of tissue fluids.

- Areas of retracted skin highlighted by faint shadowing. This may represent a tumor of the connective tissue septa extending between the skin and deep fascia of the underlying muscle. Such a tumor results in shortening of the septa and retraction or pulling of the skin inward (see Figure 15.7).

These findings can be accentuated by asking the patient to press her hands inward on her hips. This maneuver tightens the pectoralis muscles and the connective septa are further shortened, uncovering or accentuating skin defects. While the patient is still sitting, it is informative to palpate any questionable areas identified by inspection.

After noting any abnormal or questionable areas, ask the patient to lie supine with the anterior upper chest draped with a gown or cloth towel. Again, inspection is the first step during this part of the breast exam. Ask the patient to place her hands behind her head to better expose and make accessible the areas to be examined. Begin the examination by inspecting the skin, areola, and nipple just as had been done with the patient sitting.

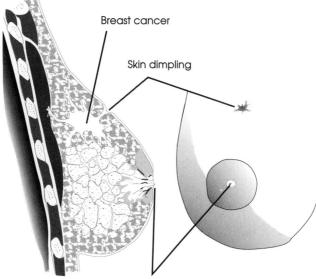

Breast cancer

Skin dimpling

Flattening of the nipple

Fig. 15.7 Nipple retraction and dimpling of the skin are clinical signs of breast cancer.

Palpation of the Breasts

Begin the palpation part of the examination by first examining the areola and nipple. Gently compress the tissue around the nipple to feel for any nodularity that might reflect involvement of the lactiferous ducts with early cancer. Evaluate the nipple being sure it is not retracted or pulled inward by an underlying cancer. Note the presence or absence of breast discharge. This is accomplished by gently trying to express ductal contents from one quadrant of the breast at a time. If a discharge is present record the quadrant from which it was expressed. This will help the surgeons identify the location of the source of the discharge if surgery is indicated. If discharge is noted, press a glass microscope slide against the nipple and before sending it to pathology for evaluation, fix the discharge on the slide with a fixing solution just as one does with a cervical pap smear.

Before beginning the examination of the mammary gland itself, palpate the supraclavicular space above each clavicle for lymph node enlargement since nodes in this area are sometimes involved with breast cancer.

To examine the glandular tissue of the breast, first ask the patient to place her hands under the back of her head. Use the fleshy, palmar side of the fingers and in an "around the clock" fashion, begin palpation of the upper inner quadrant and finish in the upper outer quadrant. Having reached the upper outer quadrant and with the patient's hands still behind her head, it is relatively easy to examine the axilla for any mammary gland tissue that might be in the axillary tail of Spence and, of equal importance, to palpate for the presence of lymph node enlargement. Gently compress the tissues of the breast between the soft part of your hand and the pectoralis muscle and bone of the chest wall beneath. It is normal for the breast tissue to have a nodular feel to it. It is only after several dozen examinations that you will begin to become comfortable with the ability to adequately examine the breast for cancer. The nodules vary in size and are rubbery in consistency, smooth, mobile, and nontender. They may be present in clumps and give the sensation of a small bunch of grapes. Lesions that are changing in size, greater than one cm in diameter, rock hard in consistency, irregular in shape, fixed to surrounding tissue and not mobile, and/or associated with any of the above discussed skin changes, are suspicious for cancer. If such findings are uncovered, a mammogram should be obtained and the patient referred to a breast cancer specialist for further evaluation.

Examination of the breast may identify two common and benign breast disorders: fibrocystic disease of the breast and fibroadenoma of the breast. Clinically identifiable in 50% of women, fibrocystic disease of the breast is the most common breast disease. This condition involves a thickening of all glandular elements which is reflected on physical exam by the presence of multiple small, nodular lesions, present in both breasts. These lesions frequently are tender and even painful to palpation, particularly in the last half of the menstrual cycle. Since these changes are stimulated by estrogen, the symptoms tend to regress in women who are postmenopausal and not on estrogen replacement. Drugs that have been used to relieve symptoms of the disease include medroxyprogesterone acetate, bromocriptine, tamoxifen, and danocrine.

Composed of fibrous and glandular tissue, fibroadenomas are the most common benign tumors found in the female breast. On examination, these adenomas are typically round, sharply circumscribed, freely mobile, and nontender. They are more commonly found in women younger than 30 years of age. Unlike fibrocystic disease, fibroadenomas are usually solitary and may reach 2 to 4 cm in diameter. Though the growth is commonly stimulated by pregnancy, the adenoma tends to regress and become calcified in postmenopausal women not on estrogen replacement. Note that a fibroadenoma and fibrocystic disease of the breast may coexist in the same women. Definitive diagnosis depends upon surgical excision and microscopic evaluation for both fibrocystic disease and fibroadenomas.

Mammograms

A mammogram is a very important part of the complete breast examination and will correctly identify cancer 85% to 90% of the time in the hands of a well-trained radiologist. Of those cancers detected by mammography, 40% are not clinically detected by breast examination. The optimal frequency for screening asymptomatic women has not been determined. The American Cancer Society Guidelines for mammography screening of asymptomatic women are as follows:

- Obtain a baseline mammogram for all women at age 35 to 40 years. The author recommends that women begin mammograms at 35 years of age if there is a history of breast cancer in a family member (i.e., sister, mother, grandmother, maternal aunt).

• Mammographic screening at one to two year intervals from age 40 to 49.

• Annual mammograms for women 50 years of age or older.

Whenever possible it is beneficial to have previous ("old") mammograms available for comparison purposes. A mammogram should not be done without a concomitant breast exam by a professional. For various reasons, some women are reluctant to have a mammogram. As health care professionals, we should be supportive and encourage screening mammograms and self-breast examination.

Breast Self-Examination

Breast self-examination is the most important part of breast screening for cancer. Women who perform breast self-examination on a monthly basis will detect breast changes and cancer earlier, at a more readily curable stage. In the menstruating woman, the exam should be performed five to seven days after the first day of menstrual flow when the glandular tissue is least affected by estrogen and progesterone. In the post menopausal woman on cyclic estrogen and progesterone, the exam should be done at the time the first estrogen pill is taken each month. Otherwise, self-breast exam should be done the first day of each month or at the same time each month. The patient should stand in front of a mirror and inspect her breasts with her arms at the side and then with her arms over her head. The supraclavicular and axillary regions should be palpated for the presence of nodes as discussed above. The tissues of the breast should then be palpated in a fashion described above in both the upright and supine position. Some women believe this part of the examination is facilitated by performing it in the shower where lathering the skin with a soapy film allows for easier palpation of breast tissues. As described above, the breast should be examined in an upright (i.e., standing or sitting) position *and* in a supine position with each quadrant of each breast and the axillary tail being carefully examined. The breast exam is completed by palpation of the areolar areas and the nipple, including gentle compression to identify the presence of any secretions.

The male has mammary gland tissue beneath each areola and nipple. This glandular tissue is capable of responding to hormonal stimulation with resultant breast enlargement. Breast cancer can also develop in this mammary gland tissue. Gynecomastia or breast enlargement is associated with genetic abnormalities, normal physiologic changes, drug administration, tumors, systemic disorders, and various miscellaneous causes. Hypogonadism (i.e., male pseudohermaphrodite) and androgen resistance syndromes (e.g., partial or complete androgen insensitivity syndromes) are typically associated with bilateral gynecomastia. Unilateral or bilateral gynecomastia may be seen as a transient physiologic phenomenon during the neonatal or pubertal

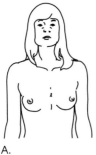
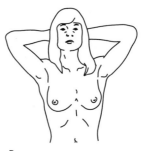

A.

B.

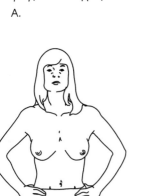
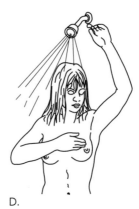

C.

D.

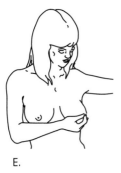
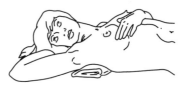

E.

F.

Fig. 15.8 Breast self examination includes inspection while standing in front of a mirror with: A. arms at the sides; B. hands clasped behind the head; and C. hands pressed firmly on the hips; as well as D. palpation of the breast in a standing position; E. palpation of the nipple; and F. palpation of the breast while in a supine position.

period. Various types of drugs that can induce gynecomastia include hormones (e.g., estrogens, aromatizable androgens), drugs that interact with estrogen receptors (e.g., marijuana, digitalis), drugs that alter androgen production or action (e.g., spironolactone, cimetidine, ketoconazole, cytotoxic agents), and central nervous system active drugs (e.g., antihypertensive agents, tranquilizers, sedatives, antidepressants, amphetamines). Estrogen secreting tumors (i.e., adrenal carcinoma, Leydig or Sertoli testicular tumors) and gonadotropin secreting tumors (i.e., testicle, lung, liver) may be associated with gynecomastia. Common systemic disorders in which gynecomastia may be seen include hepatic cirrhosis, renal failure, and thyrotoxicosis. There is also a familial gynecomastia, as well as gynecomastia associated with increased peripheral aromatization (i.e., in a morbidly obese male), and trauma to the breast tissue.

Physiologic and drug-induced gynecomastia are the most common types. Therefore, if a male complains of enlarging breasts or breast, a careful history (particularly regarding medications being taken) frequently discloses the cause of gynecomastia. Unexpected breast enlargement also occurs in women of all ages. The causes are the same or similar as those in men.

Nipple discharge is a common complaint expressed by patients and is a common finding during physical examination. Although many people associate nipple discharges with cancer of the breast, fewer than 10% of breast cancers present with nipple discharge. When discharge is present, a careful history needs to be taken noting date of onset, characteristics which have changed over time, medications being taken, past or present history of pregnancy, and characteristics of the discharge (e.g., bloody, color, thick, watery, purulent, serous). Any nipple discharge seen in post menopausal women or in men should be considered suggestive of breast cancer. Likewise, any serous or bloody discharge must be investigated. Although nipple discharge is caused by a benign intraductal papilloma over 80% of the time, it can be a harbinger of breast cancer.

The most frequent breast discharge other than breast milk in a lactating mother is the milky discharge of galactorrhea. A good history may reveal that the galactorrhea is related to a physiologic cause of hyperprolactinemia (e.g., breast stimulation, exercise, coitus, pregnancy, sleep, stress). Pathologic causes include organic etiologies such as brain tumors (e.g., craniopharyngiomas, pituitary tumors) or functional causes related to drugs. Galactorrhea has been associated with pyschotropic medications (e.g., butyphenones, phenothiazines), contraceptives, antihypertensives (e.g., reserpine, methyldopa), antigastroplegics (e.g., metoclopramide), and cannabinoids (e.g., morphine, heroin). Galactorrhea has also been reported with hypothyroidism, renal or liver failure, mastitis or breast trauma, polycystic ovary disease, and cancers of the kidney or lung.

Galactorrhea is most commonly associated with a physiologic cause or medication. Remember that the male breast contains mammary gland tissue and therefore nipple discharge, including galactorrhea, can occur in the male.

PHARMACOTHERAPEUTIC CASE ILLUSTRATION: 1

History

R.L. is a 63-year-old postmenopausal female. Her last menstrual period was at age 59. She has never been pregnant and she began menstruating at age 11. She has examined her breasts monthly for several years. She presents concerned that there is a "lump" in her left breast that has been getting larger. It is not painful to her touch and she has not noted any nipple discharge.

Past medical history (PMH) is noncontributory except for a dilation and curettement (D&C) at age 47 for heavy menstrual bleeding. She took birth control pills for 14 years. Family history (FH) revealed that she has a brother with hypertension; her sister and mother have had lumpectomies for breast cancer. R.L.'s social history (SH) indicates that she does not smoke but has used alcohol and describes herself as a moderate drinker.

Physical Examination

R.L.'s vital signs (VS) are as follows: blood pressure (BP) 136/84 mm Hg; pulse 82 beats/min; temperature 98.4° F; respiratory rate (RR) of 16/min. Examination of her head and neck showed no anterior or posterior cervical adenopathy; no supraclavicular adenopathy. Her chest was clear to auscultation and percussion. Her heart had regular rate and rhythm without murmur.

With R.L. sitting and leaning forward an examination of her breasts revealed fullness in the left upper outer quadrant of her left breast. When she pressed her hands against her hips, there was a slight skin retraction in this area of fullness. Palpation revealed a 2 x 3 cm nodular mass in left upper outer quadrant about 4 cm from the nipple at about the 1 o'clock position. No axillary adenopathy was palpated. Examination of R.L. in the supine position with her hands behind her head revealed that the lump identified in the sitting position was fixed and not movable, with a rock hard, irregular texture. It was not tender to pressure. There was no nipple discharge and no axillary adenopathy. The remainder of the exam was unremarkable.

Laboratory

A mammogram was ordered and revealed a suspicious lesion in the area described on physical examination.

Diagnosis and Management

The diagnosis of breast cancer is made by biopsy of the suspected lesion and microscopic identification of cancer in the breast tissue. If present on frozen section at the time of surgery, many surgeons will do a lymph node dissection to remove nodes so that they can be examined under the microscope. If the lymph nodes are positive for cancer, in addition to removing the cancer surgically, adjuvant therapy will be given, (i.e., radiation and/or chemotherapy).

R.L. represented several risk factors for breast cancer: age >40 years, early menarche, nulliparous (i.e., never been pregnant), late age at menopause, family history of breast cancer, and history of alcohol consumption. A risk factor R.L. did not have was exposure to ionizing radiation. A history of oral contraceptive use or fibrocystic disease of the breast does not appear to increase the risk for development of breast cancer.

As with all cancers, breast cancer diagnosis and management are based upon the extent or spread of the disease. The Tumor Node Metastases (TNM) scheme, a method of classifying the severity of the malignancy, showed stage IIIA for R.L. Decisions on breast cancer management also depend upon whether a woman is premenopausal or postmenopausal. R.L. did not show signs of metastasis and was thus not a candidate for cytotoxic chemotherapy.

Since R.L. was postmenopausal without metastases, she was treated surgically with irradiation and endocrine therapy. She was postmenopausal with positive estrogen receptors. Several hormonal drugs are effective and include tamoxifen, aminoglutethimide, estrogen, and progesterone. The endocrine choices are directed to blocking estrogen receptors which slow the cancer cell growth. Postmenopausal women with positive estrogen receptors have shown favorable responses with tamoxifen. The response is best in patients with positive estrogen receptors; a few negative estrogen receptor patients respond as well. If the tumor had not been excised, tumor reduction would take several months. R.L. should be warned about the risk of worsening symptoms with the start of tamoxifen, called a flare reaction. A flare reaction is more frequent with metastases. The most dangerous manifestation of this reaction is severe hypercalcemia that interrupts endocrine therapy. Common side effects are nausea or vomiting and hot flashes

PHARMACOTHERAPEUTIC CASE ILLUSTRATION: 2

History

L.M. is a 22-year-old female who gave birth to a 7 lb 2 oz baby girl 4 days ago by cesarean section. The mother is breast feeding and has begun to run a low-grade temperature and complains about left breast pain, swelling, and redness. The baby is sucking well and has begun to regain some of the weight normally lost the first 2 days after birth. The mother had not breast fed this last feeding because of increasing pain.

Physical Examination

L.M.'s vital signs (VS) are as follows: blood pressure (BP) 122/74 mm Hg; pulse 109 beats/min; temperature 100.4° F (38° C); respiratory rate (RR) 18/min.

A focused examination of the breast was conducted. Inspection revealed that both breasts were engorged. The skin over the lateral aspect of the left breast was slightly raised, red, and tense in appearance. Palpation of the right breast was unremarkable, including palpation in the axillary area. Palpation of the left breast revealed increased skin warmth over the affected area and marked tenderness to palpation with the tissues deep to the reddened area of the skin consolidated but not fluctuant. There was lymph node enlargement and tenderness upon examination of the left axilla. There was no abnormally appearing nipple discharge.

Laboratory

No laboratory tests were ordered. Had there been fluctuance in the infected area one might consider aspirating material and culturing it.

Diagnosis and Management

The diagnosis was mastitis or infection of the glands of the breast related to breast feeding. The most common cause of this type infection is *Staphylococcus aureus* from the skin. Because of the possibility of the *S. aureus* being coagulase positive, penicillin is usually not the first drug of choice, but rather dicloxacillin or oxacillin; however, some clinicians might prescribe a first-generation cephalosporin. If the patient is allergic to penicillin, erythromycin might be considered. In addition to the antibiotic, it would be important that the baby continue to breast feed from both breasts and that an effort be made to deplete the milk from the affected breast with each feeding. It is believed that this relieves engorgement and encourages healing. Warm packs to the breast are also used to encourage blood circulation to the area and achieve resolution of the infection before an abscess can be formed. If an abscess forms it must be drained.

Therapeutic Drug Monitoring Examples

MASTITIS

The approach to therapeutic drug monitoring by clinicians varies depending upon many factors. Some of these include preferences among clinicians in a given community or region; concurrent medical problems which dictate that certain drugs be used or avoided; the patient's response to selected medication. The following outlines of therapeutic drug monitoring offer examples which may serve to stimulate discussion and further understanding of initiating and monitoring drug use. The drugs and dosages presented should not be applied to any clinical situation without proper medical supervision.

Drug Therapy	Dicloxacillin 250 mg PO QID. Warm compresses PRN.
Monitoring	**Symptoms:** Ask the patient about the onset and severity of symptoms. Determine the treatment response by questioning about breast tenderness.
	Signs: *Gen:* Describe the degree of distress. Measure vital signs. *Breast:* Inspect and palpate the breast for swelling, fluctuance, consolidation, and tenderness. Describe the degree of inflammation. Check for nipple discharge. Examine lymph nodes in the area for signs of infection.
Laboratory Tests	The clinician may elect to order all, none, or some of these laboratory studies depending upon history and physical findings, as well as other specific clinical indications. None, unless abscess suspected [aspirated for culture/sensitivy (C&S) testing].
Adverse Drug Event Monitoring	Question about diarrhea and sign of candidiasis. If clinical status does not improve, reconsider the diagnosis or antibiotic selection.

Reproductive System: Female

*T*he female reproductive system is classically divided into external genitalia and internal genitalia (see Table 16.1). The internal genitalia (i.e., the uterus, the fallopian tubes, and the ovaries) provide a means for procreation and continuation of the species. The external genitalia provide a means of introducing sperm to achieve conception (i.e., sexual intercourse) and to serve as the birth canal through which the newborn child is birthed.

ANATOMY AND PHYSIOLOGY

Pelvis

The female reproductive system rests on and within the pelvis. The bony pelvis, along with the muscular floor of the pelvis and levator ani muscle, provides the support and protection for the internal genitalia. The pelvic bone is composed of the ilium, the ischium and the pubic bones united posteriorly by the sacrum and anteriorly at the pubic symphysis (see Figure 16.1). The uppermost aspect of the bony pelvis is composed of the iliac crest and the anterior superior iliac spine. The pubic rami descend anteriorly from the pubic symphysis to the pubic tubercle on which we sit. Stretching from the anterior superior iliac spine to the pubic symphysis is the inguinal ligament under which pass the femoral artery and vein and the femoral nerve to the lower extremities. Deep to the ischial tuberosity is the ischial spine with its sacro-spinous ligament connecting it to the sacrum. The linea terminalis or pelvic inlet plays an important role in birthing because the head of the fetus must be able to fit through it in order for vaginal birth to begin to take place. The head of the fetus is said to be engaged if its biparietal diameter fits through the pelvic inlet. The pelvic inlet and other structures mentioned are used as landmarks during physical examination and surgery.

The bony pelvis is classified into the following four general types (see Figure 16.2): The **gynecoid pelvis** has a large pelvic inlet and ischial spines that are far enough apart to allow ease of delivery of the fetus through the bony pelvis. The configuration of the **android (male) pelvis**, with its heart-shaped narrow inlet and close together spines, is the opposite of the gynecoid pelvis. Women with an android pelvis are commonly unable to birth a baby vaginally, resulting in the need for a Cesarean section delivery. The **anthropoid pelvis** is a cross between the gynecoid and android pelvis. It has a shorter transverse diameter than anterior-posterior diameter and, though it allows for delivery, a larger fetus may not engage its head as easily, necessitating a Cesarean section. The inlet of the **platypelloid pelvis** is the opposite of the anthropoid pelvis. It has a wide transverse diameter and a narrow anterior-posterior diameter of the pelvic inlet. Women generally have little trouble birthing a baby through this type of pelvis.

External Genitalia

The term vulva encompasses the organs of the external genitalia. The vulva consists of labia majora, labia minora, mons pubis, clitoris, hymen, vestibule, urethral opening, Skene's (i.e., periurethral) glands, and Bartholin's glands (see Figure 16.3).

The **mons pubis** is the most cephalad (i.e., toward the head) of these structures and consists of a fatty layer of subcutaneous tissue and skin which covers the pubic symphysis. At puberty, the mons pubis becomes covered with pubic hair which normally grows in a triangular pattern. However, a diamond-shaped pattern normally seen in males occurs in approximately 25% of normal women. The hair of the mons

Table 16.1

Female Reproductive System

External Genitalia

     Mons pubis
     Labia majora
     Labia minora
     Clitoris
     Hymen
     Vestibule
     Urethral
     Skene's (periurethral) glands
     Bartholin's (vulvovaginal) glands

Internal Genitalia

     Vagina
     Uterus
       Cervix
       Corpus (body)
     Fallopian tubes
     Ovaries

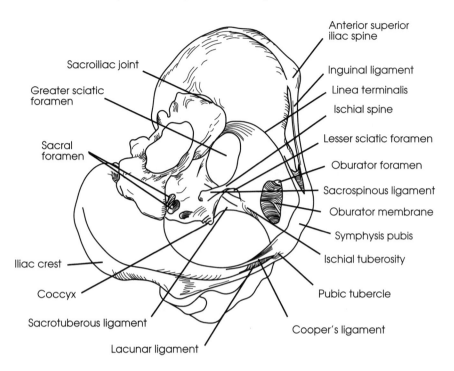

Anterior superior iliac spine

Sacroiliac joint

Greater sciatic foramen

Sacral foramen

Iliac crest

Coccyx

Sacrotuberous ligament

Lacunar ligament

Inguinal ligament

Linea terminalis

Ischial spine

Lesser sciatic foramen

Oburator foramen

Sacrospinous ligament

Oburator membrane

Symphysis pubis

Ischial tuberosity

Pubic tubercle

Cooper's ligament

Fig. 16.1 A view of the pelvis from above, illustrating the bone, joints, ligaments and foramina.

pubis spreads in a caudad (i.e., toward the feet) and posterior direction over the skin of the labia majora. The **labia majora** consists of two folds of tissue extending from the mons pubis anteriorly to blend in with the skin between the fourchette and perineal body posteriorly. The male counterpart of the labia majora is the scrotum. The outer surface of the labia majora contains hair follicles; the inner surface is absent of hair but supports many sebaceous glands. The size of the labia varies with the fat content of that area of the body.

The pinkish, smooth skin fold of the **labia minora** lies on either side of the vaginal opening, medial to the labia majora. Unlike the labia majora, the labia minora contains no adipose tissue and consists primarily of fibrous connective tissue and erectile tissue. The skin of the labia minora and the skin of the breast, are the only two areas of the body where sebaceous glands are present while hair follicles and their accompanying sweat glands are absent. The labia are homologous to the male penile urethra. They vary in size, particularly during reproductive age, but tend to be more prominent before menarche and after menopause.

The **hymen** is located at the entrance of the vagina. In a virgin woman, it is a ring of tissue with a thickened border at the opening of the vagina. In the virgin, it may be membranous with a few perforations. Otherwise, it assumes a varied appearance depending on sexual activity and number of pregnancies with vaginal births. The

clitoris, normally a short cylinder-shaped structure composed of erectile tissue, is located at the superior aspect of the vulva. The diameter of the clitoris should be noted because if it is greater than 1 cm at its base, virilization (i.e., masculinization) should be suspected and a workup begun to determine its cause. Usually the shaft or body of the clitoris is located beneath the skin with the glans, or tip, being the only part of the structure that is visible. The clitoris is the homologue of the male penis.

The vestibule of the vulva extends from the inner extent of the labia minora on either side and from the clitoris anteriorly and superiorly to the fourchette posteriorly. Four structures open into the vestibule: the vagina with its hymenal ring, the urethra, and the ducts of the two Bartholin's glands.

The **urethra** is between 3.5 and 5.0 cm in length. It carries urine from the bladder to the outside, unlike the ureters, which carry urine from each kidney to the bladder. It contains many urethral glands which may become chronically infected (i.e., chronic urethritis). A pair of relatively large urethral glands empty into the distal urethra and occasionally becomes infected (i.e., *Neisseria gonorrhoeae*). These urethral glands are called **Skene's glands** or periurethral glands, and are homologous to the prostate in the male. A second set of paired glands is called **Bartholin's** or the **vulvovaginal glands** and are located distal to the inferior aspect of the introitus with the ducts emptying into the posterior introitus. These glands secrete a lubricating material during sexual arousal and are homologous to the male bulbourethral glands.

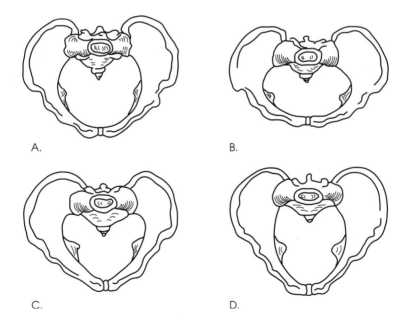

A.

B.

C.

D.

Fig. 16.2   The four general structural classifications of the bony pelvis: A. gynecoid; B. platypelloid; C. android; and D. anthropoid.

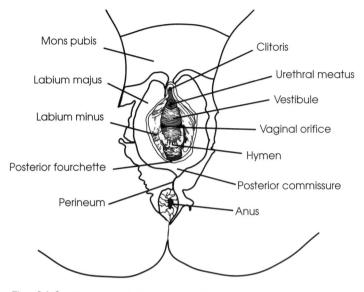

Fig. 16.3   The external female genitalia.

Posterior to the fourchette, between the anus and the fourchette, is a line where deep
and superficial tissues of the perineum come together and form the perineal body.
During childbirth it is not uncommon for an episiotomy or vertical incision to be made
through the perineum along this line to facilitate delivery of the baby. This is called a
midline episiotomy and is the most common type of episiotomy. In a midline
episiotomy, an incision is made through the fourchette, posterior hymenal ring,
posterior vagina, and into the perineal body. Occasionally the incision is carried
through the anal sphincter muscle into the anal canal and rectum. This area is quite
vascular and, because of this favorable situation, episiotomies almost always heal
without complications such as infection.

Internal Genitalia

The internal female genitalia consist of the vagina, the cervix of the uterus, the body of
the uterus, the paired fallopian tubes, and their attached, paired ovaries (see Figure
16.4). The **vagina** is a fibromuscular tube which, though distensible, is normally
collapsed. It extends from the hymenal ring externally to the cervix internally. The
urethra is located in tissues anterior to the vagina as it passes from the urinary bladder
to its external opening. Deep within the vagina near the cervix, the base of the bladder
also lies adjacent to the anterior wall of the vagina. Deep to the lateral walls of the
vagina fatty connective tissue, blood vessels, nerves and, near the cervix, the paired
ureters are found. Adjacent to the posterior wall of the vagina is the rectum as it
courses from the sigmoid colon to the anus with its encircling anal sphincter.

In a standing woman the axis of the vagina is almost horizontal. In most women an angle of at least 90° is formed between the axis of the vagina and the axis of the uterus. Under the influence of estrogen, the lining of the vagina forms hundreds of small folds or rugae. When examining the vagina, loss of rugae strongly suggests insufficient circulating estrogen. No glands are located in the vagina. During intercourse, the vagina is lubricated by a transudate produced by engorgement of the vascular plexuses that encircle the vagina and exuded through the vaginal wall.

The **cervix** is located at the deepest extent of the vagina and contains the endocervical canal through which sperm pass on their journey to the ends of the fallopian tubes where fertilization takes place (see Figure 16.5). This is also the canal through which the fetus passes during the birth process on its way to becoming a newborn. The spaces between the cervix and the vagina are called the fornices. In the adult, the length of the vagina anteriorly is between 6 and 9 cm with a posterior length of between 8 and 12 cm.

Some have likened the shape of the uterus and its vaginal extension of the cervix, to that of a pear. The globular end with its slightly flattened anterior surface is represented by the large end of the pear while the end with the stem represents the cervix. The right and left **fallopian tubes** are attached at the top of the pear-shaped uterus. Also attached anterior to the fallopian tubes are the round ligaments which support the uterus and traverse the anterior abdominal wall to imbed in the tissues of the labia majora. The outer covering of the cervix consists of flattened squamous cells. The cells lining the endocervical canal leading into the uterine cavity are tall columnar-like cells. The point at which these cells meet is known as the squamocolumnar junction and transitional zone. This is where cervical cancer begins

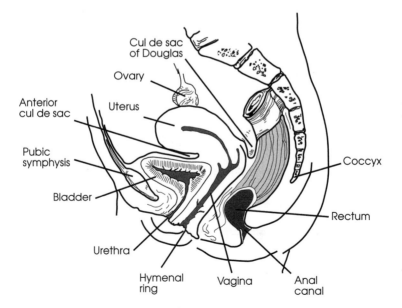

Fig. 16.4   A cross section of the internal female genitalia.

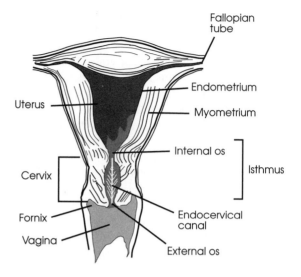

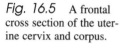

Fig. 16.5 A frontal cross section of the uterine cervix and corpus.

and it is from this part of the cervix that cells are obtained by a Papanicolaou (PAP) smear, a cervical cancer screening test. Unlike the body of the uterus which is composed mostly of smooth muscle, the cervix is made up of fibrous or connective tissue which, during birth, must allow the endocervical canal to stretch from its usual 0.5 cm diameter to 10 cm, allowing the baby's head and body to pass. The point of transition from the cervix to the body of the uterus is at the internal os or opening of the endocervical canal. The lining of the endocervical canal contains mucus secreting glands. The mucous consistency changes during the menstrual cycle and at the time of ovulation is thin and watery to facilitate sperm passage through the canal.

The body of the **uterus** has three distinct layers: the endometrium, the myometrium, and the serosal layer next to visceral peritoneum. The **endometrium** re-grows during each menstrual cycle in response to hormonal stimulation in preparation for implantation of a fertilized egg. In the absence of implantation, the endometrium is sloughed (i.e., desquamation) through the endocervical in a process called menses (also referred to as menstrual flow or the menstrual period). The layer beneath the endometrium is the much thicker **myometrium** consisting of smooth muscle. During pregnancy, this muscle layer will increase 10 to 20 fold in weight. It is this muscle's rhythmic contraction that expels the baby at the time of labor and delivery. The outermost layer is the **serosal** layer. It is a loose connective tissue layer separating the myometrium from the peritoneal lining of the pelvic cavity. The arteries, veins, and nerves that go to and from the uterus are located in this layer.

The cavity of the uterus is triangular shaped with the apex of the triangle pointed downward toward the endocervical canal and flattened in the anterior-posterior direction (see Figure 16.6). The body of the uterus is roughly one-half the size of an average man's closed fist. The dome-shaped top of the uterus is termed the fundus. The fundus is palpated to measure the changes in uterine size (i.e., fundal height) during pregnancy. Between the 20th and 36th weeks of pregnancy, each centimeter the fundus measures above the top of the pubic symphysis represents one week of fetal age. For example, if the fundal height measures 27 cm, the menstrual age of the fetus is 27 weeks. The uterus is suspended in the pelvis by a curtain of peritoneum stretching from side to side of the pelvic cavity with the uterus suspended in the middle. This curtain of tissue is termed **broad ligament**. From it hang two other curtains of tissue on either side of the uterus: the mesosalpinx and the mesovarium. At the right and left extremes of the fundus, near the attachment of the round ligaments, arise the uterine tubes or fallopian tubes (or oviducts). They extend from the uterus toward the ovary posteriorly and hang from the broad ligament by a sheet of mesentery called the mesosalpinx. Attaching at the cornua of the uterine cavity, this hollow tube continues through its fimbriated end, which opens near the ovary, where it can entrap newly released eggs. Just inside the fimbriated end of the fallopian tube is the ampulla. This is where the egg is fertilized by the sperm before it travels down the oviduct back to the uterine cavity. During this process, the egg divides several times before it implants in the endometrial wall of the uterus. These oviducts are susceptible to injury by sexually transmitted diseases, specifically *N. gonorrhoeae* and *Chlamydia trachomatis*. These infections commonly result in infertility or ectopic pregnancy secondary to damage to the tube and/or ovary.

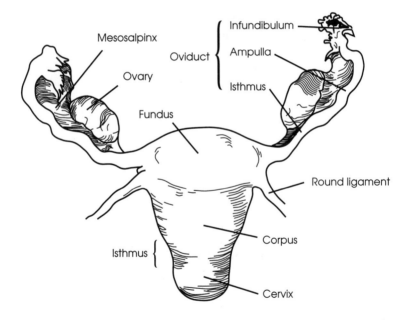

Fig. 16.6   An anterior view of the uterus.

The paired ovaries hang from the broad ligament by a curtain of mesentery called the **mesovarium** and sit on a "shelf" of tissue in the pelvic sidewall termed the ovarian fossa. During the reproductive years the **ovary** is about the size of a large almond (i.e., 1.5 cm x 2.5 cm x 4.0 cm). Once hormonal stimulation of the reproductive years ceases, the ovaries become much smaller and, during the postmenopausal years, should not be palpable. The ovary contains primary follicles (about 500,000 at the time of menarche) each with its own yet-to-mature egg. This ovarian follicle can become quite large in size and palpable during physical examination.

Physiology

The physiology of the female reproductive system supports procreation of the species and sexual enjoyment. Physiologic activity begins to be manifest at puberty, is cyclical, and ceases at the time of menopause. The controls or triggers for this monthly cyclical activity, the menstrual cycle, are found in the brain, the hypothalamus, and adjacent structures. During puberty (i.e., secondary sexual maturation), biological and physiological changes occur which make sexual reproduction possible. Puberty has four stages of development which typically occur in a specific order taking place over a period of 1.5 to 6 years (average 4.5 years). The first stage of puberty is breast development (i.e., **thelarche**) which is first noted as breast budding as early as age nine (see Chapter 15: Reproductive System: Breast Examination). Pulsatile secretions of gonadotropin releasing hormone (GnRH) from the hypothalamus stimulate secretion of luteinizing hormone (LH) and follicle stimulation hormone (FSH) from the anterior pituitary. This in turn stimulates secretion of estrogen and progesterone from the ovary. Circulating estrogen and progesterone facilitate the process of secondary sexual maturation, puberty, and, after it is complete, support the periodic menstrual cycle and ovulation. After breast budding has begun and around the age of 10 years, pubic and axillary hair (i.e., **adrenarche** or **pubarche**) are first noted, stimulated by androgens secreted from the adrenal glands. Following the onset of thelarche and adrenarche a maximal growth spurt occurs (i.e., that time in grade school where the girls are taller than the boys whose growth spurt is yet to come). For girls, this growth spurt peaks around 11 years of age. The last stage in pubertal development is menstruation (i.e., **menarche**). Menarche is normally first noted between the ages of 12.5 and 14 years. Ovulation may occur before menstruation. Thus, it is possible to become pregnant without ever having had a menstrual period. But normally, the first several menstrual cycles are either anovulatory or display random ovulation (e.g., occurring one cycle, but not the next). In North America, abnormally early onset of puberty (i.e., precocious puberty) occurs if sexual development (i.e., any sign of secondary sexual maturation) begins before 8 years of age in females. The causes of precocious puberty are many and some are listed in Table 16.2.

At the other extreme, failure to experience menarche, or primary amenorrhea, is diagnosed when a woman fails to experience spontaneous uterine bleeding by age 16.5. The causes of primary amenorrhea are multiple and varied (see Table 16.3). Evaluation should be initiated as soon as precocious puberty or primary amenorrhea is recognized. Secondary amenorrhea is the absence of menses for six months or longer in a person who has previously had spontaneous menstrual periods.

The menstrual cycle for most women is 28 days (plus or minus 2 days) from the start in one month to the start in the following month. However, the interval may vary from

Table 16.2
Causes of Precocious Puberty

Heterosexual Precocious Puberty

      Virilizing tumor of ovary or adrenal gland
      Congenital adrenal hyperplasia
      Exogenous estrogen exposure (e.g., birth control pills)

Isosexual Precocious Puberty

      Complete isosexual precocious puberty
        Constitutional (ideopathic, unknown cause)
        Organic brain disease
      Pseudosexual precocious puberty
        Ovarial tumor
        Adrenal tumor
        Hypothyroidism, advanced
        McClune-Albright Syndrome
        Peutz-Jegher's Syndrome

---

21 to 35 days and still be considered normal. The cycle is divided into two parts for purposes of understanding basic physiology: the period from the beginning of menses, or flow, to the time of ovulation and the period from ovulation to the beginning of the next period, normally 14 days regardless of the length of the total cycle. When considering ovarian function, the first part of the cycle is termed the **follicular phase** (i.e., the period of egg development in the ovarian follicle before ovulation). The second part is the **luteal phase** (i.e., the period of change in the follicle to support implantation of the fertilized egg). When considering uterine endometrial function, the first part of the cycle is called the proliferative phase (i.e., a time of buildup of the endometrial lining) and the second part is termed the secretory phase. This period lasts 14 days and represents a change in the endometrium to support implantation of the fertilized egg.

Estrogen is the primary hormone that, together with progesterone, drives the ovarian changes necessary for ovulation and the uterian lining changes necessary to support implantation. The ovary, the hypothalamus, and the pituitary gland are involved in this preparation. In the first few days of the menstrual flow, estrogen and progesterone levels circulating in the blood are low. These low levels feed back to the hypothalamus in the brain and the pituitary gland which signals an increase in production of estrogen and progesterone, as well as release of follicle stimulating hormone (FSH). Increased circulating FSH stimulates the ovary to produce estrogen through maturation of ovarian follicles in preparation for ovulation.

At the same time the follicle matures, the endometrium of the uterus thickens. The estrogen production from the ovary continues to rise and peaks just before ovulation. Estrogen peak triggers the very important luteinizing hormone (LH) surge or rapid rise in LH which, in turn, triggers ovulation. The LH surge is accompanied by a drop in circulating estrogen and a rise in circulating progesterone. Progesterone is produced by the cells remaining after the follicle ruptures. Once ovulation has occurred and the egg is released, the remaining cells in the follicle change their function and, instead of producing only estrogen, now produce large amounts of progesterone (i.e., corpus luteum). This progesterone is necessary for implantation and support of the fertilized egg up to the tenth week (i.e., menstrual age) when the placenta takes over the production of progesterone.

During the first part of the cycle increasing amounts of estrogen are produced and the egg in the follicle is being prepared to be "hatched" into the fallopian tube. The estrogen circulating in the blood reaches a "peak" that triggers a rapid rise (i.e., spike) in LH secretion from the anterior pituitary. This spike triggers ovulation, which is followed by a fall in the circulating levels of estrogen and a rise in levels of progesterone. Once ovulation has occurred, the luteal phase (i.e., ovary) and the secretory phase (i.e., endometrium of uterus) begin. With failure of implantation 7 to 8 days after release, the levels of circulating progesterone and estrogen fall. The endometrium is no longer supported by adequate levels of estrogen and progesterone and is sloughed off as menstrual flow, and the next menstrual cycle begins. The low estrogen level triggers increased FSH production and secretion by the anterior pituitary which stimulates the ovary to produce estrogen and the cycle starts again.

Table 16.3

Causes of Primary Amenorrhea

Breast Development/Absent Uterus

Testosterone in normal female range (ovary present)
Congenital absence of uterus
Testosterone in normal male range (testicle present)
Androgen insensitivity (testicular feminizing syndrome)

No Breast Development/Uterus Present

FSH normal or low
Hypogonadotropic hypogonadism
Kallmann's Syndrome
Pituitary tumor (craniopharyngioma)
FSH high (postmenopausal range, need Karyotype)
Gonadal dysgenesis
Turners' Syndrome

No Breast Development/Absent Uterus

FSH and LH elevated, testosterone male range
Noonan's Syndrome (46XY female)
Vanishing Testicles Syndrome

Breast Present/Uterus Present

Prolactin normal
Polycystic ovary disease
Hypothalamic dysfunction
Hypothalamic-pituitary failure
Ovarian failure
Prolactin elevated
Prolactinoma (tumor) of pituitary

In preparation for implantation and support of the fertilized egg, the endometrium changes during the menstrual cycle. Day one of the cycle is by definition the first day of menstrual flow. During the first two to four days of the cycle, the endometrium is sloughed (i.e., desquamation) down to the basal layer. As circulating estrogen begins to rise, the cells of this basal layer begin to divide and within days rebuild the thickened endometrium. A few days before ovulation at midcycle, glands begin to appear in this thickened lining. At the time of ovulation and increasing progesterone levels, the glands develop material that will be secreted to support the fertilized egg before, during, and following implantation. If the LH surge does not occur causing ovulation, there will not be a significant rise in progesterone and the endometrium will not be prepared to receive a fertilized egg. Estrogen will continue to thicken the endometrium, menstrual flow will begin, usually at the expected time, and the flow may be heavy, generally without cramping. Since there has been no ovulation and no, or minimal, progesterone effect, the endometrium has not been prepared for implantation. Birth control pills, with their varying levels of estrogen and progesterone, mimic pregnancy by circulating high estrogen levels and suppressing ovulation. The progesterone component of the birth control pill prepares the endometrium for desquamation which follows the rapid fall in estrogen and progesterone after the last pill is taken.

PHYSICAL ASSESSMENT

History

In any clinician-patient encounter, the first contact with the patient is critical. This is particularly true when evaluating problems of the reproductive tract where the sharing of sensitive information, feelings, and anxiety is important to reaching a proper diagnosis. A gynecologic history includes a complete general history, which has been discussed in previous chapters, plus a history focused on the female reproductive tract. Begin by observing nonverbal clues reflected by facial expression and posture. These observations will help guide you in gathering additional historical information and prepare you to approach the physical examination.

A tense facial expression with a tight mouth and darting eyes, the presence of perspiration, a dry mouth, or a forward, leaning posture with endless hand activity suggests a frightened patient. Frequently, an angry patient has narrow tight lips, a furrowed brow, narrowed eyes, and sits on the edge of her chair leaning forward as if to pounce. The angry patient radiates aggression in her posture, harsh voice, and tendency to overreact to questions, often answering in short, defensive phrases. However, the patient with a smile, eyes that sparkle, sitting relaxed and offering the clinician a warm friendly greeting is the patient who is happy, self-assured, and in good personal control. Nonverbal communication of the apathetic patient includes a bland facial expression, minimal muscular movement of the face, a neutrally positioned thin mouth, a slouched posture, and weak handshake. The apathetic patient often answers verbal questions with short and unemotional responses. The sad patient, like the apathetic patient, sits with shoulders slouched, but the eyes are large and sad and the mouth is turned down at the corners. The sad patient is also usually depressed and her voice may echo hopelessness and remorse.

When taking a history from a patient with a reproductive system problem, direct specific questions in the following areas: menstrual history; pregnancy history; history of vaginal or pelvic infection; gynecologic surgery; urologic history; pelvic pain; abnormal vaginal bleeding; sexual status; birth control status; and a general review of systems with questions regarding sexual abuse, past surgical history, social history, allergies, current medications and family history (see Table 16.4).

The patient's menstrual history is the cornerstone for the evaluation of the woman with reproductive system concerns. Gather information about the patient's menstrual cycle, its regularity, frequency, duration of flow, and any changes in the pattern of menstrual flow, as well as the age of onset of menarche and if and when the patient has gone through menopause. Important in itself, this information also indicates a level of risk for ovarian cancer. Women with early menarche and late menopause are at higher risk for ovarian cancer.

Questioning should determine whether or not the pattern of vaginal bleeding is outside the expected norm. Note the relationship between vaginal bleeding and the patient's expected menses. The absence of a period or periods that occur at times other than expected is termed abnormal vaginal bleeding. Missed or absent menses is called amenorrhea or oligomenorrhea, and is most often associated with pregnancy and menopause. Ask the patient if the bleeding associated with the normal menstrual cycle is heavier than usual and lasts longer than normal with, or without, clots, and with, or without, uterine cramping. If the patient has been menopausal, ask if she has had an episode of unexpected bleeding or postmenopausal bleeding, that may be associated with endometrial cancer. Table 16.5 lists the risk factors for endometrial cancer. Determine if vaginal bleeding occurred before the age of eight, signaling precocious puberty. Bleeding of genital or extragenital origin that has been greater than normal without any obvious organic cause is termed dysfunctional uterine bleeding. If vaginal bleeding is unexpected and occurs between normal menses it is called intermenstrual bleeding. Menometrorrhagia is prolonged uterine bleeding occurring at irregular intervals. If this uterine bleeding lasts longer than seven days or is excessive in amount (i.e., >80 ml), but occurs at regular intervals, it is termed menorrhagia or hypermenorrhea. However, if the uterine bleeding is not at regular intervals but is frequent and varying in amount, it is labeled metrorrhagia. Polymenorrhea is uterine bleeding occurring regularly but at less than 21-day intervals. In oligomenorrhea, the intervals between periods are greater than 35 days but less than 6 months, whereas amenorrhea is the term used to described the absence of menses for more than six months.

Pregnancy history provides information about a woman's ability to become pregnant and problems with past pregnancies that may raise concerns about future pregnancies or increased risk for chronic illnesses. This information is recorded as **gravidity** (i.e.,

Female Reproductive System History

Table 16.4

Menstrual History

Last normal menstrual period (LNMP):
Previous menstrual period (PMP):
Menstrual cycle (interval, duration, regularity):
Age of menarche:
Age of menopause:

Vaginal Bleeding, Abnormal

Timing relative to period (first or last half of cycle):
Amount (how many pads soak in one hour):
Duration (how long did it last: hours, days, weeks):
Frequency (number of episodes in set time period: hours, days, weeks):
Onset (gush of blood, slow bleed):

Pregnancy History

Gravidity (number of pregnancies):
Parity [number of term births, preterm births, abortions, living children (TPAL)]:
Age of first pregnancy:
Age of first birth:
Method of birth (vaginal, Cesarean section):
Pregnancy complications [preterm labor (PTL), gestational diabetes mellitus (GDM), preeclampsia, premature rupture of membranes (PROM), preterm premature rupture of membranes (P-PROM)]:
Labor and devlivery complications (intrauterine fetal demise (IUFD), cervical lacerations, postpartum hemorrhage):

History of Vaginal or Pelvic Infections

Vaginitis (yeast, bacterial vaginosis):
Sexually transmitted disease (*Neisseria gonorrhoeae, Chlamydia trachomatis,* trichomonas):
Pelvic inflammatory disease:

History of Gynecologic Surgery

Hysterectomy:
Oophorectomy:
Vaginal surgery:
Laparoscopic surgery (list reason for surgery):
Bilateral tubal ligation:
Salpingostomy for ectopic pregnancy:

Table 16.4

Female Reproductive System History (continued)

Urologic History

Surgery on bladder, ureters, kidney:
Urinary tract infections (UTI):
Urinary incontinence:

Pelvic Pain

Location of pain:
Onset/duration (in relation to menstrual cycle; sudden, gradual):
Character/intensity (e.g., sharp, dull, cramping, moderate, severe):
Frequency of pain (e.g., with each cycle):
Aggravation of pain (e.g., urination, defecation, dyspareunia, walking down stairs):
Relief of pain (e.g., period begins, after menstrual flow stops):
Radiation of pain (e.g., into labia majora, down back of leg):

Sexual Status

Enjoyment or concerns about sexual intercourse:
Age of first sexual intercourse:
Number of partners:
How long with current partner:

Birth Control Status

Not using any method of birth control:
Type of birth control used
   Oral contraceptive pill (name):
   Barrier method (condoms):
   Norplant implants (date implant was placed):
   Depo-provera injections (date of last injection):
   Tubal ligation (type):
   Intrauterine device (type and date device was placed):

Review of Systems

Chronic or acute illnesses:
Hospitalizations:
Bleeding problems:
History of cancer (colon, breast, endometrium, ovary):

Table 16.4

Female Reproductive System History (continued)

Past Surgical History

Surgeries, non gynecologic (types and dates):
Blood transfusions:
Reaction to anesthesia:

Social History

Smoker [pack(s) per day, age began]:
Alcohol use (frequency and amount):
Drugs of abuse (type, frequency, amount):
Marital status:
Vocation and avocation:

Allergies

Medications:
Environmental allergens:
Tapes (e.g., adhesive tape, elastoplast):

Medications (effect on sex drive, libido)

Oral contraceptive pills:
Fertility medications:
Prescription drugs:
Over the counter drugs:

Family History

Congenital malformations:
Mental retardation:
Reproductive wastage:
Diabetes, hypertension, cancer (type):

---

number of pregnancies) and **parity** (i.e., having given birth to a child, alive or stillborn). Four aspects of parity are recorded: TPAL (i.e., Term births, Preterm births, Abortion, and Living). A woman who has been pregnant three times and has two living children, one born at term and one born preterm, and one miscarriage would be recorded as G3P1112. Women with a history of preterm labor (PTL) or premature rupture of membranes (PROM or P-PROM) are at increased risk for these problems during subsequent pregnancies. Women who have had pre-eclampsia (PET) or gestational diabetes mellitus (GDM) with pregnancy are at increased risk of developing hypertension or diabetes mellitus later in life, respectively. A history of complications during labor and/or delivery may suggest the potential for similar problems in subsequent pregnancies. A history of intrauterine fetal demise (IUFD) suggests increased risk for IUFD in subsequent pregnancies. A history of cervical laceration that had to be surgically repaired alerts the clinician to the possibility of an incompetent cervix during subsequent pregnancies with the risk of early labor or pregnancy loss.

Obtaining a history of previous vaginal or pelvic infections is very helpful in anticipating future medical problems. Past yeast infections and bacterial vaginosis signals the clinician to be alert for signs and symptoms of similar infections in the future. A history of sexually transmitted diseases (STDs) alerts the clinician to the possibility of ectopic pregnancy or infertility secondary to damage of the fallopian tubes caused by *N. gonorrhoeae* or *C. trachomatis* infections. It also suggests patient education is necessary regarding use of barrier methods (i.e., condoms) and the need for examination of the sexual partner or partners. Pelvic inflammatory disease (PID) is almost always caused by *N. gonorrhoeae* or *C. trachomatis*; and therefore, is an STD. Like *N. gonorrhoeae* or *C. trachomatis* infection of the cervix, pelvic inflammatory disease is associated with increased risk of ectopic pregnancy and infertility.

A history of gynecologic surgery not only alerts the clinician to past medical problems with the female reproductive system, but helps the clinician plan for future medical care. A woman who has had a hysterectomy may no longer be at risk of developing cervical cancer, but continues to be at risk for ovarian cancer (see Table 16.6). A woman who has had a hysterectomy and bilateral oophorectomy requires ongoing surveillance to manage estrogen replacement therapy (ERT) to minimize the risk for osteoporosis, fractures, and heart disease. A history of previous surgery for ectopic pregnancy alerts the clinician that the patient is at increased risk for subsequent ectopic pregnancy and its potentially life-threatening hemorrhage.

A urologic history is helpful in considering the possibility of future gynecologic surgeries and assessing pelvic and abdominal symptoms. Symptoms caused by

Table 16.5

Risk Factors for Cancer of the Endometrium[a]

Factors that Increase Risk[b]

        Unopposed estrogen
            Exogenous: estrogen without opposing progesterone
            Endogenous: tumors
        Polycystic Ovary Syndrome
        Obesity
        Nulliparity
        Late menopause (onset after 52 years of age)
        Diabetes mellitus
        Caucasian race

Factors that Decrease Risk

        Ovulation
        Progestin therapy
        Combination birth control pills
        Early menopause (before 49 years of age)
        Normal weight
        Multiparity

[a]Endometrial cancer is the most common cancer of the female genital tract.
[b]Risk factors also apply to endometrial hyperplasia.

Risk Factors for Ovarian Cancer[a,b] *Table 16.6*

Factors that Increase Risk

        Late menopause
        Nulliparity
        Late onset of child brearing
        Early menarche

Factors that Decrease Risk

        Several pregnancies
        Early menopause
        Late menarche
        Use of birth control pills

---

[a] Ovarian cancer is the second most frequent cancer of the female genital tract.
[b] Ovarian cancer has the highest mortality rate of cancers of the female genital tract.

problems with the urinary system may mimic symptoms related to female reproductive system problems. Severe pelvic pain can be and is often confused with the pain of a ureteral (i.e., kidney) stone. Urinary incontinence may be associated with weakness in the support tissues of the vagina (i.e., urethrocele, cystocele) or previous pelvic surgery (i.e., hysterectomy) and is commonly a result of inadequate estrogen in the postmenopausal woman (often corrected by administration of estrogen).

Pelvic pain is one of the most challenging aspects in evaluating the female reproductive system. Its assessment requires a detailed history which includes a definition of the pain. Gather information regarding the type, location, onset, frequency, and radiation of pain, along with a description of things that aggravate, and relieve the pain. Ask about its association with the menstrual cycle, sexual intercourse (i.e., dyspareunia), and urination or defecation. One common type of pelvic pain is that associated with a ruptured follicular cyst which is sharp and cramping in nature, often causing the patient to double over in pain; sudden in onset and lasting hours to days, it occurs around midcycle. It can mimic the pain of appendicitis, ruptured ectopic pregnancy, spastic colon, and other diseases involving organs of the lower abdomen and pelvis.

Evaluation of sexual status is helpful in assessing and diagnosing acute conditions, as well as in determining the risk for future medical problems. Use nondirected questioning to ascertain the patient's concerns regarding normal sexual intercourse. Determine whether the patient finds intercourse satisfying, enjoyable, painful, or frightening. The age of first intercourse, the number of partners, and the length of time with the current partner provide information identifying risks for such problems as ectopic pregnancy, sexually transmitted diseases, pelvic inflammatory disease, human immunodeficiency virus or acquired immunodeficiency syndrome (HIV/AIDS), and cervical cancer. Early, frequent intercourse with multiple partners increases the risk for each of these as well as the risk of cervical cancer (see Table 16.7).

Ask the patient if she is using any birth control methods. If no birth control methods are being used and there has been unprotected intercourse on a regular basis for over a year without pregnancy, consider the possibility of infertility of male or female origin. If birth control is being used, ask the patient what type she is using; oral contraceptives or birth control pills (record the specific type/brand name); levonorgestrel implants; Depo-Provera injections every three months; tubal ligation (e.g., the most common type of sterilization); intrauterine device (IUD); barrier method (i.e., condoms; cervical cap; or diaphragm). Ask if other techniques such as spermicidal gels, foams, or sponges are being used. If a woman is taking oral contraceptives, is over the age of 35, and smokes or has hypertension, she should be taken off this type of birth control because of the increased risk to her health. If she is using subcutaneous implanted levo-norgestrel (Norplant), be aware that these have a finite life for usage and must be replaced every five years.

A general review of systems should be completed not unlike that done on any other patient being seen for the first time or presenting with a new medical problem. Following the review of systems approach (see Chapter 1: Physical Assessment and Interviewing the Patient), question chronic and acute illnesses, hospitalization, bleeding problems, and a history of cancer. This review is helpful in uncovering contraindications to use of birth control pills (see Table 16.8). Because of the tendency for cancer of the colon, breast, endometrium, or ovary to occur in the same patient, questions regarding a history of these cancers should be specifically addressed. A woman having one of these four cancers has an increased risk (i.e., greater than the general population) of developing one of the others. Special attention should be directed at obtaining a history of abuse (e.g., physical, sexual such as incest or rape, and emotional). This tends to be a very sensitive and protected area of a person's life and must be approached carefully, with sensitivity, concern, and empathy.

A history of past surgeries can be very helpful. A woman presenting with vaginal bleeding who has had a hysterectomy presents a uniquely different problem than if

Risk Factors for Cancer of the Cervix[a]

Table 16.7

Factors that Increase Risk

Early intercourse
Multiple sex partners
Early marriage
Early childbearing
Prostitution
Venereal infections (papillomavirus)
Use of birth control pills
Cigarette smoking
Previous radiation in the area of the cervix
Diethylstilbestrol (DES) exposure *in utero*

[a]Cervical cancer is the third most common cancer of the female genital tract.

Table 16.8

Contraindications to the Use of Birth Control Pills

Absolute Contraindications

> Vascular disease (present or past)
>> Thromboembolism
>> Thrombophlebitis
>> Atherosclerosis
>> Cerebrovascular accident (CVA)
> Systemic lupus erythematosis (SLE)
> Sickle cell disease (not the trait)
> Cigarette smoking plus age 35 or older
> Hypertension
> Diabetes mellitus with vascular disease
> Hyperlipidemia
> Cancer of endometrium or breast[a]
> Pregnancy (masculinization of female genitalia *in utero*)
> Congestive heart failure (CHF)
> Mitral valve prolapse
> Liver disease (active)

Relative Contraindications

> Heavy cigarette smoking at any age
> Migraine headaches
> Amenorrhea (not until the cause has been determined)
> Depression
> Insulin dependent diabetes mellitus without vascular disease

---

[a]Listed by the FDA as an absolute contraindication, but no data to indicate that birth control pills are harmful to women with these cancers.

that same woman had not had her uterus surgically removed. Since the diagnosis and management of medical problems involving the female reproductive system frequently involve some type of diagnostic or definitive surgical procedure, information regarding previous blood transfusions and any adverse reactions to such transfusions, as well as a history of adverse reaction to anesthesia are important.

Determining whether or not a woman smokes and how long she has smoked, is important for evaluating risk for certain reproductive organ-related illness, contraindications for use of birth control pills, as well as added risk for certain types of anesthesia. Similarly, information regarding alcohol use (frequency and amount) and/or drug abuse (type, frequency, and amount) helps the clinician anticipate present and future medical problems. Exposure to certain toxic substance at work, or when participating in an avocation, also provides helpful information, particularly in the pregnant woman.

Just as in any other medical history, the types of allergies and associated response to the allergen should be determined. Certain medications may affect libido, menstrual periods, the ability to ovulate, or the health of an embryo in the uterus. Questions should be directed at identifying these medications as well as the use of contraceptives, fertility medications, and over the counter (OTC) medications.

The usual family history of chronic disease (e.g., cancer, diabetes, hypertension) should be obtained. In addition, determine if there is a family history of congenital malformations, mental retardation, or reproductive wastage (i.e., miscarriage of a pregnancy).

Physical Examination

Having obtained a complete and detailed history from the patient, direct your attention to the physical examination. Conduct the exam in a warm examination room. Ask the patient to disrobe and put on a gown that is warm and protects her modesty. Leave the examination room while the patient undresses. It is important during this examination that the patient be allowed to be in control whenever possible. This can be done by allowing the patient to have options. One of the first options is whether or not the patient would like a support person in the room with her. This person can provide support during potentially uncomfortable or embarrassing parts of the examination. Regardless of whether the examiner is male or female, it is recommended that a female chaperone/helper be present during the examination.

General Examination. Observe the patient's posture and review vital data such as height, weight, and blood pressure. Declining height can be an indication of postmenopausal osteoporosis with vertebral compression fractures. As has been discussed in previous chapters, a general examination, including a breast examination (see Chapter 15), should be completed before beginning the pelvic examination.

Pelvic Examination. Having completed the general examination, place the patient in a supine position with her feet in the stirrups. If the stirrups do not have cloth coverings, allow the patient to wear her socks. Drape the patient's abdomen and lower extremities with a sheet and slightly elevate the patient's head. A hand mirror may be used if the patient wishes to view the examination with the clinician. Ask the patient to relax as much as possible, and to allow her relaxed legs to fall apart. Have her relax her abdominal muscles.

Begin the examination with an orderly inspection of the external genitalia. Inspect the external genitalia or perineum beginning with the mons pubis. Examine the quality and pattern of hair and note whether the distribution is male or female pattern. Record the presence of any body lice or crabs. Specifically examine the skin for evidence of redness, excoriation, discoloration, and pigment loss which can be associated with cancerous or noncancerous conditions. Look for the presence of vesicles, ulcerations, pustules, warty or neoplastic growths, or pigmented nevi. Record the presence and location of scars from previous surgery. Any questionable lesion discovered on the vulva should be evaluated by laboratory tests. A punch biopsy should be performed and the tissue sent to a pathologist for diagnosis.

Systematically examine specific perineal structures beginning with the clitoris, noting its size, shape, and length. Carefully examine the labia minora and majora for evidence of trauma, abnormal hair distribution patterns, and skin changes that might suggest early cancer. Begin the examination of the introitus with the hymen; note if it is intact or marital, or if it is imperforate (a cause of primary amenorrhea or failure to have menses). Examine the perineal body and associated muscles of support. Lastly, inspect the perineal area for the presence of hemorrhoids, sphincter incontinence, anal fissures, or condyloma (i.e., venereal warts).

The next step in the exam is to palpate certain areas of the vulva. With gloved hands, separate the labia minora and inspect the urethra. Placing your index or middle finger gently in the vagina, palpate the length of the urethra and "milk" it by pressing anteriorly against the urethra as you withdraw your finger. Near the opening of the urethra, specifically palpate for the presence of enlarged or infected Skene's glands. If milking the urethra results in pus coming out the urethral opening, the pus should be sent for Gram stains and to be cultured (usually *Neisseria gonorrhoeae*). Next, leaving the index finger in the vagina and placing the thumb on the outside of the labia minora, palpate the lower third of the labia minora where the Bartholin's gland is located. Check for infection of the Bartholin's gland and drainage of pus from its opening.

Now hold the labia apart and inspect the vaginal opening. The anterior or posterior vaginal wall may be abnormally visible, suggesting the presence of a cystocele, urethrocele, or rectocele. A bulge at the mid or high posterior vagina may represent a herniation of bowel in the tissue space between the rectum and the vagina. If there is marked weakening of the pelvic floor and support structures of the uterus, the cervix may be seen. Prolapse into the upper aspect of the vagina is termed mild, first degree, or stage I descensus of the uterus. With moderate, second degree, or stage II descensus, the cervix and uterus have fallen or prolapsed to the level of, but not through, the hymenal ring of the vagina. When the cervix and uterus are protruding through the vaginal opening, the term marked, third degree, or stage III descensus is used. Have the patient bear down as if trying to have a bowel movement to see if these bulges are further accentuated or if new ones are seen indicating relaxed pelvic support.

Speculum Examination. The most commonly used speculum is called a Grave's speculum and it is available in three sizes. The small speculum is used for young children, a virginal female who has not used tampons, a woman with a tight perineal repair, or the aged where in the absence of estrogen stimulation, the vaginal opening has become contracted. The medium sized speculum is most commonly used. The large speculum is longer and wider and reserved for use with large obese women and/or grand multiparous women. There is also a Pedersen's speculum which is made in the same lengths as the Grave's speculum, but is more narrow. This speculum might be used in the woman who is not active sexually, has not become pregnant, does not use tampons, or has had surgery narrowing the vagina. It is important to select a speculum that will provide the patient the greatest comfort and yet allow for adequate visualization of the vagina and cervix.

After warming the speculum, tell the patient that you will place it against her thigh to be certain that it is not too warm. With one or two fingers, depress the posterior vagina over the perineal body asking the patient to try and relax the muscle that you are touching. Gently insert the speculum so that the transverse diameter is in the anterior-posterior direction. Once inserted, carefully turn the speculum so that the transverse diameter is now horizontal. During the entire examination, tell the patient what you are doing and what to expect. This helps her to be less uncomfortable and better cooperate with the examination. Insert the full length of the speculum directing it toward the rectum and posterior fornix. When the tip is in the posterior fornix, gently open the speculum so that the cervix comes into view between the two blades of the speculum. Tighten the screw on the speculum so that the blades of the speculum will be held open while you obtain a Papanicolaou (PAP) smear and more closely examine the cervix.

Inspect the walls of the vagina as the speculum is being inserted and as it is being removed. Look for areas of discoloration, the presence or absence of rugae, raised areas, or cystic structures, and any areas that are suspicious and may need to be biopsied by a gynecologist. If a vaginal discharge is present, describe it. Note its color (e.g., gray, yellow, red, green, brownish), consistency (e.g., watery, thick, bubbly, cottage-cheese like), the presence or absence of odor, and amount. Obtain a specimen to send to the laboratory for examination if it is other than a normal clear to slightly white, thin, odor free discharge.

Inspection of the cervix should reveal a normal pink, shiny, clear appearance with a round external os in the nulliparous, and fishmouth-like opening in the parous woman. There are often slightly raised clear to white cystic structures or Nabothian cysts that are normal findings. Particularly in older women, a fleshy, bulbous structure may be seen protruding from the cervix. This is a cervical polyp and is commonly associated with postmenopausal bleeding. Any areas that are white or raised, irregular, or bleeding should be noted and the patient seen by a gynecologist because of the possibility of cancer. Next, obtain a PAP smear. After gently removing excess mucus from the cervix with a cotton-tipped swab, obtain two specimens. Collect the first specimen with a cytobrush, a long plastic stick with bristles arranged in a circular fashion on the end (see Figure 16.7A). Insert the cytobrush into the endocervical canal, rotate it a quarter turn, and remove it. Roll the brush on a slide. The slide must be sprayed with fixative within 30 seconds, before the cells dry and become distorted (i.e., uninterpretable by the pathologist). Obtain the second specimen with an Ayre's spatula, a long piece of wood resembling a popsicle stick that has a configuration on one end to allow it to fit snugly against the cervix. Place the spatula firmly against the cervix and rotate it in a clockwise fashion with the cervix as the pivot point, moving over the extent of the squamocolumnar junction (see Figure 16.7B). The cells on the lead side of the spatula are then smeared in a thin film on a slide and fixative added as with the cytobrush specimen.

Since their introduction, routine PAP smear screenings have reduced the incidence of cervical cancer by 50%. Currently accepted guidelines for obtaining PAP smears are:

- The first PAP smear should be obtained when a woman is 18 years of age or when she first becomes sexually active;

- If a woman is at high risk (e.g., early sexual activity, multiple partners), she should have annual PAP smears;

- If a woman is at low risk (e.g., late exposure to coitus, one sex partner), after two successive negative annual smears, PAP smears can be done every one to three years at the discretion of the clinician. Most gynecologists recommend no less than once every two years.

If a woman is experiencing menorrhagia, menometrorrhagia, metrorrhagia, or postmenopausal bleeding, an endometrial biopsy should be done after the PAP smear is completed so that cells from the endometrium do not contaminate the PAP test. This is done by inserting a small cannula into the endometrial cavity, pulling back the plunger to create a vacuum within the cannula, and twisting the cannula as it is being pulled out to collect endometrial cells.

Bimanual Examination. The purpose of the bimanual examination of the pelvis is to palpate the uterus and the adnexa (fallopian tubes and ovaries). With gloves on and water soluble lubricant on the ends of the index and middle finger of your dominant hand, place these two fingers in the vagina with the thumb of your dominant hand tucked under the palm. Insert to the depth of the posterior fornix. To steady your examining hand, place your corresponding foot (i.e., your right foot if you are right-handed) on the footrest of the examining table and rest your elbow on your knee.

Fig. 16.7 Methods for collecting specimens for Pap smears. A. To collect the first specimen, insert a cytobrush into the endo-cervical canal, rotate it a quarter of a turn, and remove it. B. Cells for the second sample are obtained by placing an Ayre's spatula firmly against the cervix and rotating it in a clockwise fashion.

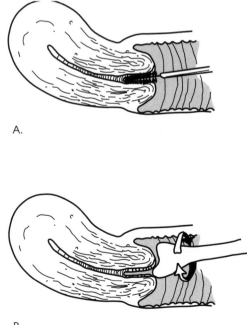

A.

B.

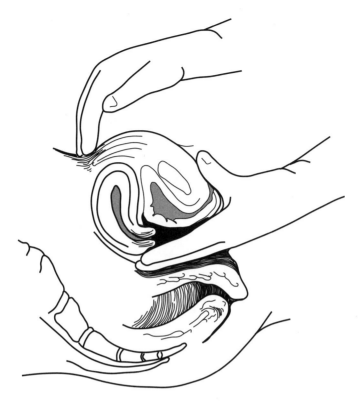

Fig. 16.8 Internal examination of the uterus. The two examining figures elevate the uterus out of the pelvis toward the anterior abdominal wall. The uterus is then palpated between the two fingers of the examining hand in the vagina and the fingers of the hand on the abdomen.

Elevate the usually anteflexed uterus out of the pelvis toward the anterior abdominal wall and place your other hand on the patient's lower abdomen. The uterus can now be palpated between the fingers of your examination hand in the vagina and the fingers of your hand on the abdomen. In examining the uterus, note the position (e.g., centered in the pelvis, anteflexed, retroflexed, anteverted, retroverted), size (e.g., normally about 6 cm by 4 cm and weighing 70 gm), shape (e.g., smooth, pear shaped, no irregular or nodular areas), consistency (e.g., firm, not rock hard or boggy, no areas of tenderness), mobility (i.e., the uterus and adnexa should be easily mobile without pain). Any observations out of the normal should be recorded. With the anteflexed uterus, the abdominal hand can palpate the posterior wall of the uterus. The uterus is said to be in a first degree retroversion if it lies in a straight line with the vagina, second degree retroversion if it lies back in the cul-de-sac posterior to a straight line with the vagina, and third degree retroversion when the uterus is flexed deeply into the cul-de-sac pressing toward the rectum. Loss of mobility reflects pelvic adhesions usually associated with previous pelvic surgery or infection such as pelvic inflammatory disease. Nodular irregularities on the uterus usually represent uterine fibroids. An enlarged, boggy, perhaps tender uterus in a nonpregnant patient, who gives a history of menorrhagia or menometrorrhagia, may indicate adenomyosis where the endometrium becomes buried in the myometrium.

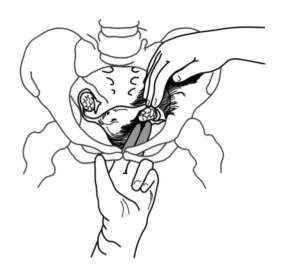

Fig. 16.9 Palpation of the adnexal areas. The examiner places the vaginal examination fingers deep in the lateral fornix with the abdominal hand just medial to the anterior superior iliac crest.

Bimanual examination of the adnexa is begun by placing the vaginal examination fingers deep in the right lateral fornix with the abdominal hand just medial to the anterior superior iliac crest. Bring your fingers together and sweep them downward toward the introitus. The ovary is walnut-sized (3 x 2 cm) and smooth. It is mobile and has a firm rubbery consistency. It tends to be tender to palpation. Note its size, mobility, and consistency. Importantly, the ovary should not ever be palpable in the postmenopausal woman. If palpable, pathology must be suspected. In menstruating women, the ovaries will not be palpable all of the time.

The last part of the pelvic examination is the rectovaginal examination. Change gloves on the vaginal examination hand and lubricate the index and middle finger again. Place your index finger in the vagina and your middle finger in the rectum. Examine the rectovaginal septum (i.e., tissue between the rectum and vagina) for defects, masses, or thickened areas. Palpate the uterosacral ligaments that extend from the posterior wall of the cervix to the sacrum on the right and left side. Thickening, beadiness, tenderness, or pain may signal inflammatory reactions or endometriosis. If the uterus is retroflexed (i.e., third degree retroversion), use your abdominal hand to examine it and determine its size, shape, consistency, and mobility.

Complete the rectovaginal examination by palpating of the rectum in all directions to identify any masses that might be associated with rectal polyps or cancer, the frequency of which begins to increase after age 35. Recall that 50% to 70% of colon cancers occur within reach of this rectal examination. Record the tone of the anal sphincter, the presence of hemorrhoids, fissures, or masses. If stool is present, check it for occult blood.

The examination being completed, assist the patient out of the stirrups to a sitting position and offer facial tissues to help remove the jelly from the perineum. Leave the room so the patient may get cleaned up and dressed.

PHARMACOTHERAPEUTIC CASE ILLUSTRATION

History

J.J. is a 22-year-old-female who has been pregnant twice; she has one living child and has had one abortion (G2 P1011). Her last normal menstrual period (LNMP) was 30 days ago. She presents at the emergency room late one evening complaining of lower abdominal pain which has gradually worsened over the past two days. She has begun to have a fever without chills. She describes the pain as diffuse, located in the lower abdomen and bilateral. It is a dull constant pain that does not wax and wane. It is relieved by sitting or lying still and aggravated by jerking motions such as walking down stairs. Dyspareunia is also present. She has experienced an increase in the vaginal discharge which is described as yellowish white and thick with small amounts of blood occasionally present. There is no odor to the discharge. She said she feels tired and has a poor appetite. She has a sexual history of four different partners in the last five months without a previous history of sexually transmitted disease. She does not know if her partners have had sexually transmitted diseases. Currently not using birth control pills, J.J. began participating in sexual intercourse at age 13.

Physical Examination

J.J.'s vital signs were as follows: blood pressure (BP) 114/64 mm Hg; pulse 82 beats/min; respiratory rate (RR) 18/min; temperature 100.8° F. Her tympanic membranes were normal; her throat was without erythema and there was no tonsillar enlargement. Her thyroid was not enlarged, and there was no sign of anterior or posterior cervical adenopathy. Her chest was clear to auscultation and percussion; no CVA tenderness was detected. Her heart had a regular rate and rhythm without enlargement or extra heart sounds. An examination of J.J.'s abdomen revealed the following: normal bowel sounds; not distended; no masses or megaly; generalized tenderness to deep palpation in the lower right and left quadrants without rebound tenderness; no tenderness located over McBurney's point. Examination of J.J.'s extremities revealed negative heel tap and negative psoas sign. A pelvic exam revealed that J.J.'s external genitalia were normal. Her Bartholin's gland, urethra, and Skene's glands (BUS) were normal without evidence of purulent discharge or infection. Her vagina was pink with abundant rugae present and no discharge. Her cervix was multiparous with mild ectropion and purulent discharge from cervical os. J.J.'s uterus was of normal size, shape, and consistency, mobile but with marked uterine and cervical motion tenderness. Her adnexa felt full and there was marked tenderness with bimanual palpation bilaterally.

Laboratory

A complete blood count (CBC) returned the following results: hemoglobin (Hgb) 14.2, hematocrit (Hct) 43.0, white blood cell (WBC) count 13.2 with polys 84, bands 8, lymphs 6, monos 2. A pregnancy test was negative. A Gram's stain of the cervical discharge showed too numerous to count white blood cells, and the presence of gram-negative intracellular diplococci present. A culture of cervix was taken; results will be available in 24 hours. J.J.'s erythrocyte sedimentation rate (ESR) was elevated to 27 mm/hr.

Diagnosis and Management

Because of the acuteness of onset; the absence of infection anywhere except the cervix and internal female genitalia; the elevated temperature and white blood cell count with a left shift (i.e., increased polys and bands); an elevated ESR; and Gram's stain positive for what are probably *Neisseria gonorrhoeae*. J.J. was diagnosed as having cervicitis with pelvic inflammatory disease (PID) with at least salpingitis and parametritis with possible endometritis.

It was decided to treat her with antibiotics as an outpatient. After an initial dose of ceftriaxone 250 mg IM, she was prescribed Doxycycline hyclate 100 mg BID for 14 days.

Discussion

Disease. Pelvic inflammatory disease presents with a wide range of signs and symptoms. It can be an incidental finding in an asymptomatic patient or present as an acute life-threatening illness. When the diagnosis is based upon clinical assessment, it has a high false negative rate and a high false positive rate. When in question, the definitive diagnosis is made by diagnostic laparoscopy. The differential diagnosis of acute pelvic inflammatory disease includes: appendicitis, ectopic pregnancy, torsion of ovary or rupture of adnexal mass, and endometriosis.

In appendicitis, the exam would demonstrate localized pain to McBurney's point; also heel tap and psoas sign would have been positive. Pelvic exam would have been negative except for possible tenderness and fullness in the right iliac fossa area. Ectopic pregnancy would have had a positive pregnancy test, and abdominal examination would have been similar to J.J.'s except that there would have been localized pain to one or the other adnexum, whichever one held the pregnancy. Torsion of ovary or ruptured adnexal mass would be similar to ectopic pregnancy except that the pregnancy test would have been negative. Endometriosis is a diagnosis which can mimic any of the above and is made by diagnostic laparoscopy.

Though PID has been associated with infection by Bacteroides species, Enterobacteriaceae species, and Streptococci, the two most common etiologies are

Chlamydia trachomatis and *Neisseria gonorrhoeae* (the most common, >50%). *N. gonorrhoeae* can infect any part of the body (e.g., pharynx, urethra, Skene's or Bartholin's glands, eye, anus, skin, joints, cervix, vagina, fallopian tubes, ovaries, peritoneum). Fifteen percent of women with *Neisseria gonorrhoeae* of the cervix will have PID. Infertility occurs in 10% to 20% of women after their first PID involving *Neisseria gonorrhoeae* or *Chlamydia trachomatis* infection of fallopian tube (i.e., salpingitis). Infertility rate rises to 75% after three or more episodes of salpingitis. There is a 7 to 10 fold increase in ectopic pregnancies in women who have had salpingitis.

Management. Unless a causative organism is isolated, antibiotic management is empiric and directed primarily at the two major pathogens: *N. gonorrhoeae* and *C. trachomatis*. Patients with severe PID should be hospitalized and treated with parenteral antibiotics after appropriate cultures have been obtained. Mild cases of PID can be treated in a primary care setting (see Table 16.9).

Table 16.9

Antimicrobial Regimens
Recommended by the Centers for Disease Control
for Treatment of Acute Pelvic Inflammatory Disease

Treatment Setting, Drugs, Schedule	Advantage	Disadvantage	Clinical Considerations
Inpatient			
Cefoxitin[b] plus doxycycline[a] Administer cefoxitin (2 gm IV Q 6 hr) plus doxycycline (100 mg IV Q 12 hr) for a total of at least 4 days and for at least 48 hr after defervescence. Continue doxycycline (100 mg PO BID) after discharge to complete 10–14 days of therapy.	Optimal coverage of *Neisseria gonorrhoeae* (including resistant strains) and *Chalmydia trachomatis*	Possible suboptimal anaerobic coverage	Penicillin-allergic patients may also be allergic to cephalosporins. Tetracycline use in pregnant patients may cause discoloration of teeth and reversible inhibition of skeletal growth in the fetus.
Clindamycin plus an aminoglycoside Administer clindamycin (900 mg IV Q 8 hr) plus gentamicin or tobramycin (1.5–2 mg/kg IV Q 8 hr) for a total of at least 4 days and for at least 48 hr after defervescence. Continue clindamycin (450 mg PO QID) after discharge to complete 10–14 days of therapy.	Optimal coverage of anaerobes and gram-negative enteric rods	Possible suboptimal coverage of *N. gonorrhoeae* and *C. trachomatis*	Patients with decreased renal function may not be good candidates for aminoglycoside treatment or may need a dose adjustment.
Outpatient			
Cefoxitin plus probenecid or ceftriaxone and doxycycline[a] Administer cefoxitin (2 gm IM once) plus probenecid (1 gm PO once) or ceftriaxone (250 mg IM once). Concomitantly administer doxycycline (100 mg PO Q 12 hr) for a total of 10 days.	Good to excellent coverage of *N. gonorrhoeae* and optimal coverage of *C. trachomatis*	Possible suboptimal anaerobic coverage	Considerations outlined above with regard to penicillin-allergic patients and tetracycline use in pregnant patients apply.

J.J. was given a 250 mg intramuscular dose of ceftriaxone (Rocephin) and doxycycline 100 mg PO BID for 14 days. If J.J. cannot tolerate the doxycycline, she can be treated alternatively with ofloxacin (Floxin) 400 mg PO BID, plus either clindamycin (Cleocin) 450 mg PO QID for 14 days or metronidazole (Flagyl) 500 mg PO BID for 14 days. A single oral dose of 1 gm azithromycin (Zithromax) also is an alternative to doxycycline for treatment of chlamydia; however, it is considerably more expensive and its role less clear. If J.J. is pregnant, doxycycline, tetracyclines, and ofloxacin are contraindicated; and the safety of azithromycin in pregnancy has not been adequately studied. Erythromycin 500 mg PO QID for 10 days (or 250 mg for 14 days) can be safely used in J.J. as an alternative to doxycycline, for the management of her chlamydia if pregnancy is a complicating variable.

Since J.J. is not pregnant, the practitioner should assess whether she uses an intrauterine device (IUD) for contraception and should remove it if present. An alternative to IUD contraception is necessary because the IUD is a foreign object and can serve as a nidus for her PID. J.J. should avoid intercourse until after the completion of her therapy and her sexual partners should be examined and treated as necessary. J.J. must be re-examined to insure compliance and cure. Treatment failure or re-infection can lead to infertility or ectopic pregnancy which can still occur despite adequate treatment.

If J.J. fails to respond to outpatient therapy within 72 hours, she should be hospitalized. The indicators of failure are no improvement of worsening of initial symptoms. Intravenous cefoxitin 2 gm IV Q 6 hr or cefotetan 2 gm IV Q 12 hr plus doxycycline 100 mg IV Q 12 hr or clindamycin 900 mg IV Q 8 hr, plus gentamicin 1.5 mg/kg IV Q 8 hr are empiric choices. When the patient has received four days of intravenous antibiotics and has been afebrile for at least 48 hours and is without symptoms, parenteral therapy can be changed to oral antibiotics. Either oral doxycycline or clindamycin should continue after hospital discharge for 14 days, especially for *C. trachomatis* or anaerobic infection.

Therapeutic Drug Monitoring Examples

POSTMENOPAUSAL ESTROGEN REPLACEMENT THERAPY (ERT)

The approach to therapeutic drug monitoring by clinicians varies depending upon many factors. Some of these include preferences among clinicians in a given community or region; concurrent medical problems which dictate that certain drugs be used or avoided; the patient's response to selected medication. The following outlines of therapeutic drug monitoring offer examples which may serve to stimulate discussion and further understanding of initiating and monitoring drug use. The drugs and dosages presented should not be applied to any clinical situation without proper medical supervision.

Drug Therapy
: **With Uterus:** Conjugated equine estrogen 0.625 mg/day, days 1 to 25 each month and medroxyprogesterone acetate 10.0 mg/day, days 16 to 25 each month; or conjugated equine estrogen 0.625 mg/day and medroxyprogesterone acetate 2.5 mg/day.

Without uterus: conjugated equine estrogen 0.625 mg/day.

Monitoring
: **Symptoms:** Ask the patient if she is experiencing hot flushes, emotional lability, loss of or decreased libido, history of fractures, intermenstrual bleeding, or breast tenderness.

Signs: Check for elevated blood pressure, breast nodule, and absent or decreased rugae in vaginal mucosa.

Laboratory Tests
: The clinician may elect to order all, none, or some of these laboratory studies depending upon history and physical findings, as well as other specific clinical indications. Serum cholesterol, LDL, HDL, mammogram before beginning ERT, PAP before beginning ERT and at regular intervals, EMB if abnormal uterine bleeding is present.

Therapeutic Drug Monitoring Examples

POSTMENOPAUSAL ESTROGEN REPLACEMENT THERAPY (ERT)
(continued)

Adverse Drug Event Monitoring	Ask the patient if she smokes cigarettes. If she does, ask how many. Ask the patient if she has experienced any of the following symptoms: breast pain or tenderness, spotting or breakthrough bleeding, gallbladder pain, breast lumps, nausea, or headaches (especially migraine headaches).

Therapeutic Drug Monitoring Examples

ENDOMETRIOSIS

The approach to therapeutic drug monitoring by clinicians varies depending upon many factors. Some of these include preferences among clinicians in a given community or region; concurrent medical problems which dictate that certain drugs be used or avoided; the patient's response to selected medication. The following outlines of therapeutic drug monitoring offer examples which may serve to stimulate discussion and further understanding of initiating and monitoring drug use. The drugs and dosages presented should not be applied to any clinical situation without proper medical supervision.

Drug Therapy	Leuprolide depot 3.75 mg IM monthly for 6 months.
Monitoring	**Symptoms:** Ask the patient about the onset and severity of symptoms. Ask about the following symptoms and any change if they were previously present: pelvic pain or tenderness, dyspareunia, and dysmenorrhea. Tell the patient that initial flare-up of symptoms is normal. Determine if she has reached the treatment of goal of amenorrhea.
	Signs: *Gen:* Describe the degree of distress. Measure the patient's weight. *MSE:* Describe the patient's appearance and behavior (note motor restlessness, facial expression, and posture). *Breast:* Inspect and palpate the breast for swelling, tenderness, and consistency. *Genitalia:* Inspect/palpate the external genitalia. Note any discharge or lesions. Using a speculum, inspect the vagina and cervix. Describe any lesions or bleeding. If indicated, obtain a PAP smear. Palpate the uterus and adnexa for tenderness.
Laboratory Tests	The clinician may elect to order all, none, or some of these laboratory studies depending upon history and physical findings, as well as other specific clinical indications. Laparoscopy, if indicated.

Therapeutic Drug Monitoring Examples

ENDOMETRIOSIS
(continued)

Adverse Drug Event Monitoring	Question about leuprolide-induced postmenopausal effects. Is the patient experiencing hot flashes? Does she report headache, depression or emotional lability, or nausea/vomiting?

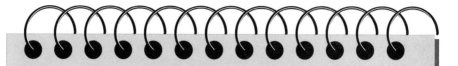

Therapeutic Drug Monitoring Examples

VAGINITIS, TRICHOMONAL

The approach to theraputic drug monitoring by clinicians varies depending upon many factors. Some of these include preferences among clinicians in a given community or region; concurrent medical problems which dictate that certain drugs be used or avoided; the patient's response to selected medication. The following outlines of therapeutic drug monitoring offer examples which may serve to stimulate discussion and further understanding of initiating and monitoring drug use. The drugs and dosages presented should not be applied to any clinical situation without proper medical supervision.

Drug Therapy | Metronidazole 2 gm PO as a single dose.

Monitoring

Symptoms: Ask the patient to describe her symptoms at the start of treatment. Are they still present to the same degree? If vaginal discharge was present, ask if she still has a vaginal discharge with or without vulvar itching. If a discharge is present, is it malodorous or distressing to the patient? Is her partner having symptoms and has he been treated?

Signs: *Genitalia:* Inspect the external genitalia for sign of discharge and inflammation. If discharge is seen, note the odor, amount, and color. Inspect the vagina for inflammation and red granular or petechial spots on the fornix. Look for cervical drainage. Obtain a vaginal smear.

Laboratory Tests

The clinician may elect to order all, none, or some of these laboratory studies depending upon history and physical findings, as well as other specific clinical indications. Vaginal smears for bacteria, *Trichomonas vaginalis*, and *Candida albicans*.

Adverse Drug Event Monitoring

Ask the patient if she has experienced nausea or an unpleasant metallic taste since starting treatment. Instruct the patient to avoid ingesting alcohol, including nonprescription drugs that contain alcohol, while taking this medication.

Therapeutic Drug Monitoring Examples

ORAL CONTRACEPTION

The approach to therapeutic drug monitoring by clinicians varies depending upon many factors. Some of these include preferences among clinicians in a given community or region; concurrent medical problems which dictate that certain drugs be used or avoided; the patient's response to selected medication. The following outlines of therapeutic drug monitoring offer examples which may serve to stimulate discussion and further understanding of initiating and monitoring drug use. The drugs and dosages presented should not be applied to any clinical situation without proper medical supervision.

Drug Therapy	Lo/Ovral-28 One tablet daily, beginning on the first Sunday after menstruation begins.
Monitoring	**Symptoms:** Ask if the patient has experienced any breakthrough bleeding or spotting. If she has, determine when it occurred in the cycle. Ask if she has experienced any of the following: breast tenderness, nausea, weight changes, bloating, depression, or headaches (especially migraine).
	Signs: *Gen:* Check the patient's blood pressure and weight. *Breast:* Inspect and palpate for lumps and tenderness. Note any discharge. *Genitalia:* Inspect the external structures. Using a speculum, inspect the vagina for color, areas of discoloration, and discharge. Next inspect the cervix and obtain a PAP and other smears as indicated. Using the bimanual method, palpate the uterus and adnexa.
Laboratory Tests	None.
Adverse Drug Event Monitoring	Question about new onset headaches (e.g., migraine), bloating, nausea, cramping, edema, depression or irritability, weight changes, spotting, breakthrough bleeding (BTB), changes in menstrual flow, dysmenorrhea, or amenorrhea.

Therapeutic Drug Monitoring Examples

ORAL CONTRACEPTION
(continued)

Adverse Drug Event Monitoring	Immediately refer the patient to her physician if she has any complaints of acute, severe pain associated with the eyes, chest, head, abdomen, or legs. Pain in these areas may indicate a blood clot.

Reproductive System: Male

*T*he male reproductive system consists of the penis, the prostate, seminal vesicles, ductus deferens (i.e., vas deferens), epididymis, and testes. As with the female reproductive system, there is a period of embryological differentiation which, in the male, is controlled by the Y chromosome and a period of pubescence normally beginning after the age of nine. The period of pubescence in the male on average lags about one year behind that of the female. Precocious puberty is said to be present in the male if the development of secondary sex characteristics appears before nine years of age (see Table 17.1).

ANATOMY AND PHYSIOLOGY

Penis

The penis is an oblong organ composed of erectile tissue arranged in three tube-like structures: the corpus spongiosum, the tip of which is the glans of the penis, and the two corpora cavernosa. In a cross section of the penis, the **corpora cavernosa** lie side by side in the dorsal aspect of the shaft of the penis. They are suspended proximally from the pubic symphysis by the suspensory ligament of the penis (see Figure 17.1). They divide at the pubic symphysis into a right and left crus and attach to the right and left ischiopubic rami.

The corpora cavernosa are surrounded by a thick fascial sheath (i.e., **Buck's fascia**) which is separated from the corpora cavernosa by another fascial sheath (i.e., the **tunica albuginea**). The ischiocavernosus muscle overlies the fascia of the corpora cavernosus proximally and also attaches to the ischiopubic rami. The **corpus spongiosum** is located ventral to the paired corpora cavernosa in the depression between them. Proximally, it connects to the under surface of the urogenital diaphragm and is surrounded by fascial layers similar to those of the corpora

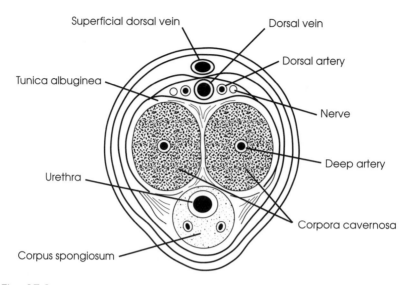

Fig. 17.1 A cross-sectional view of the internal structures of the penis.

cavernosa. Outside these fascial layers at the base of the corpus spongiosum is the **bulbocavernosus muscle** (also called bubospongiosus muscle). Each of these three cavernous structures contain erectile tissue and large arteries. External to Buck's fascia is **Colles' fascia** which is a continuation of Scarpa's fascia of the anterior abdominal wall. Colles' fascia encircles the penis and attaches to the base of the penis ventrally. Connecting with Colles' fascia near its caudal attachment to the base of the penis is **Dartos fascia** which provides support to the scrotal sac and lies beneath the skin of the scrotum (see Figure 17.2). External to Colles' fascia is a covering of skin which is devoid of fat and is loosely applied to the erectile bodies of the penis. At birth, the skin of the penis extends over the glans of the penis as the prepuce or foreskin. It is this foreskin that is removed during a circumcision. If not removed, it can be retracted proximal to the glans in the uncircumcised adult male. It should not be forcefully retracted in newborns, infants, or young children (see Table 17.2).

The corpora cavernosa, corpus spongiosum, and attached glans penis are specialized tissues composed of septa of smooth muscle and erectile tissue enclosing vascular cavities which, when filled with blood allow the penis to become firm and erect. The **urethra** located in the corpus spongiosum on the ventral side of the penis normally opens through a meatus at the tip of the glans penis. Failure in embryologic development may result in the opening being more proximal on the ventral or dorsal surface of the penis. When this is identified it is termed hypospadius or epispadius and may require surgical repair when the child gets older.

Infections or cancers of the skin of the penis are carried by lymphatics that drain into the inguinal nodes beneath the inguinal ligament causing enlargement of these nodes. Infections involving structures deep within the penis such as urethritis (i.e.,

Table 17.1

Sexual Maturity Rating Scale for Boys

Stage	Pubic Hair	Genital	
		Genital	Testes and Scrotum
Stage 1	Preadolescent: no pubic hair except for the fine body hair (vellus hair) similar to that on the abdomen	Preadolescent: same size and proportions as in childhood	Preadolescent: same size and proportions as in childhood
Stage 2	Sparse growth of long, slightly pigmented, downy hair, straight or only slightly curled, chiefly at the base of the penis	Slight or no enlargement	Testes larger; scrotum larger, somewhat reddened, and altered in texture
Stage 3	Darker, coarser, curlier hair spreading sparsely over the pubic symphysis	Larger, especially in length	Further enlarged
Stage 4	Coarse and curly hair, as in the adult; area covered greater than in Stage 3 but not as great as in the adult and not yet including the thighs	Further enlarged in length and breadth, with development of the glans	Further enlarged; scrotal skin darkened
Stage 5	Hair adult in quantity and quality, spread to the medial surfaces of the thighs but not up over the abdomen	Adult in size and shape	Adult in size and shape

inflammation of the periurethral glands) drain by lymphatics to the lymph nodes near the external iliac, internal iliac, and common iliac arteries deep in the pelvis and lower abdomen and, therefore, are not usually palpable on routine clinical examination. If cancer of these penile structures has metastasized to the nodes, the nodes are not palpable during a general physical exam.

At the base of the penis the penile urethra continues as the prostatic urethra surrounded by the **prostate gland**. Lying above the base of the penis, the prostate sits on the urogenital diaphragm just behind the pubic symphysis. The bladder sits on top of the prostate gland emptying into the prostatic urethra. This relationship explains how enlargement of the prostate [e.g., benign prostatic hypertrophy (BPH) or prostatic cancer] might compress the prostatic urethra resulting in difficulty starting urination, decreased force of urinary stream, and other signs of urinary outflow obstruction.

Table 17.2

Age at which Foreskin can be Retracted

Age	Foreskin Retraction (%)
at birth	4% of boys
6 months old	15%–20%
1 year old	50%
3 years old	80%–90%
17 years old	97%–99%

Prostate Gland

The prostate gland is a fibromuscular and glandular organ which weighs about 20 gm and is about the size of a large chestnut. It is surrounded by a fibrous prostatic capsule and supported anteriorly by the puboprostatic ligament attached to the bone of the pubic symphysis. On the posterior floor of the 2.5 cm long prostatic urethra is a slightly raised area called the urethral crest into which the prostate gland and each of the ejaculatory ducts empty. The ejaculatory ducts are an intraprostatic continuation of the vas deferens into which the seminal vesicles empty. The prostate is made up of several lobes, not all of which can be examined by rectal examination. Each lobe is composed of several glands (about 25) which empty into the floor of the prostatic urethra at the urethral crest. Located in the urogenital diaphragm just distal to the

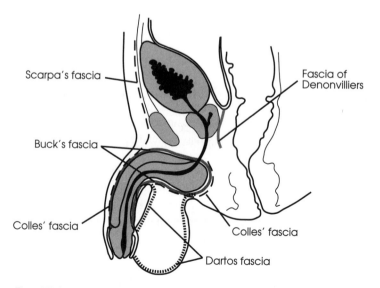

Fig. 17.2   Fascial planes of the male lower genitourinary tract.

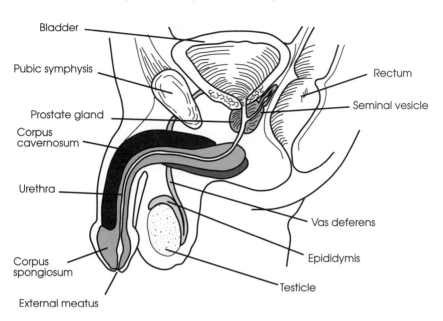

Fig. 17.3   A diagram showing the relations of the bladder, prostate, seminal vesicles, penis, urethra, and scrotal contents.

prostate and emptying into the proximal penile urethra are the bulbourethral or **Cowper's glands** which secrete a mucoid lubricant during sexual arousal.

Seminal Vesicles

The **seminal vesicles** are found cephalad to the prostate, but still beneath the bladder lying just lateral to the vas deferens on either side. At the point at which the right and left seminal vesicles join the right and left vas deferens, the vas deferens changes in name to become the **ejaculatory duct** which in turn empties into the prostatic urethra at the level of the lower urethral crest. The seminal vesicles can usually be palpated on rectal exam as they lie superior and lateral to the prostate on the posterior bladder. With infection they may be tender, swollen, and enlarged to palpation. A mucus membrane lines the vesicle outside of which a thin layer of fascia and smooth muscle is found. When this layer of smooth muscle contracts, seminal vesicle contents are extruded into the ejaculatory duct. The **vas deferens** is a long tubular structure connecting the epididymis of the testes with the ejaculatory duct which then empties into the prostatic urethra. The vas deferens travels in a circuitous route from the testes in the scrotal sac to the external inguinal ring in the lower anterior abdominal wall just below the inguinal ligament. It continues through the abdominal wall structure in the inguinal canal to the internal inguinal ring where it enters the abdominal cavity. It then remains behind the peritoneum on its way to the base of the bladder and the ejaculatory duct. Direct and indirect inguinal hernias occur in the lower anterior abdominal wall medial to the internal inguinal ring and the inguinal canal or through the internal inguinal ring into the inguinal canal respectively.

Spermatic Cord

From the internal inguinal ring to the testes, the vas deferens is enclosed in a structure called the **spermatic cord**. The thin fascia of this cord surrounds its contents, which are the vas deferens, the internal and external spermatic arteries, the artery of the vas deferens, the venous pampiniform plexus and its superior continuation, the spermatic vein, lymphatic vessels, and nerves. This thin fascia layer contains muscle fibers (i.e., the cremasteric muscle). The close proximity of the pampiniform plexus of veins and the testicular artery provides the opportunity for counter current mechanisms to lower the temperature of blood (34° C) going to the testicle (maintaining it at an optimal temperature for spermatogenesis). This configuration of blood vessels also facilitates the exchange of androgens coming from the testicular Leydig cells and the veins to the testicular artery where the androgens are in low concentration. The androgens can then return to the testicle to stimulate and support spermatogenesis. The presence of a varicocele (i.e., enlarged varicose veins of the pampiniform plexus secondary to incompetence of venous valves) results in a rise in the temperature of the blood flowing to the testicles and, thereby, compromises spermatogenesis.

Located on the backside and lateral to the testes, the **epididymis** is important to the maturation and storage of sperm. A coiled, tubular structure, it is connected to the testes by multiple efferent ducts and, at its lower pole, is continuous with the vas deferens. Anatomically, it is divided into a head (i.e., caput), a body (i.e., corpus) and a tail (i.e., caudal) portion, each having a different function with regard to the maturation and storage of sperm. The epididymis can be palpated during physical examination and may be found to be swollen and markedly tender when infected (i.e., epididymitis).

Testicles

The **testicle** is located in the scrotum having descended during embryologic development from near the kidney on the posterior abdominal wall down and through the inguinal canal into the scrotum. At birth, the process of descent may be incomplete and the testicle may be palpated in the inguinal canal or may still be in the abdominal cavity. If the testicle fails to descend out of the abdomen, the risk of cancer is high. It must be surgically removed if it cannot be brought into the scrotal sac. Importantly, the testicle has a dense fascial covering, the tunica albuginea. In the adult male, the testicle weighs 30 to 45 gm and measures 2.5 by 5 cm. One third of the volume of the testicle is interstitial tissue containing Leydig cells where androgens such as testosterone are made. On the posterior surface of the testes, this fascia penetrates deep into the substance of the testes dividing it into over 200 lobules. Each lobule contains one to three seminiferous tubules. As the testis descended through the inguinal ring into the scrotal sac it carried with it an evagination, (i.e., **processes vaginalis**) of the abdominal wall peritoneum (i.e., somewhat like sticking your finger into a balloon and carrying with it the rubber of the balloon). Adjacent to the testis, the processes vaginalis becomes the tunica vaginalis. The part of the tunica vaginalis peritoneum that rests against the testis is called the **visceral peritoneum** of the testes. The part that is not attached to the testis is termed the **parietal peritoneum** of the testes. It is separated from the testes by a fluid-filled space. Most often the connection between the abdominal cavity and the abdominal peritoneum's evagination into the scrotum is closed off preventing abdominal fluid from entering this space. If this closure does not occur or is incomplete, a hydrocele will develop. A hydrocele is produced when the tunica vaginalis is filled with abdominal peritoneal fluid. Due to the force of gravity, the amount of abdominal fluid in the tunica vaginalis increases when the patient stands (see Figure 17.5). When the patient lies down, the fluid flows out of the tunica vaginalis and returns to the abdominal cavity.

Each of the more than 200 lobules contains seminiferous tubules which connect with the epididymis via the efferent ducts. The seminiferous tubule consists of two types of cells: Sertoli or supporting cells and spermatogonia. The Leydig cells are found in the interstitium between the seminiferous tubules. Under the microscope it can be seen that the seminiferous tubule is lined by

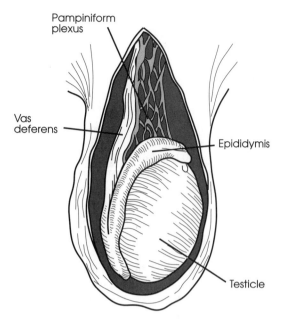

Fig. 17.4 Anatomy of the testicle and epididymis.

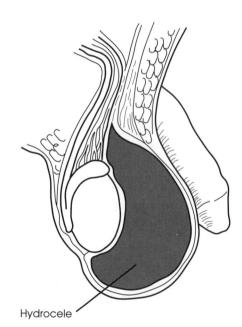

Fig. 17.5 A cross-sectional view of a hydrocele.

Sertoli cells to which sperm are attached as they develop from spermatogonia to spermatocytes, to spermatids, and finally to spermatozoa (i.e., sperm). Importantly, near the membrane on which the Sertoli cell sits there is a "tight junction" between Sertoli cells. The tight junction forms a blood-testis barrier which helps protect the antigenically different developing sperm from the body's immune system, and helps prevent the development of an autoimmune response which usually results in infertility. The primary function of these various components will be discussed below under the section on physiology. Reflecting its place of origin near the kidneys, the testicular artery arises from the aorta just below the origin of the renal artery. The right testicular vein empties into the inferior vena cava near the renal vein. However, the left testicular vein empties into the left renal vein.

The scrotal sac or **scrotum** in which the testes are located hangs from the perineum posterior and inferior to the base of the penis and anterior to the perineal body and anus. On the outside, the scrotum appears to be one sac; however, internally it is divided into two sacs, one for each testicle. At the superior extent of each sac is the external inguinal ring leading into the inguinal canal. Beneath the rugated skin covering the scrotum in the Dartos fascia are fibers of the dartos muscle. Helping to maintain proper temperature for spermatogenesis, the dartos muscle, along with the cremasteric muscle, is capable of contracting to pull the scrotum and testicle closer to the warmth of the body when exposed to cold or to relax and allow the testicles to move further from the body when exposed to excessive heat.

Physiology

The male reproductive system has two functions. First, it acts as an endocrine organ involved in the synthesis and secretion of male hormones or androgens (the

Table 17.3

Function of Testosterone and Dihydrotestosterone

Spermatogenesis
Sperm maturation in epididymis
Genitalia growth (penis, testes)
Masculine hair pattern
   Beard growth
   Male baldness pattern
   Pubic hair pattern/growth
Bone maturation, closure of epiphyses
Production of sebum from sebaceous gland
Sexual behavior (libido)
Increase muscle mass (male distribution)

Table 17.4

Hormones Produced by the Testes

Sertoli Cells

          Inhibin
          Androgen binding protein

Leydig Cells

          Testosterone
          Androgens other than testosterone

---

predominant androgen is testosterone). Secondly, it acts as an exocrine organ producing sperm (i.e., male gametes). Androgen is synthesized by the **Leydig** cells found in the interstitial space, whereas the seminiferous tubules contain the various cell types responsible for production of sperm (i.e., spermatogenesis). Both the endocrine and exocrine function are under the influence of the anterior pituitary and the gonadotropins it secretes. These gonadotropins, [i.e., follicular stimulating hormone (FSH) and luteinizing hormone (LH)] modulate testicular function. The luteinizing hormone (LH) participates in the anterior pituitary-Leydig cell axis. Follicle stimulating hormone (FSH) interacts with the Sertoli cells of the seminiferous tubule epithelium, the anterior pituitary-seminiferous tubule axis, to influence sperm development. Participants in the pituitary-Leydig cell axis include gonadotropin releasing hormone (GnRH) from the hypothalamus, LH, testosterone, and prolactin. Excess prolactin inhibits biosynthesis of testosterone resulting in impotence. Therefore, if a clinician sees a male patient with gynecomastia who is complaining of impotence, one possible etiology is an anterior pituitary prolactin-secreting adenoma (tumor). LH acts on the Leydig cell to promote testosterone synthesis from cholesterol. The testosterone produced is released into blood capillaries which lie close by. This interaction begins in the seventh week of intrauterine life and participates in the development of male features, testicles, scrotum, and the descent of testes. Following birth, the LH-Leydig axis remains rather quiet until puberty when it is reactivated and the resultant increased production of LH stimulates the Leydig cells to produce testosterone which, in turn, stimulates the development of secondary male sex characteristics, pubic and axillary hair growth, penile and testicular enlargement, and growth toward the male's habitues or body features.

Testosterone in the blood feeds back to the hypothalamus where it decreases the frequency of pulsatile release of GnRH which in turn decreases the release of LH from the anterior pituitary with resultant decreased testosterone production by the Leydig cells. In the male, about 95% of testosterone in the blood is derived from the Leydig cells of the testes. Much of the testosterone circulating in the blood is bound to testosterone binding globulin (TeBG) which is produced in the liver, androgen binding protein (ABP) which is produced by the Sertoli cells, and serum albumin. About 3% to 5% of circulating testosterone is unbound and active. Exogenously administered drugs such as estrogen increase the amount of TeBG; whereas, testosterone decreases TeBG production. Over half of the plasma testosterone is cleared (i.e., metabolized) by the liver with a single pass, a function which is altered by the administration of various drugs. The primary extracellular androgen is testosterone. The principal intracellular androgen is dihydrotestosterone (DHT). Testosterone is responsible for fetal development of male gonads and gonadotropin secretion. Dihydrotestosterone stimulates differentiation of external genitalia, male secondary sex characteristics, and spermatogenesis.

Participants in the pituitary-seminiferous tubule axis include the Sertoli cells found in the seminiferous tubules, FSH from the anterior pituitary, and inhibin. In response to GnRH released from the hypothalamus, FSH is released from the anterior pituitary. FSH works in concert with LH and testosterone to maintain spermatogenesis. Once initiated, most of the FSH-induced events can be maintained by testosterone alone. Inhibin is produced by Sertoli cells and feeds back to the anterior pituitary to decrease the secretion of FSH.

In the male, throughout adult life and with the support of Sertoli cells, the sperm cells in the seminiferous tubule multiply (i.e., mitosis) and mature (i.e., meiosis) from spermatogonia. Somewhat like an assembly line, the sperm cells migrate from the basal lamina of the seminiferous tubules toward the tubule lumen as they mature from spermatogonia to spermatocytes to spermatids to spermatozoa. Initially, spermatocytogenesis (i.e., mitosis) takes place to increase the numbers of spermatocytes which then undergo meiosis to form spermatids, each containing a haploid number of chromosomes (23 chromosomes). The process is termed spermiogenesis. Recall that in the female, all mitotic division occurs before birth and all the ova a woman will ever have are present at birth. In the male, spermatogonia are continually dividing and forming more spermatogonia to develop into sperm. Eighty- and ninety-year-old men have been reported to have fathered children.

The development of a sperm takes about two and one-half months in the testes and one month in the epididymis for maturation. During this period of development and maturation, sperm are susceptible to alteration by outside influences such as mutagenic drugs, irradiation, and environmental toxins that may not only affect chromosome content and structure, but may also alter the ability of sperm to impregnate the egg or ovum. The last change in the sperm that takes place to enable the sperm to fertilize the egg or ovum occurs in the female reproductive tract. This change is called capacitation and alters certain characteristics in the head of the sperm so that it can penetrate and fertilize the egg. The normal range for the number of sperm in an ejaculate is around 20 to 80 million with 60% of these being motile. Male infertility can be related not only to too few sperm, but also to inadequate numbers of motile sperm. In couples who are infertile, the infertility is due to a male factor as high as 40% of the time.

During sexual intercourse (i.e., coitus), semen is deposited in the vaginal vault of the female. The semen contains material from four different organs or glands: the epididymis, the seminal vesicle, the prostate gland, and the bulbourethral glands (i.e., Cowper's glands). As previously noted, the epididymis is where sperm mature and are stored in preparation for ejaculation. During ejaculation, as sperm leave the vas deferens and enter the ejaculatory duct, secretions from the seminal vesicles join with the sperm. Making up about 60% of the ejaculate volume, with a slight yellow color, these seminal vesicle secretions contain fructose and other nutrient substances used by the sperm, as well as prostaglandins and fibrinogen.

The prostaglandins aid in fertilization by interacting with the mucus from the cervix to make it more receptive to sperm. Some also believe that the prostaglandins produce reverse peristalsis in the uterus and fallopian tube to aid in moving sperm toward the distal tube near the ovary where fertilization will take place. Sperm can reach this part of the fallopian tube in as little as five minutes after being deposited in the posterior fornix of the vagina.

During a process called emission, secretions from the prostate gland are joined with the soon-to-be ejaculate. Making up about 30% of the total ejaculate volume, these prostatic secretions further add to the bulk of the semen. In synchrony with the vas deferens, the capsule of the prostate contracts producing secretions that are thick, milky in color, and alkaline, containing citric acid, calcium, acid phosphatase, a fibrinolysin, and a clotting enzyme. The alkaline nature of this material is important in successful fertilization by neutralizing the acidic nature of the vas deferens fluid and the acidic vaginal secretions (pH <4.5). Sperm fertility is inhibited in an acidic medium. Optimal motility requires a pH of surrounding fluids of between 6.0 and 6.5.

As the semen passes out of the prostatic urethra into the penile urethra, mucus from the bulbourethral gland is added to the mix. The seminal vesicle fluids are the last to be emitted to form semen. It is believed that the large amount of seminal vesicle fluid serves to wash the sperm out of the ejaculatory duct and urethra. The prostatic fluid gives the semen a milky color and raises the pH to approximately 7.5. The mucoid consistency of the semen is provided by the mucus secretions from the seminal vesicles and the bulbourethral glands. The clotting enzymes of the prostatic fluid combine with the fibrinogen of the seminal vesicle to give a viscous nature to the semen which holds the sperm relatively immobile for a few minutes after ejaculation.

Products of Male Reproductive Glands

Table 17.5

Seminal Vesicles

        Fructose
        Phosphorylcholine
        Ascorbic acid
        Prostaglandin

Prostate Gland

        Spermine
        Cholesterol
        Fibrinolysin
        Zinc
        Acid phosphatase

Table 17.6

Phases of Male Orgasm

Phase One: Emission

> Adrenergic control
> Semen formed in the prostatic urethra

Phase Two: Ejaculation

> Contraction of bulbocavernosus muscle
> Forceful expulsion of semen from the penile urethra

Subsequently, the ejaculate become less viscous and the sperm are highly active. At body temperature the maximum life span of sperm is 24 to 48 hours. At lower temperatures they live longer and, in fact, can be preserved for years at temperatures below −100° C.

Maximum fertility for males is gauged by several different factors. These include: the volume of the ejaculate, approximately 3.5 mL (normal range: 1 to 5 mL); the total number of sperm, greater than 20 million/mL as a minimum (normal range: 20 to 400 million per mL); percentage of sperm that are motile, greater than 60% of sperm demonstrate motility; and the morphology of the sperm, fewer than 40% of the sperm are morphologically abnormal. If leukocytes are present in the semen, this may represent infection which can adversely affect fertilization.

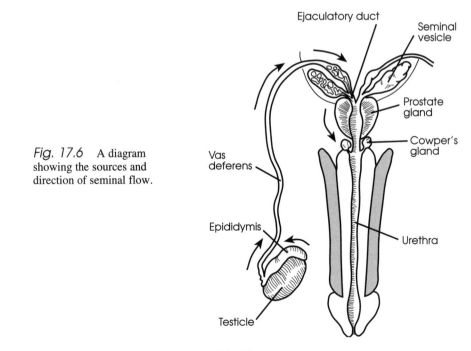

Fig. 17.6 A diagram showing the sources and direction of seminal flow.

The sexual act (i.e., coitus) is the result of emotional excitement and sensory input generating sexual arousal. Sensory input for sexual arousal travels through the sacral plexus of nerves to the spinal cord. Though the man's source of sensory input is primarily from the penis, other areas innervated by the sacral plexus such as scrotum, anal epithelium, and perineal structures can add to the sexual arousal. Through over-filling or through infection, irritation of internal organs such as the urethra, bladder, prostate, seminal vesicle, testes, and vas deferens can also stimulate arousal. Aphrodisiac drugs such as cantharides irritate the bladder and urethral mucosa and, thereby, increase sexual desire.

The male erection is the first effect of sexual stimulation and is proportional to the degree of psychic and/or physical stimulation. It results when parasympathetic impulses pass from the sacral portion of the spinal cord to the penis and dilate arteries filling the erectile tissue (i.e., large, cavernous, venous sinusoids) of the corpus spongiosum and corpora cavernosa. This occurs because the venous outflow from the erectile tissue remains unchanged and, therefore, in a relative manner, is partially occluded. The parasympathetic nerves also act to lubricate the urethra through stimulation of secretion from the urethral glands and bulbourethral glands. These secretions also contribute to lubrication during coitus by adding to the female lubrication secretions from the vaginal wall and the Bartholin's glands. If coitus is painful, the pain may inhibit rather than excite sexual arousal. Whereas preparation (erection) is parasympathetically directed, emission and ejaculation are mediated through the sympathetic nerves which arise higher in the spinal cord at L1–L2 level.

Injury to the spinal cord at or above that level can affect the ability of the male to ejaculate and, thereby, procreate. Emission begins with contraction of the vas deferens to expel semen into the prostatic urethra. Contraction of the muscular coat of the prostatic gland, followed by contraction of the seminal vesicle expels the fluid forcing sperm forward. The prostatic urethra, sensing that it is full, signals the beginning of rhythmic contraction of the internal organs (i.e., the ischiocavernosus and bulbocavernosus muscles compress the base of the penile erectile tissue to move semen from the urethra to the exterior, producing ejaculation). The act of emission and ejaculation is referred to as male orgasm. In the female, a plateau of sexual excitement can be maintained from which repeated orgasm can occur. Within one or two minutes following orgasm in the male, sexual excitement disappears and erection ceases.

PHYSICAL ASSESSMENT

History

In any clinician-patient encounter, the first contact with the patient is critical. This is particularly true when evaluating problems of the reproductive tract where the sharing of sensitive information, feelings, and anxiety is important to reaching a proper diagnosis. A male reproductive history includes a complete general history, which has been discussed in previous chapters, plus a history particularly focused on the male reproductive tract. Begin by observing nonverbal clues reflected by facial expressions and posture. These observations will help guide your subsequent gathering of historical information and your approach to the physical examination. (See Chapter 16: Female Reproductive System, for further discussion of nonverbal clues.)

The clinician should also be alert for certain verbal clues. Men may have certain sexual difficulties (e.g., difficulty in achieving or maintaining an erection, premature ejaculation). For many men in our society, loss of sexual power is not to be admitted, even to a physician. Therefore, the patient frequently presents with other complaints, and the aware clinician will key on these complaints. Most often these other complaints are related in some way to the genital area. For example, the patient might say "My prostate is bothering me." It is important to be alert to these indirect clues. Common sexual act-related complaints include: loss of desire (i.e., libido) for sexual intercourse, orgasm without ejaculation (i.e., retrograde ejaculation into bladder), premature ejaculation, inability to maintain an erection once achieved, or the inability to achieve an erection.

When taking a history focused on the male reproductive system, it is necessary to separate those symptoms relating to the urinary tract (e.g., kidney, ureters, bladder, and urethra) and those related to the reproductive tract (e.g., testicles, epididymis, vas deferens, spermatic cord, seminal vesicles, prostate, urethra, penis, and scrotum). This separation is not always possible. The following discussion primarily focuses on the male reproductive tract.

Questions regarding **urination** should be asked and specifically directed at problems with starting or stopping urination (i.e., terminal dribbling), urinary incontinence, loss of force and caliber of stream, symptoms of chronic or acute urinary retention, or interruption of urinary stream. Difficulty in starting urination or hesitancy is an early symptom of bladder outlet obstruction (i.e., prostate enlargement or urethral stricture). As the narrowing of the outlet worsens, hesitancy is prolonged, frequently causing the patient to have to strain to force urine through the narrowed outlet. Terminal dribbling or difficulty stopping urination is also associated with obstruction and becomes more and more noticeable as the obstruction worsens. Though these symptoms are most frequently associated with benign prostatic hypertrophy, they can also be associated with acute prostatitis or prostatic cancer. A prostate symptom index prepared by the American Urologic Association is presented in Table 17.7 (prostatism: mild ≥ 7, moderate 8–18, severe >18). The results are scored and the score determines the risk for prostatic cancer.

Urinary incontinence is a subject within itself. There are four types of incontinence described which a good history can help to distinguish. Loss of urine without warning (periodically or consistently) is associated with injury to the urethra and muscular sphincter or a congenitally-acquired neurologic disease which may also be associated with sexual dysfunction. This condition is termed true incontinence. Urge incontinence and stress incontinence are related to dysfunction of the urinary system. Paradoxic (i.e., overflow) incontinence is commonly associated with chronic urinary

Table 17.7

American Urologic Association
Urinary Symptom Index for Prostatism

Symptom	Score					
	Not at all	Less than 1 time in 5	Less than half the time	About half the time	More than half the time	Almost always
1. Over the past month or so, how often have you had a sensation of not emptying your bladder completely after you finished urinating?	0	1	2	3	4	5
2. Over the past month or so, how often have you had to urinate again less than two hours after you finished urinating?	0	1	2	3	4	5
3. Over the past month or so, how often have you found you stopped and started several times when you urinated?	0	1	2	3	4	5
4. Over the past month or so, how often have you found it difficult to postpone urination?	0	1	2	3	4	5
5. Over the past month or so, how often have you had a weak urinary stream?	0	1	2	3	4	5
6. Over the past month or so, how often have you had to push or strain to begin urination?	0	1	2	3	4	5

7. Over the last month or so, how many times did you most typically get up to urinate from the time you went to bed at night until the time you got up in the morning?

    0 times   1 time   2 times   3 times   4 times   5 times

AUA Symptom Score = sum of questions 1–7 = _____

Interpretation of AUA Symptom Index

    Mild prostatism ≤7

    Moderate prostatism 8–18

    Severe prostatism >18

    Highest possible score = 35

retention such as in prostatic obstruction of urine outflow. Urine is lost when pressure of a large volume of retained urine in the bladder exceeds the pressure of the urethral obstruction.

Change in caliber of the stream and loss of force of the stream is related to outflow obstruction most commonly associated with prostate enlargement. Acute prostatism may be associated with an acute onset of the inability to urinate, increased suprapubic pain, and a sense of urgency. The patient may experience a resultant dribbling of small amounts of urine as a result of acute urinary retention caused by the obstruction of outflow. In contrast, patients with chronic urinary retention symptoms associated with prostatic obstruction present with painless, constant dribbling of urine (i.e., paradoxic incontinence) with marked hesitancy of urination and decreased caliber and force of urinary stream. A sudden interruption of the stream with associated pain radiating down the penis is not prostate related, but rather, associated with a ureteral calculus that is now in the bladder and acutely obstructs the outflow of urine.

Urethral discharge is a very common complaint and most commonly is associated with urethritis, though it can be seen with prostatitis. Usually it is first noted by the patient as a yellowish stain of the underwear and on closer inspection the patient notes drainage from the urethral meatus at the tip of the penis. *Neisseria gonorrhoeae* is the most common cause of purulent urethral discharge.

Ask about changes in the skin of the penis and scrotum. Note whether the patient is circumcised and ask if he has noticed ulcers of the skin. If so, ask if these ulcers have been painful (e.g., herpes genitalis) or not painful (e.g., syphilis). Are warts present on the skin and if so, have they changed in size and are they increasing in number? Are there noticeable enlargements around the base of the penis and anterior abdominal wall or inguinal area (i.e., groin), testicles, or epididymis that might be associated with penile tumors, lymphadenopathy from chancroid, syphilis, lymphogranuloma venereum, hydrocele, varicocele, spermatocele, hernia, chronic epididymitis, or testicular tumor. To detect early cancer, all males should begin to self examine their testicles on a regular monthly basis beginning in their mid-thirties. Swelling of the legs can be a symptom of compression of the veins and/or lymphatics draining the legs as a result of metastases from penile cancer. If the patient complains of swelling of the scrotum consider hydrocele, indirect inguinal hernia, chronic ascites, and filariasis. Infection of the prostate or seminal vesicle should be considered when the patient states that there is blood in the ejaculate (i.e., hematospermia). If a male gives a history of gradually worsening enlargement of the breast, even though common in the elderly and often idiopathic, consider a source of exogenous estrogen (e.g., treatment for prostatic cancer) or endogenous estrogen (e.g., Leydig and/or Sertoli cell tumors of the testes).

Physical Examination

Having obtained a complete and detailed history from the patient, direct your attention to the physical examination. In a warm examination room, ask the patient to disrobe and put on a gown that is warm and protects his modesty. Leave the examination room while the patient undresses. It is important during this examination that the patient be allowed to be in control whenever possible. This can be done by allowing the patient to have options. One of the first options is whether or not he would like a support person in the room with him. This person can provide support during potentially uncomfortable or embarrassing parts of the examination. Whether the examiner is male or female, some clinicians recommend that a male chaperone be present during the examination.

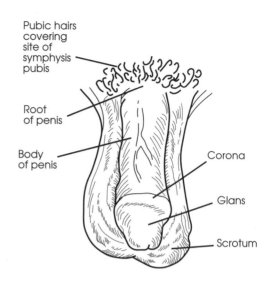

Fig. 17.7 The external structures of the penis.

Though the physical examination of the male reproductive system should focus on the organs of reproduction, remember that disease of this system can be reflected by and/or through changes in other parts of the body. The lymphatic system should be examined with particular care to assess the lymph nodes of the neck, supraclavicular, and inguinal areas. Testicular cancer can metastasize to nodes of the neck and supraclavicular area.

The presence of gynecomastia is common, particularly around puberty, and is related to physiologic changes in hormones. Gynecomastia in the young man can be associated with testicular tumors or Klinefelter's syndrome. [see Chapter 16: Female Reproductive System: Breast Exam for further discussion of exogenous factors (e.g., certain drugs and endogenous factors such as liver disease) that are associated with gynecomastia.]

Inspect the penis for changes in the skin. If lesions are present, record their location, size, consistency (e.g., rubbery, rock hard), smooth or rough surface, fixed or mobile, and whether single or multiple. If multiple, record whether lesions are separate or coalescing. If ulcers are present, note if they are painful when touched. Note the pattern of hair distribution on the mons pubis (i.e., male or female distribution patterns) and the size of the penis. A small penis (i.e, micropenis) is seen with low or inadequate levels of circulating androgen. A larger than normal penis (i.e., megalopenis) is seen with androgen producing interstitial (Leydig) cell tumors of the testis or over-activity of the adrenal cortex (i.e., adrenal hyperplasia). Similar attention should be paid to the skin of the scrotum. It is important to retract the foreskin of the uncircumcised male and look for irregular raised growths which may be squamous cell carcinoma or for ulcers of syphilis or herpes genitalis. The retracted foreskin may reveal purulent material set on a base of erythematous skin suggesting infection or balanitis.

The position of the opening of the urethra at the tip of the penis should be noted. Examine the urethral meatus for stenosis or discharge and the glans for phimosis or paraphimosis. If the meatus is abnormally located proximal to the tip of the penis it is usually on the ventral or under side of the penis (i.e., hypospadias). Infrequently, the meatus may open on the dorsal side of the penis (i.e., epispadias). These more proximal openings may be associated with abnormal curvature of the penis in the direction of the opening. Though the meatus may occasionally be stenotic with hypospadias or less frequently epispadias, it may also be stenotic in its normal anatomic position at the tip of the glans. Any evidence of urethral meatus stenosis should be noted and referral to a urologist considered. If urethral discharge is present, record the color, consistency, and presence or absence of odor and blood. Whereas the discharge of nongonococcal urethritis (often due to **Chlamydia trachomatis**) is yellow to gray, thin or watery and scant, the discharge of gonococcal urethritis is profuse, yellow to gray-brown and thick. In gonococcal urethritis, a Gram's stain of the discharge viewed under the microscope will reveal the typical gram-negative stained diplococci inside the white blood cells. If the discharge is bloody, the presence of urethral stricture (anywhere along the course of the urethra), a foreign body in the urethra, or tumor must be considered. If the patient has voided just before the exam, discharge may not be evident. In this situation, examination of the patient's underwear may reveal the tell-tale yellowish stain of the urethral discharge.

Examination of the skin of the scrotum may demonstrate small sebaceous cysts. The skin of the fold between the base of the scrotum and proximal thigh may appear irritated and occasionally even broken down and weeping in areas where it is cracked. If small, erythematous satellite lesions surround these larger areas of breakdown and erythema, one must suspect a candidiasis (i.e., yeast) infection. Candidiasis is an infection common to areas of the body that are moist and warm (e.g., diaper rash) particularly in persons who are diabetic (diagnosed or not diagnosed). The scrotal sac may be distended or swollen at the time of inspection. If both the right and left sides are distended, consider edema of congestive heart failure (CHF). If one side is distended, palpation and transillumination may reveal hydrocele or hernia. Hydroceles tend to surround the testis completely and can be differentiated from a testicular tumor because they will transilluminate and a testicular tumor will not. Cysts may also be palpated, separate from the testis, in the regions of the upper pole of the testis.

If palpation of the spermatic cord reveals a worm-like structure, it is often the dilated, varicose veins of the pampiniform plexus (i.e., varicocele). A varicocele is commonly palpated above and behind the testes and is associated with incompetent venous valves. A Valsalva maneuver may enlarge the "mass." Lying supine may reduce the size of a varicocele as gravity helps empty the dilated veins by allowing for easier return of blood to the heart. Examination of the mons pubis should not only determine if the hair distribution pattern is male or female, but may also identify "crabs" or lice present on the pubic hairs or on the skin at the base of the hairs. Inspect for thickening of the skin with scaling. If this pattern is generalized, consider the possibility of seborrheic dermatitis (i.e., dandruff). If focal and the scales have a purplish hue to them, think more along the lines of psoriasis.

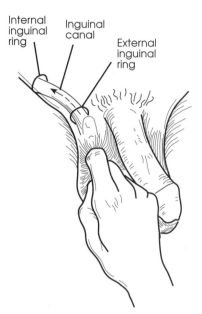

Internal inguinal ring

Inguinal canal

External inguinal ring

Fig. 17.8 The position of the examining finger in the inguinal canal during palpation for inguinal hernias.

No exam of the area is complete without an evaluation for the presence of a hernia and an examination of the testes and associated epididymis. To evaluate for a hernia, both an internal and external examination must be conducted. The internal examination is accomplished by placing your gloved index finger below the base of the scrotum and gently pushing your finger with scrotal sac before it through the external inguinal ring and into the inguinal canal to the level of the internal inguinal ring. Ask the patient to turn his head away from the side being examined and cough. If the inguinal ring is intact, it will stay tight and abdominal contents will not protrude against the tip of the finger into the inguinal canal. Repeat the same procedure on the opposite side to check the competency of the contralateral internal inguinal ring. This examination excludes the diagnosis of indirect inguinal hernia, but does not evaluate for a direct inguinal hernia. The external exam helps with this differentiation. With your left index finger still in the left inguinal canal, place the middle finger of your right hand on the skin over the internal inguinal ring and proximal inguinal canal. Place your index finger above and medial to the inguinal canal, and your fourth finger below and lateral to the inguinal canal. Again, ask the patient to cough. A bulge medial to your middle finger, under your index finger, suggests a direct inguinal hernia; a bulge under your middle finger suggests an indirect inguinal hernia; and a bulge under your fourth finger suggests the presence of a femoral hernia. Record your findings.

Examine each testis and epididymis with the patient either supine with thighs slightly spread or in the standing position. Place the testis between your thumb and second and third fingers. The testicle, like the ovary, is very sensitive and should be examined with a gentle touch. Marked sensitivity or pain to touch, with associated swelling or enlargement of the testicle, may be associated with orchitis or torsion of the testes. Some examiners conduct this examination by placing the testis between the fingers of both hands. Any smooth or nodular enlargement of the testis must be regarded as a tumor until demonstrated otherwise. The mass should be transilluminated in a darkened room to rule out the presence of a hydrocele; a hydrocele will transilluminate. The testis may be small and somewhat boggy, which is a normal finding in the elderly male. The testis may also be small if there is a history of mumps orchitis or torsion of the spermatic cord with subsequent loss of blood supply to the testis. In both of these cases, endocrine function is generally maintained and sperm production is lost. The testis may be absent and found intra-abdominally (i.e., true cryptorchidism), or it may be physiologically retracted into the inguinal canal (i.e., false cryptorchidism). Palpation of the groin in the area of the inguinal canal may identify the retracted testis which sometimes can be milked out of the inguinal canal into the upper scrotum. If the testis is absent, the patient should be referred to an urologist. Intra-abdominal testis tend to have a higher risk for development of testicular cancer and the heat of the intra-abdominal site adversely affects normal sperm production.

Next, palpate the epididymis which most often is closely attached to the posterior surface of the testis. Palpate to discern the presence of a cystic structure or induration which, if present, indicates a spermatocele or infection. Infection is often associated with marked tenderness during palpation. The three organisms which commonly cause epididymitis are *Neisseria gonorrhoeae, Chlamydia trachomatis*, and *Escherichia coli*. Marked epididymitis may affect the testis and adjacent scrotal wall which becomes erythematous. If the induration is painless and chronic, suspect tuberculosis which may be associated with palpable beading of the vas deferens, a thickened seminal vesicle, a nodular prostate, and purulent discharge which is sometimes blood-tinged and sterile when cultured.

Examination of the prostate should be preceded by collection of a urine specimen if there is a question of bladder or kidney infection. During the prostate examination, it is common for prostatic secretion to be expelled into the prostatic urethra. These secretions would contaminate a subsequent urinalysis specimen. The prostate exam should determine its size, shape, consistency, and nodularity.

The prostate is wider at its cephalad end near the bladder and narrower inferiorly. Approximately 4 cm in length, the prostate has a palpable central depression or furrow running from cephalad to caudad, dividing it into right and left posterior lobes. Laterally, there is a sulcus on each side which becomes deeper as the prostate becomes enlarged. As the lateral sulcus becomes deeper, the median depression or furrow becomes more shallow to palpation. These are two signs of benign prostate hypertrophy. The size of the prostate does not determine the clinical significance of the benign prostatic hypertrophy. This diagnosis is more often related to a complex of

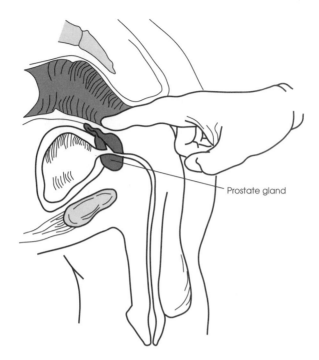

Fig. 17.9   Palpation of the prostate gland.

symptoms, including the amount of urine residual in the bladder after voiding (i.e., post-void residual) and a decrease in the force and caliber of the urine stream. Remember that the rectal prostate exam only evaluates the posterior aspect of the prostate, a relatively small portion of the total volume of prostate tissues.

To examine the prostate, have the patient stand at the end of the examination table facing the table with his back to you. Placing his hands on the examination table, he should bend at the waist 90° and lean forward until his forehead is resting on the table. With a gloved hand and water-based lubricating gel on the tip of your examining index finger, spread the cheeks of the buttocks with the fingers of your other gloved hand and identify the anal opening. When first placing your finger against the anal opening there will be an involuntary reflex tightening of the anal sphincter. Wait until the anal sphincter is felt to relax. Gently and slowly insert your finger through the anal canal until the base of the prostate can be palpated behind the anterior wall of the rectum. In an orderly manner, examine the prostate by applying gentle pressure against it from cephalad to caudad and from the lateral sulcus on one side to the lateral sulcus on the other side, identifying the median furrow in the process.

To develop a sense of the consistency of the prostate, oppose the thumb tightly to the little finger and feel the contracted thenar eminence muscle mass. This is the consistency of a normal prostate, a rubbery sensation. Chronic infection or lack of frequent intercourse may result in the prostate having a boggy consistency (i.e., thenar eminence without the muscle contracting). In acute prostatitis, because of the severity of pain it is often difficult to access and evaluate the prostate by digital palpation. If the gland has a rock hard feel, like the sense one gets when pressing the end of the finger against the knuckle, consider the possibility of prostate cancer until proven otherwise. In addition to early stages of cancer, the differential diagnosis for firm areas identified upon palpation of the prostate includes: fibrosis from past infection, granulomatous disease of the prostate (i.e., tuberculosis), and prostatic calculi. Firm to rock hard areas identified during prostatic examination should be referred to an urologist for further evaluation.

Mobility of the gland is often difficult to assess because it may vary from time to time in the same patient. Local extension of cancer into surrounding tissues tends to fix the prostate to these tissues and reduce its mobility.

Massage of the prostate is achieved by moving the examining finger from cephalad to caudad in a lateral to medial direction toward the median sulcus or furrow. This "milking" of the prostate can also be achieved by a rolling motion of the finger from lateral to medial and may be better tolerated by the patient. As secretions move into the prostatic urethra they cause the sensation of having to void urine (i.e., urinate). If these secretions are sufficient enough in volume, they flow down the penile urethra and are present at, or drip from, the meatus and can be easily obtained for Gram's stain and cultures. This exam may reveal an asymptomatic prostatitis. Because of this, some physicians recommend that this milking procedure be done whenever the prostate is examined. If no secretions are obtained, immediately after the prostate exam collect the first part of a voided urine in a sterile cup and submit this specimen, properly labeled, for Gram's stain of the cellular components and for culture if indicated (e.g., presence of bacteria or white blood cells on microscopic examination).

Seminal vesicles may be palpated at the cephalad end of the prostate where they diverge upward and laterally (usually not easily palpated unless the patient is quite thin and the examination finger long). If palpated easily, suspect over-distention which

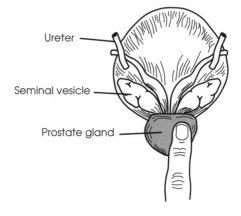

Fig. 17.10 The relationship between the size of the normal prostate gland and the examining finger.

Ureter

Seminal vesicle

Prostate gland

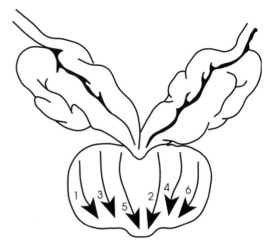

Fig. 17.11 Prostatic massage. The arrows indicate the areas of the prostate that are massaged and the sequence and direction of the massage.

may be associated with chronic infection (e.g., tuberculosis, schistosomiasis) or advanced carcinoma of the prostate that has involved the seminal vesicles. When "milking" the prostate, if the seminal vesicles are accessible, it is advisable to also "milk" them in a similar fashion. If the prostate is infected, the seminal vesicle is also usually infected. The reverse is also true. If the seminal vesicle is infected, the prostate is also usually infected.

In the woman, self-examination of the breast is an important part of early diagnosis of cancer of the breast. In the man, self-examination of the testicles is an important part of early diagnosis of cancer of the testicle. Beginning in their mid-thirties, all males should self-examine their testicles on a regular monthly basis. This can be accomplished while bathing. The testicles are normally smooth except for the area of the epididymis. The exam should be sufficiently complete to identify and "outline" the epididymis. Any change in this smooth feeling, or the presence of a raised, firm, pea-sized area may represent early testicular cancer and needs to be brought to the attention of a health care professional. Testicular cancer may be cured if identified and treated early.

If a prostate specific antigen (PSA) test is to be obtained, the blood should be drawn before digital examination of the prostate. Manipulation of the prostate may give a falsely high and abnormal result. Prostate specific antigen is the most useful tumor marker available for diagnosing, staging, and monitoring prostate cancer. PSA is a serine protease which is produced exclusively by epithelial cells of all types of prostatic tissue: normal, hyperplastic, and cancerous. PSA can be detected in the serum of young men with small, nonhyperplastic prostates, older men with benign prostatic hypertrophy (BPH), and men with localized or metastatic prostate cancer. If prostatic cancer is suspected, a transrectal ultrasound can be done which will allow for suspected tumor localization and for ultrasound-guided biopsy of the suspicious area and pathologic diagnosis.

PHARMACOTHERAPEUTIC CASE ILLUSTRATION

History

W.R. is a 37-year-old male who presents with a history of acute onset of fever, chills, low back pain, and a burning sensation with urination. Further symptom history revealed that W.R. experienced the low back pain particularly over the sacrum and the chills and fever were worsening. Along with the dysuria, he has experienced symptoms of urinary urgency, frequency, nocturia, and more difficulty starting the urine stream. The urine stream has been smaller than usual and less forceful, and there was dribbling at the end of urination. Though the symptoms began four days ago, he has experienced muscle aches (i.e., myalgias) and joint pain (i.e., arthralgias) for the past day and a half. W.R. denies any previous history of urinary tract infections (UTIs), ureteral stones, or prostate infections. He has no symptoms suggestive of epididymitis or orchitis. Bowel movements have been regular and unchanged.

Past medical history and review of systems (ROS) is otherwise noncontributory and reveals an otherwise healthy young man. He has no known drug allergies. W.R.'s family history (FH) is negative except for a maternal uncle who has non-insulin-dependent diabetes mellitus. His social history (SH) indicates that he smokes one pack of cigarettes a day, drinks alcoholic beverages socially, and denies use of illegal drugs. He is married with children and works as a long distance truck driver.

Physical Examination

W.R.'s vital signs (VS) were as follows: blood pressure (BP) 138/82 mm Hg; pulse 84 beats/min; respiratory rate (RR) 18/min; temperature 38° C (100.8° F).

W.r.'s tympanic membranes were normal. His throat was without erythema and no tonsillar enlargement was noted. His thyroid was not enlarged; and there was no sign of anterior or posterior cervical adenopathy. His chest was clear to auscultation and percussion, with no CVA tenderness. His heart had regular rate and rhythm with no enlargement or extra heart sounds. An examination of his abdomen revealed no evidence of distention. He had normal bowel sounds and his abdomen was soft to palpation without direct or rebound tenderness. He had no evidence of edema.

External genitalia examination revealed a circumcised male. The urethral meatus was neither stenotic nor erythematous and there was no evidence of discharge. There were no other positive findings on inspection. A yellowish discharge was noted on W.R.'s underwear on the front inside. Examination of each testicle and epididymis was unremarkable as was the examination for inguinal hernia. The prostate exam was accomplished with gentleness on the part of the examiner and minimal discomfort on the part of the patient. The prostate was exquisitely tender to direct palpation, swollen, firm, indurated, and warm to the touch. The prostate gland was not milked because of the pain. The seminal vesicle could not be reached. Following the exam there was a small amount of discharge from the urethra which was sent to the lab for Gram's stain and culture and sensitivity (C&S).

Laboratory

A complete blood count (CBC) returned the following results: white blood cell (WBC) count 15,250, Poly 77%, Bands 8%, Lymphs 13%, Monos 2%m, hemaglobin (Hgb) 13.2, hemocrit (Hct) 40.1.

Urinalysis before prostate examination was entirely negative except for infrequent red blood cells (RBCs) and white blood cells (WBCs). Urinalysis on first voided specimen after prostate examination revealed a few red blood cells and many white blood cells. A specimen prostate secretion was collected for Gram's stain and culture and sensitivity.

Diagnosis and Management

Discussion. W.R. was diagnosed as having acute bacterial prostatitis. He was empirically prescribed TMP/SMX 1 tablet PO BID.

Disease. W.R.'s symptom complex is similar to that of an acute urinary tract infection of the bladder or kidneys. However, the kidney pain of pyelonephritis occurs in the costovertebral angle area, or perhaps in the flank; W.R. experienced pain over the sacrum. W.R.'s symptoms of urinary tract obstruction (e.g., difficulty starting stream, prolonged urination, dribbling at the end of urination) also point to a partial obstruction of the prostatic urethra. The absence of costovertebral angle tenderness and the presence of positive physical findings from the prostate exam point to a diagnosis of prostatitis. Laboratory studies support this diagnosis with an elevated white blood cell count with a shift to the left, a urinalysis without any evidence of infection prior to prostate examination and evidence of infection following prostate examination. The cultures will most probably come back positive for *E. coli* or Pseudomonas, the two most common bacteria causing acute bacterial prostatitis.

One complication of acute prostatitis is urinary retention resulting from swelling of the prostate and obstruction of the prostatic urethra. This usually resolves with proper antibiotic therapy and rarely requires surgical intervention. One or more abscesses may form which tend to be more resistant to therapy. Since acute bacterial cystitis occasionally accompanies bacterial prostatitis, pyelonephritis may become a complication. Acute bacterial epididymitis may also develop. Of all complications, the most serious is bacteremia and the possibility of septic shock. Needless to say, early and aggressive treatment of acute bacterial prostatitis is indicated.

Management

Several antibiotics are effective against gram-negative enteric organisms. Pending culture results and assessment of infection severity, empiric treatment could be initiated with oral or parenteral antibiotics. The choices are an oral fluoroquinolone, oral trimethoprim/sulfamethoxazole (TMP/SMX), or a parenteral combination of an aminoglycoside plus ampicillin. In the acutely inflamed prostate gland, all these agents penetrate the tissue and eradicate the bacteria. However, many clinicians prefer oral trimethoprim/sulfamethoxazole (160 mg/800 mg BID) because of the good trimethoprim penetration of prostatic tissue, its lower per dose cost, and its lower side effect profile. To reduce the risk of relapse or re-infection, treatment should continue for at least four weeks at full, daily dosage levels. Also, males with acute prostatitis are at risk of developing chronic prostatitis if treatment is not long enough.

In the systemically septic patient, parenteral therapy with an aminoglycoside and ampicillin should be begun immediately upon hospitalization. Based upon urine culture and antibiotic sensitivity testing, the parenteral therapy is continued or changed. When the patient becomes afebrile for 48 hours, appropriate oral therapy may be started in the hospital. If the patient remains afebrile for an additional 24 hours, he may be discharged and instructed to continue treatment for a total of 30 days at home. If at all possible, selection of the oral antibiotic should be based on pre-antibiotic treatment culture and sensitivity results.

Success in the treatment of acute prostatitis is measured by monitoring symptoms of perineal pain, ability to freely urinate (i.e., no evidence of partial obstruction), and fever. Once these indicators are stable and antibiotic therapy has been administered for several days, the prostate gland can more easily be examined with less risk of precipitating bacteremia and septicemia. Over several weeks, the enlarged inflamed gland should become less tense and should return to its normal size, shape, and consistency. A prostate examination should be conducted at that time to evaluate the prostate for a cancer that may have been masked by the prostatic infection.

Therapeutic Drug Monitoring Examples

PROSTATE CANCER (STAGE 2D)

The approach to therapuetic drug monitoring by clinicians varies depending upon many factors. Some of these include preferences among clinicians in a given community or region; concurrent medical problems which dictate that certain drugs be used or avoided; the patient's response to selected medication. The following outlines of therapeutic drug monitoring offer examples which may serve to stimulate discussion and further understanding of initiating and monitoring drug use. The drugs and dosages presented should not be applied to any clinical situation without proper medical supervision.

Drug Therapy	Leuprolide depot 7.5 mg IM monthly.
Monitoring	**Symptoms:** Ask the patient about the severity of symptoms since starting treatment. Ask about the following symptoms and their change if previously present: urinary hesitancy, poor urine stream, dribbling on urination, hematuria, nocturia, and bone pain. Tell the patient that an initial flare-up of symptoms is normal at the start of therapy.
	Signs: *Gen:* Measure the patient's weight. *Rectal Exam:* Palpate the prostate for size, tenderness, nodules, and consistency. Check the pelvic lymph nodes.
Laboratory Tests	The clinician may elect to order all, none, or some of these laboratory studies depending upon history and physical findings, as well as other specific clinical indications: serum acid phosphatase, prostate specific antigen, transrectal ultrasonography.
Adverse Drug Event Monitoring	Ask the patient if he is experiencing hot flashes and explain that this is normal at the start of treatment. If the patient experienced bone or tumor pain, ask if the pain has become worse. Ask about rare side effects such as impotence, nausea/vomiting, or headache.

Therapeutic Drug Monitoring Examples

BENIGN PROSTATIC HYPERTROPHY

The approach to therapuetic drug monitoring by clinicians varies depending upon many factors. Some of these include preferences among clinicians in a given community or region; concurrent medical problems which dictate that certain drugs be used or avoided; the patient's response to selected medication. The following outlines of therapeutic drug monitoring offer examples which may serve to stimulate discussion and further understanding of initiating and monitoring drug use. The drugs and dosages presented should not be applied to any clinical situation without proper medical supervision.

Drug Therapy	Finasteride 5 mg/day PO.
Monitoring	**Symptoms:** Compare the degree of change in the following obstructive symptoms: nocturia, urinary daytime frequency, hesitancy, terminal dribbling, urgency, dysuria, sensation of incomplete voiding, and bladder incontinence.
	Signs:*Rectal Exam:* Palpate the size, shape and consistency of the prostate; feel for any nodules and note any tenderness.
Laboratory Tests	The clinician may elect to order all, none, or some of these laboratory studies depending upon history and physical findings, as well as other specific clinical indications: baseline urinalysis (UA), serum creatinine, and prostate specific antigen. If indicated, cystoscopy, urography studies, and urodynamic studies.
Adverse Drug Event Monitoring	Ask the patient about the following rare side effects: impotence, decreased libido, and reduced ejaculation volume. Caution the patient about the teratogenic effects of the drug. Since finasteride has been found in the semen of patients taking the drug, the patient should not expose his partner to his semen if she is or may become pregnant. Women who are or may become pregnant should avoid direct contact with broken finasteride tablets.

Terminology

Abscess. Localized accumulation of purulent material in the dermis or hypodermis.

Accommodation. Adjustment of the vision for various distances.

Adnexa. The uterine appendages, ovaries, and fallopian tubes.

Adrenarche. Development of pubic and axillary hair during puberty in females, generally begins after thelarche and before the maximum growth spurt.

Allergic rhinitis. Pale-bluish swelling of the nasal mucosa associated with sneezing and watery discharge.

Alopecia. Excessive hair loss; may be circumscribed or diffuse.

Amenorrhea. Absence or abnormal cessation of menses for a period of time greater than 6 months.

Anasarca. Generalized massive edema.

Anastomose. A connection between vessels by collateral channels: artery to artery, vein to vein, or artery to vein.

Androgens. Hormones that stimulate activity of the accessory sex organs of the male and encourage development of male sex characteristics.

Aneurysm. A sac or dilation formed by the weakening of the wall of an artery, a vein, or the heart.

Angle of Louis. Point of union where the manubrium meets the body of the sternum at the level of the second costal cartilage.

Anisocoria. A normal variation in which the pupils may be of unequal size, but both react normally to light accommodation.

Anterior axillary line. An imaginary line extending vertically from the anterior fold of the axilla toward the waist.

Anterior serrati muscles. Chest wall muscles joining the scapula to the anterior rib cage.

Aphasia. A defect or loss of expression and/or understanding of speech, writing, or signs caused by injury to the brain, especially in stroke.

Apnea. Cessation of breathing.

Apraxia. Loss of the ability to perform familiar tasks, especially the inability to make use of familiar objects.

Arcus senilis. Lipid deposits in the iris frequently seen in aged patients or younger patients who have hyperlipidemia.

Ascites. Effusion and accumulation of serous fluid in the abdominal cavity.

Asterixis. A motor disorder marked by intermittent lapse of an assumed posture, as a result of alternating contraction and relaxation of muscle groups. A characteristic of hepatic coma, but also seen in numerous conditions; also known as liver flap.

Asthenia. Lack or loss of strength and energy; weakness.

Atelectasis. Incomplete expansion of the lung; a collapsed lung segment.

Athetosis. Involuntary movement of the hands in a continuous, slow pattern.

Atrial diastolic gallop (S_4). Caused by a rushing of blood into the ventricles. It is associated with hypertensive heart disease, chronic heart failure, or coronary heart disease.

Atrophy. Thinning of the skin due to loss of its substance. This may be epidermal, where the skin appears transparent.

Auscultatory gap. Time in which sound is not heard in the auscultatory method of sphygmomanometry, occurring particularly in hypertension and in aortic stenosis.

Bartholin's glands. Vulvovaginal glands located in the lower third of the labia minora.

Beau lines. Transverse depressions of the fingernails.

Benign prostatic hypertrophy. Enlargement of the prostate gland with increasing age. The process is not cancerous and affects a very large percentage of older men.

Bezoar. A concretion of various compositions sometimes found in the stomach or intestines of man. It may consist of hair, plants, or fibers.

Bilateral tubal ligation. Surgical ligation of the fallopian tubes to prevent pregnancy.

Borborygmi. Rumbling noises made by the propulsion of gas through the intestines.

Brachiocephalic veins. Large veins collecting blood from the head and neck and emptying into the superior vena cava.

Bradycardia. A heart rate of 60 beats per minute or less.

Bradypnea. Decreased rate of breathing.

Broad ligament. The uterus is suspended in the pelvis by a curtain of peritoneum stretching from side to side of the pelvic cavity with the uterus suspended in the middle.

Bronchi. Large airways of the lung branching from the trachea to subdivide into smaller bronchioles.

Bruit. A sound or murmur heard in auscultation, generated by turbulent blood flow.

Bulbocavernosus muscle. Muscle overlying the proximal end of the corpora spongiosum which contracts during orgasm, expelling the semen from the penile urethra.

Bulbourethral glands. Glands at the base of the urethra that, along with the urethral glands, secrete mucus in response to sexual arousal which acts as a lubricant during sexual intercourse.

Bulla. A circumscribed area of separation of the epidermis, due to the presence of clear serum (blister); > 0.5 cm in diameter.

Capacitation. Changes in sperm after they are deposited in the vagina which allow the head of the sperm to penetrate into the ovum.

Caput medusae. Dilated cutaneous veins around the umbilicus, seen mainly in newborns and in patients suffering with cirrhosis of the liver.

Carbuncle. A deep necrotizing form of folliculitis involving several adjacent hair follicles (also see furuncle).

Cesarean section. Surgical removal of the fetus through the anterior abdominal wall.

Chalazion. An infection or granuloma of the meibomian gland.

Cheilitis. Inflammation of the lips.

Cheilosis. A condition of the lips and angles of the mouth characterized by dry scales and fissuring. Cracking of the angles of the mouth is termed perlèche.

Cheyne-Stokes respiration. Abnormal, rhythmic variations of depth of respiration with regular periods of apnea.

Chorea. Involuntary jerky movements of the body in rapid, highly complex patterns as in dancing.

Circumstantiality. A term used to describe speech that is indirect and delayed in reaching the point because of unnecessary, tedious details and parenthetic remarks.

Clanging. Speech in which sound, rather than meaningful, conceptual relationships govern word choice; it may include rhyming and punning.

Click. An extra heart sound heard during mid- or late systole.

Clonus. Rapid, alternating muscle contraction and relaxation.

Clubbing. Increase in the angle between the nail bed and the base of the finger to greater than 180°. A fusiform enlargement of the distal digit may also occur.

Cogwheel rigidity. Abnormal muscle stiffness which gives way to brief jerks during passive motion.

Collecting ducts. The ducts which carry milk from the alveoli and secretory ducts to the nipple.

Coma. A state of unconsciousness from which the patient cannot be aroused.

Common carotid artery. Major artery off of the aortic arch carrying blood to the head and neck.

Compulsion. Repetitive and purposeful behavior performed according to certain rules or in a stereotyped fashion.

Confabulation. Fabrication of facts or events in response to questions about situations or events that are not recalled because of memory impairment.

Confusion. Disturbed orientation to person, place, or time.

Consolidation. The condition of being solid, as when the lung becomes firm as air spaces are filled with exudate in pneumonia.

Corneal arcus. Lipid deposits in the periphery of the iris.

Coryza. An acute inflammation of the nasal mucous membranes with a watery discharge of the nostrils.

Cowper's glands. Synonymous with bulbourethral glands. See bulbourethral glands.

Crackles. Moist breath sounds heard with the stethoscope during inspiration. Similar to the "crackle" of Rice Krispies or paper being crumpled. Some classify as "moist" or "dry." Synonymous with rales.

Crepitation. A sound similar to that caused by rubbing the hair between the fingers; a crackling sound.

Crepitus. A crackle-like sensation felt during palpation caused by air misplaced to subcutaneous tissues beneath the skin.

Crust. Dried serum, blood, or purulent material on the skin surface.

Cyanosis. A bluish discoloration of the skin.

Cystocele. Weakness in the anterior vaginal wall such that the base of the bladder bulges into the vagina.

Dacryocystitis. Inflammation of the lacrimal sac.

Death rattle. Loud, gargling sounds heard over the mouth of a stuporous or comatose patient. A sign of thick secretions in the trachea and large bronchi. Often a sign of impending death.

Delirium. A short course of mental disorientation, illusions, restlessness, delusions, incoherence, and hallucinations.

Delusion. A false personal belief based on incorrect inference about external reality and firmly sustained in spite of what everyone else believes.

Dementia. A loss of intellectual functions such as memory, judgment, abstract thinking, and other higher cortical functions.

Depersonalization. An alteration in the perception or experience of the self so the feeling of one's own reality is temporarily lost.

Descensus. Weakness of the pelvic floor such that the uterus falls into the vagina.

Desquamate. Shedding, peeling, or scaling off the outer layer of cells from any surface (e.g., shedding of the endometrium at the time of menses).

Diastasis recti. Separation of the rectus muscles of the abdominal wall.

Diastole. The period between the second and first heart sounds in the cardiac cycle.

Diplopia. Perception of two images of a single object.

Disorientation. Confusion about the date or time of day, where one is (place), or who one is (identity).

Dizziness. A term to describe faintness, giddiness, unsteadiness, light-headedness. A vague sensation of insecurity and unsteadiness. It is reported with non-vestibular diseases such as arrhythmias.

Ductus deferens. Tubular structure that transports sperm from the epididymis to the ejaculatory duct.

Dysarthria. Impaired speech caused by a disturbance of muscle control from damage of central or peripheral nerves.

Dysfunction uterine bleeding. Greater than normal uterine bleeding without obvious organic cause, genital or extragenital.

Dyskinesia. Impairment of the power of voluntary movement, resulting in incomplete movements.

Dyspareunia. Female pelvic pain during the act of sexual intercourse.

Dysphagia. Difficulty in swallowing.

Dysphonia. Difficulty in speaking.

Dyspnea. Subjective sensation of difficulty in breathing.

Dyspnea on exertion. Shortness of breath associated with exercise.

Dystonia. Disordered tonicity of muscle; involuntary, irregular clonic contortions.

Ecchymosis. A large purpuric lesion, usually >0.5 cm in diameter.

Echolalia. Echoing of the words or phrases of others.

Ectopic pregnancy. Pregnancy established outside the uterine cavity, usually in the fallopian tubes.

Ectropion. Outward turning of the eyelid.

Egophony. Usually auscultated over an area of compressed or consolidated lung. The spoken letter "e" sounds like "aaaaa."

Ejaculation. Expulsion of semen out of the penile urethra during orgasm.

Ejaculatory duct. Continuation of the vas deferens through the prostate to end as it empties into the prostatic urethra. Contents from the prostate gland and the seminal vesicles empty into the ejaculatory duct.

Emission. Process of forming semen.

Endocervical canal. Canal leading from the inside of the uterus to the outside of the cervix.

Endometrium. Cellular lining of the endometrial cavity that receives the fertilized egg and, in the absence of fertilization, is shed as menstrual flow (menses).

Entropion. Inward turning of the eyelid toward the eyeball.

Epididymis. Convoluted tubule connecting the testis to the vas deferens in which sperm mature and are stored prior to ejaculation.

Epididymitis. Infection of the epididymis.

Episiotomy. During delivery, a surgical incision of the vulva on the perineum that allows delivery of a baby and prevents laceration at the time of delivery.

Epispadias. Meatus may open on the dorsal side of the penis.

Erythema. Pink to red blanchable discoloration of the skin (secondary to dilation of blood vessels).

Estrogen. The primary female hormone responsible for breast and female genitalia development, menarche, and ovulation.

Excoriation. Superficial linear or punctuate excavation in the skin that results from scratching.

Exophthalmos. Protrusion of the eye.

Exostosis. A benign bony growth projecting outward from the surface of a bone, characteristically capped by cartilage.

External carotid artery. A branch of the common carotid artery carrying blood to the superficial structures of the head and neck.

External jugular veins. Superficial veins in the neck which return blood from the head and neck to the internal jugular vein.

Facial nerve. Cranial nerve 7; it is the motor nerve to the facial muscles of expression.

Fasciculation. Localized small muscle contractions.

Fetus. Name given to the baby when it is in the uterus.

Fissure. Linear cleavage in the skin.

Flight of ideas. A nearly continuous flow of accelerated speech with abrupt changes from topic to topic.

Follicle stimulating hormone. Gonadotropin secreted by the anterior pituitary under the influence of GnRH. In the female, it stimulates the ovary to produce a follicle containing an egg and to secrete estrogen. In the male, it stimulates Sertoli cells and sperm production.

Follicular or proliferative phase. The first half of the menstrual cycle when the uterine endometrium thickens under the influence of estrogen produced during the development of the ovarian follicle.

Fordyce's spot. Enlarged sebaceous glands that appear as small yellow papules on the buccal surface.

Foreskin. That skin loosely covering the glans at the tip of the penis.

Fovea centralis. Central point of vision located in the center of the macula.

Friction rub. An auscultatory sound caused by the rubbing together of two serous surfaces.

Furuncle. Deep necrotizing form of folliculitis involving a single hair follicle.

Gametes. Containing a haploid number of genes (23); in the male these are called sperm and in the female they are called ova.

Gestational diabetes mellitus. Diabetes precipitated by pregnancy that resolves with completion of pregnancy.

Goiter. An enlargement of the thyroid gland, causing a swelling in the front of the neck.

Gonadotropin releasing hormone. A substance produced in and released by the hypothalamus of the brain that stimulates gonadotropin (FSH and LH) release.

Gonadotropins. Produced by the anterior pituitary, the two gonadotropins affecting male and female reproductive systems are FSH and LH.

Grandiosity. An inflated appraisal of one's worth, power, knowledge, importance, or identity.

Gravidity. Number of pregnancies.

Hallucination. A sensory perception without external stimulation of a sensory organ.

Hematospermia. The presence of blood in semen, intermixed with sperm.

Hemianopsia. Defective vision or blindness in half of the visual field of an eye.

Hemiparesis. Muscle weakness affecting one side of the body.

Hemiplegia. Paralysis of one side of the body.

Hepatojugular reflux. Distention of the jugular vein induced by applied pressure below the liver in the mid abdomen; suggests insufficiency of the right heart; formerly called hepatojugular reflex.

Hernia. The protrusion of a loop of intestine through the abdominal wall.

Hyperesthesia. Increased skin sensitivity to stimulation such as touch or pin prick.

Hypermenorrhea. See menorrhagia.

Hyperopia. Farsightedness.

Hyperpnea. An abnormal increase in the depth of breathing.

Hyperventilation. An abnormal increase in the rate and depth of breathing.

Hypospadias. A condition in which the meatus is abnormally located proximal to the tip of the penis, located on the ventral or under side of the penis.

Hypothalamus. Several structures in the base of the brain, where GnRH is released to stimulate FSH and LH release by the anterior pituitary.

Hysterectomy. Surgical removal of the uterus either through the vagina or through the anterior abdominal wall.

Icterus. Jaundice.

Ileus. Obstruction of the intestines.

Illusion. A misperception of a real external stimulus.

Implantation. Attachment of the fertilized egg to the endometrial lining with subsequent embedding in the endometrium.

Inhibin. Produced by the Sertoli cell, this substance feeds back to the anterior pituitary and decreases the production of FSH.

Intercostal muscles. Muscles of the rib cage which connect adjacent ribs.

Intercostal space. The space between the ribs occupied by intercostal muscles, intercostal nerve, artery, and vein. The intercostal spaces are numbered according to the rib above (i.e., the second intercostal space is located between the second and third ribs).

Intermenstrual bleeding. Unexpected bleeding occurring between normal menstrual periods.

Internal jugular veins. Veins that carry blood from the head and neck to the brachiocephalic veins.

Intrauterine fetal demise. Death of the fetus inside the uterus prior to labor and delivery.

Ischiocavernosus muscle. A muscular layer which overlies the corpora cavernosus on the ischiopubic rami.

Jaundice. A syndrome characterized by hyperbilirubinemia and deposition of bile pigment in the skin, mucous membranes, and sclera with resulting yellow appearance of the patient.

Korotkoff sounds. Sounds heard during auscultatory determination of blood pressure, produced by sudden distention of the artery, the walls of which were previously relaxed because of the proximally placed pneumatic cuff.

Kyphosis. An abnormal convexity of the thoracic spine.

Labyrinthitis. Inflammation of the vestibular system. A cause of vertigo.

Lactiferous ducts. The ducts that carry milk from the alveoli and secretory ducts to the nipple.

Laparoscopic surgery. Surgery where a laparoscope is used to evaluate the condition of the pelvic reproductive organs and assist with surgery; also known as "band-aid surgery."

Lethargy. A condition of drowsiness or indifference.

Leukoplakia. Development of white thickened patches under the mucous membranes of the gums, tongue, or cheeks that have a fissured surface and cannot be rubbed off. It is regarded as precancerous; also called smoker's patches, smoker's tongue, or leukoma.

Leydig cells. Found in the interstitium of the testicle, these cells produce testosterone and other androgens when stimulated by LH.

Lichenification. Thickening of the epidermis with accentuation of the normal skin lines.

Lid-lag. A condition in which a rim of sclera is visible between the upper lid and iris as the lid lags behind the eyeball when rapidly looking downward; a sign in hyperthyroidism.

Loosening of association. Thinking characterized by speech in which ideas shift from one subject to another, completely unrelated or only obliquely related, without the speaker showing any awareness that the topics are unconnected.

Luteal or secretory phase. The second half of the menstrual cycle when the uterine endometrium shows development of secretory glands under the influence of progesterone and estrogen.

Luteinizing hormone. Hormone secreted by the hypothalamus that increases progesterone production in females and testosterone production in males.

Lymphadenopathy. Enlargement of the lymph nodes.

Major depressive episode. A dysphoric mood with loss of interest or pleasure in all, or most usual activities and pastimes.

Manubrium. The upper-most bony part of the sternum. The clavicles and the first and second ribs articulate with it.

Masculinization. The attainment of male sexual characteristics.

Membranous urethra. That part of the urethra located within the urogenital diaphragm.

Menarche. The onset of menstruation which signals the completion of puberty.

Menometrorrhagia. Bleeding occurring at irregular intervals that is prolonged.

Menorrhagia. Uterine bleeding longer than 7 days or excessive (i.e., greater than 80 mL) occurring at regular intervals.

Menstrual cycle. Periodic buildup and sloughing of the endometrium at the time of menses, usually 28 days in duration but can normally vary from 21 to 35 days.

Mesosalpinx. Curtain of peritoneum attached to the broad ligament and suspending the fallopian tube.

Mesovarium. Curtain of peritoneum attached to the broad ligament and suspending the ovary.

Metorrhagia. Uterine bleeding of varying amounts occurring at frequent but irregular intervals.

Mid axillary line. An imaginary line drawn from the mid axilla vertically toward the waist, dividing the axilla into an anterior half and a posterior half.

Midclavicular line. An imaginary vertical line drawn from the mid point of the clavicle to the waist.

Middle meningeal artery. A branch of the external carotid artery carrying blood to the lining of the brain.

Midsternal line. An imaginary vertical line drawn from the mid point of the sternal notch toward the waist, dividing the sternum into a right and a left half.

Moniliasis. Infection with Candida species, especially *Candida albicans*. Such an infection of the mouth is termed thrush.

Mons pubis. A fatty layer of subcutaneous tissue and skin which covers the pubic symphysis. At puberty, it becomes covered with pubic hair which normally grows in a triangular pattern in females and in a diamond pattern in males.

Mood. A prolonged emotion that colors the whole psychic life; it generally involves either depression or elation.

Multiparity. Indication that a woman has been pregnant several times.

Murmur. A cardiac sound resulting from vibrations secondary to turbulent blood flow.

Myoclonus. Strong rhythmic jerking of muscle groups of usually one part of the body.

Myometrium. Smooth muscle making up the wall of the uterus.

Myopia. Nearsightedness.

Myringitis. Inflammation of the eardrum.

Myringotomy. Incision and drainage of the eardrum.

Neologism. New words invented by the subject, distortions of words, or standard words to which the subject has given new, highly idiosyncratic meaning.

Neurotic disorder. A mental disorder in which the predominant disturbance is a symptom or group of symptoms that is distressing to the individual and is recognized by him or her as unacceptable and alien.

Newborn. Name used to identify a child age birth to 28 days of life; neonatal.

Nodule. Palpable, solid lesion that may extend above the surrounding skin; usually >0.5 cm in diameter.

Nulligravida. Having never conceived a child.

Nulliparity. Having given birth to no children alive or stillborn.

Nystagmus. Involuntary, rapid movement of the eyeball, which may be horizontal, vertical, rotatory, or mixed.

Obsession. Recurrent, persistent ideas, thoughts, images, or impulses that invade consciousness.

Occipital lymph nodes. A group of lymph nodes located in the back of the neck at the base of the occipital bone.

Oligomenorrhea. Prolonged interval between uterine bleeding greater than 35 days but less than six months.

Oophorectomy. Surgical removal of one or both ovaries.

Ophthalmoscopy. Inspection of the internal eye structures using an ophthalmoscope.

Otaglia. Ear pain.

Otitis externa. Infection of the external ear canal.

Otitis media. Infection of the middle ear.

Otitis. Inflammation of the ear.

Otorrhea. Ear discharge.

Oviducts. See fallopian tubes.

Pallor. Lack of normal skin color; whitish color.

Pampiniform plexus. Plexus of veins which are found in the spermatic cord and drain the testicle. Proximally, they come together to form the testicular vein.

Papanicolaou smear. Cells obtained from the cervix to screen for cervical cancer.

Papule. Circumscribed solid elevation of the skin <0.5 cm in diameter.

Paranoid ideation. Of less than delusional proportions, it involves suspiciousness or the belief that one is being harassed, persecuted, or unfairly treated.

Paraplegia. Paralysis of the legs and lower body.

Paresis. Weakness of a muscle group or extremities.

Paresthesia. An abnormal sensation such as tingling or burning.

Parietal pleura. That part of the lining of the pleural cavity which is attached to the chest wall.

Parity. Having given birth to a child or children; recorded as number of term births, preterm births, abortions, living children.

Paroxysmal nocturnal dyspnea. Severe shortness of breath that awakens the patient from sleep.

Pectoriloquy. Transfer of spoken sounds through the chest wall.

Pelvic inflammatory disease. Infection of female reproductive organs, uterus, fallopian tubes, ovaries.

Penile urethra. That part of the urethra located within the penis.

Pericardial friction rub. A scratching noise caused by inflammation of the pericardial sac.

Periurethral glands. See Skene's glands.

Phobia. A persistent, irrational fear of a specific object, activity, or situation that results in a compelling desire to avoid the object, activity, or situation.

Phrenic nerves. Paired motor nerves that innervate the diaphragm.

Pinguecula. A yellow spot of tissue on the bulbar conjunctiva near the sclerocorneal junction, usually on the nasal side.

Pleural cavity. Fluid-filled space between the lung and the chest wall, lined by parietal pleura (chest wall) and visceral pleura (lung).

Pneumothorax. An accumulation of air in the pleural space.

Polymastia. The presence of ancillary breast tissue along the milk line.

Polymenorrhea. Uterine bleeding occurring at regular intervals of less than 21 days.

Polyp. A protruding growth from a mucous membrane.

Polythelia. The presence of ancillary nipples along the milk line.

Posterior axillary line. An imaginary vertical line drawn from the posterior aspect of the axillary fold (latissimus dorsi muscle) toward the waist.

Postmenopausal bleeding. Vaginal bleeding after menopause has begun.

Postpartum hemorrhage. Vaginal bleeding within 2 hours following delivery.

Precocious puberty. Development of secondary sexual characteristics prior to age 8 years in the female and prior to age 9 years in the male.

Preeclampsia. In pregnancy, development of high blood pressure, protein in the urine, and other symptoms and signs which place the mother and fetus in danger.

Premature rupture of membranes. Rupture of fetal membranes prior to onset of labor after 37 weeks' gestation.

Prepuce. The foreskin overlying the glans of the penis.

Presbyopia. Impairment of vision due to advancing age; diminution of the power of accommodation from loss of elasticity of the lens, causing the patient to hold close objects farther from the eye in order to see them clearly.

Preterm labor. Onset of labor prior to 38 weeks' gestation.

Preterm premature rupture of membranes. Rupture of fetal membranes prior to 38 weeks' gestation.

Primary amenorrhea. Failure to have spontaneous uterine bleeding by age 16.5 years.

Progesterone. A hormone secreted by the ovary under the influence of luteinizing hormone which acts on the follicle, the breast, and the endometrium of the uterus to prepare for implantation and support of the embryo.

Prolactin. Secreted by the anterior pituitary, it stimulates the production of milk in the alveolar cells of the mammary gland.

Proprioception. Sensation of body position and movements.

Prostate gland. Resting on the urogenital diaphragm, the prostate gland is situated between the base of the bladder and the penile urethra which begins at the urogenital diaphragm. Surrounding the prostatic portion of the urethra, its contents empty into the urethra and contribute to semen as well as the nurture of the sperm therein.

Prostatic urethra. That part of the urethra found within the prostate gland and connecting the bladder to the penile urethra.

Psychomotor agitation. Excessive motor activity associated with a feeling of inner tension.

Psychomotor retardation. Visible generalized slowing down of physical reactions, movements, and speech.

Psychotic. Gross impairment in reality testing.

Ptosis. Drooping of the upper eyelid.

Pubarche. Onset of development of secondary sexual characteristics.

Puberty. See secondary sexual maturation, development of secondary sexual characteristics.

Rectocele. Weakness in the posterior vaginal wall such that the rectum bulges into the vagina.

Regurgitation. A backward flowing of blood into the heart or between chambers. Insufficiency and incompetence are synonyms.

Respiratory excursion. A measure of chest and lung expansion.

Rhinitis. Inflammation of the nasal mucous membranes.

Rhinophyma. A form of rosacea characterized by redness, sebaceous hyperplasia, and swelling of the nose.

Rhinorrhea. A profuse discharge of thin nasal mucosa from the nasal mucous membranes.

Rigidity. Abnormal muscle stiffness.

Ronchi. Coarse breath sounds heard during auscultation of the lung, usually representing collection of mucoid material in the large airways.

Salpingostomy. Surgical incision in the fallopian tube usually for the purpose of removing an ectopic pregnancy.

Scale. A small thin plate of horny epithelium.

Scalene muscles. Muscles of the anterior neck. Considered a group of accessory respiratory muscles.

Scaphoid. Shaped like a boat.

Scoliosis. An abnormal lateral curvature of the spine.

Sebaceous glands. Holocrine glands, oil glands that open into the base of hair follicles.

Secondary amenorrhea. The absence of menses for six months or longer in a person who has previously had spontaneous menstrual periods.

Secondary sexual maturation. Point in the development of the female or male at which secondary sexual characteristics begin to develop.

Semen. Composed of sperm, secretions from the prostate gland, the bulbourethral glands, and the seminal vesicles.

Seminal vesicles. Glands attached to the base of the bladder. They empty into the ejaculatory duct, secreting substances which contribute to the semen and nurture the sperm therein.

Seminiferous tubules. Long tubular structures found in the septated testicle in which sperm are formed and pass into the epididymis.

Senile macula degeneration. Impairment of central vision; a common problem in the elderly.

Sertoli cells. Cells found in the seminiferous tubules which facilitate the development of sperm from spermatogonia.

Sexually transmitted disease. Infection transmitted between partners through sexual intercourse.

Sinusitis. Inflammation of the lining of any sinus, especially of one of the nasal sinuses. It may be purulent or nonpurulent and acute or chronic.

Skene's glands. Urethral glands that open into the distal urethra and may become infected with *Neisseria gonorrhoeae* bacteria.

Spasm. A sudden, painful, violent, involuntary muscle contraction.

Spasticity. Abnormal muscle tone with hyperactive reflexes.

Spermatic cord. The thin fascia of this cord surrounds the vas deferens, the internal and external spermatic arteries, the artery of the vas deferens, the venous pampiniform plexus and its superior continuation, the spermatic vein, lymphatic vessels, and nerves.

Spermatids. Cells arising from spermatocytes that are haploid (i.e., contain 23 chromosomes).

Spermatocytes. Cells arising from spermatogonium.

Spermatocytogenesis. See spermatogenesis.

Spermatogenesis. The process of development and formation of the mature sperm.

Spermatogonia. Primary diploid cell (i.e., containing 46 chromosomes) from which sperm develop.

Spermatozoa. Synonymous with fully developed sperm.

Spermiogenesis. The development of spermatozoa from spermatids.

Spider nevi. A telangiectasis composed of small vessels a few millimeters long radiating from a central arteriole; it resembles a spider.

Splinting. Protecting one side of the chest by limiting the amount of air breathed into that side.

Squamocolumnar junction. Point at which the columnar cell lining of the endocervical canal meets the squamous cell lining of the cervix. Area where cervical cancer is believed to begin.

Stereognosis. Understanding the shape of objects by the sense of touch.

Sternocleidomastoid muscles. Muscles of the anterior neck joining the mastoid process of the skull to the sternum.

Sternum. Sometimes called the "breast plate." Ribs are attached to it anteriorly. It is composed of three parts: the manubrium, the body, and the xiphoid process.

Strabismus. A muscular defect of the eye resulting in one eye turning inward or outward.

Stridor. A loud, shrieking abnormal breath sound caused by large airway or tracheal spasm.

Stupor. Partial or nearly complete unconsciousness, manifested by responding only to vigorous stimulation.

Supraclavicular lymph nodes. A group of lymph nodes located in the base of the posterior triangle of the neck above the clavicle.

Systole. The cardiac period between the first and second heart sounds.

Tachycardia. A heart rate of 100 beats per minute or more.

Tachypnea. Abnormal increase in the rate of respiration.

Tardive dyskinesia. Involuntary, repetitive movements of the facial, buccal, oral, and cervical musculature.

Thrill. A vibration felt on the precordium or over a blood vessel.

Thyroid storm. A sudden and life-threatening increase in the symptoms of thyrotoxicosis.

Tic. Involuntary, stereotyped movement which is repetitious, and appears to be purposeful, frequently involving the face or shoulders.

Tinnitus. A buzzing or humming sound in one or both ears associated with diseases of the middle ear, the inner ear, or the sensory cortex.

Tonic pupil (Addie's pupil). A benign condition in which one pupil reacts to light more slowly than the other.

Tonometry. The measurement of pressure within the eye.

Trachea. Primary large airway connecting the larynx with the primary bronchi, right and left.

Transitional zone. That area of the cervix where columnar cells of the endocervical canal are transitioning into squamous cells of the cervix. Area where cervical cancer is believed to begin.

Tremor. Involuntary quivering or shaking.

Trigeminal nerve. Cranial nerve 5 which has three branches: the ophthalmic, the maxillary, and the mandibular. A sensory nerve from the forehead, face, and upper anterior neck.

Tumor. An elevated, solid mass of tissue usually >2 cm in diameter.

Turgor. Rapidity with which skin returns to its original shape when pinched together.

Tympanite. Distention of the abdomen due to the presence of gas or air in the intestine or in the peritoneal cavity.

Ulcer. A lesion of the skin surface caused by superficial loss of tissue.

Ureter. Muscular tube connecting the kidney with the urinary bladder; it carries urine from the kidney to the bladder.

Urethra. Muscular tube extending from the urinary bladder to an opening just above the vaginal orifice in the female and at the tip of the glans penis in the male.

Urethrocele. Weakness in the anterior vaginal wall such that the urethra bulges into the vagina.

Urinary incontinence. Uncontrolled loss of urine.

Urinary tract infection. Bacterial or viral infection of the kidney and/or urinary bladder.

Uterine tubes. Synonymous with the oviduct of the fallopian tube. See fallopian tube.

Valsalva maneuver. A maneuver to increase intrathoracic pressure by forcible exhalation effort against the closed glottis.

Varicocele. Enlarged varicose veins of the pampiniform plexus secondary to incompetence of venous valves.

Varicose veins. Swollen veins caused by improper valve function.

Vas deferens. See ductus deferens.

Venous hum. A continuous blowing, singing, or humming murmur heard on auscultation over the right jugular vein in anemia, cirrhosis, and occasionally in healthy patients.

Ventricular diastolic gallop (S_3). Heard in the middle third of diastole, a heart sound caused by oscillation of blood back and forth between the walls of the ventricle.

Vertigo. A sensation of irregular or whirling motion. A person with vertigo may describe a room as spinning while standing still. A symptom of a balance disorder.

Vesicle. A small circumscribed elevation of the skin, containing serum (blister); <1 cm in diameter.

Vestibule. Entrance to the vagina; area between the labia minora and the vaginal opening.

Virilization. Masculine changes in a female, increased size of clitoris, male hair distribution, lower voice, male balding pattern.

Visceral pleura. That part of the lining of the pleural cavity which is attached to the lung.

Visual acuity. The ability of the eye to focus on both near and far objects.

Vocal/tactile fremitus. A vibration perceptible on palpation of the chest as the patient speaks.

Vulvovaginal glands. See Bartholin's glands.

Wheeze. Heard during auscultation of the lung, primarily during expiration, as a continuous musical sound produced by air flowing through a narrowed bronchi.

Xanthelasma. A papule, nodule, or plaque of yellow skin affecting the eyelids, due to deposits of fat.

Xerosis. Dry skin.

Xiphoid. A short cartilagenous structure found at the tip of the sternum in the epigastrium.

Abbreviations

A

A₂ Aortic second sound

A₂P₂ Second aortic sound greater than second pulmonic sound

A & O Alert and oriented

A & O x 3 Awake and oriented to person, place, and time

A & P Auscultation and percussion

A & W Alive and well

AAA Abdominal aortic aneurysm

AAL Anterior axillary line

AB Abduction *or* abortion

Abd Abdomen

ABG Androgen binding globulin *or* arterial blood gases

AC Air contrast *or* acromioclavicular *or* before meals

AC/C Accommodative convergence/accommodation

AC>BC Air conduction greater than bone conduction

ACC Accommodation

accel Acceleration

ACDF Anterior cervical discectomy and fusion

ACTH Adrenocorticotropic hormone

AD Right ear

ad lib As desired

ADD Adduction

ADH Antidiuretic hormone

ADL Activities of daily living

ADM Admission

AE Above elbow

AF Atrial fibrillation

A-flutter Atrial flutter

AICD Automatic implantable cardiac defibrillator

AIDS Acquired immune deficiency syndrome

AIVR Accelerated idioventricular rhythm

AJ Ankle jerk

AK Above knee

AKA Above knee amputation

ALA Acromion left anterior position

Alb Albumin

A-line Arterial line

alk Alkaline

ALP Acromion left posterior position

alt Alternate

AM Before noon

AMA Against medical advice

amb Ambulatory

amnio Amniocentesis

AMP Ampicillin *or* ampule *or* amputation

amt Amount

ANA Antinuclear antibody

A-n-DNA Anti-native deoxyribonucleic acid

anes Anesthesia

ANT Anterior

AO Anterior occiput position

A-paced Atrial paced rhythm

A-PD Anteroposterior diameter

AP Anterior posterior *or* apical pulse

APC Aspirin, phenacetin, caffeine

A phos Alkaline phosphatase

APL Anteroposterior and lateral

approx Approximate

aPTT Activated partial thromboplastin time

aq Aqueous

AR Aortic regurgitation

ARA Acromion right anterior position

ARDS Adult respiratory distress syndrome

ARF Acute renal failure

AROM Artificial rupture of membrane *or* active range of motion

ARP Acromion right posterior position

art Arterial, artery

AS Anterior sacrum position *or* aortic stenosis *or* left ear

ASA Acetylsalicylic acid (aspirin)

ASAP As soon as possible

ASHD Arteriosclerotic heart disease

ASMA Anti-smooth muscle antibody

ASO Antistreptolysin-O titer

ATA Thyroid autoantibodies

ATC Around the clock

ATR Achilles tendon reflex

AU Both ears

ausc Auscultation

av Arteriovenous

AV Atrioventricular

1°AVB First degree atrioventricular block

2°AVB Second degree atrioventricular block

3°AVB Third degree atrioventricular block

AV nicking Arteriovenous nicking

A-V paced Atrial-ventricular paced rhythm

ax Axillary

B

BAER Brainstem auditory evoked response

BAM Brain auditory mapping

baso Basophilic leukocyte

BBB Bundle branch block

BC Blood culture *or* bone conduction

BC>AC Bone conduction greater than air conduction

BCP Birth control pills

BE Barium enema *or* below elbow

BEE Basal energy expenditure

BID Twice a day

bilat Bilateral

Bili Bilirubin

BiVAD Biventricular assist device

BJ Bone and joint

BK Below knee

BKA Below knee amputation

bl vol Blood volume

BLA Brow left anterior position

BLP Brow left posterior position

BLT Brow left transverse position

BM Bowel movement

BO & P Blood, ova, parasites

BOM Bilateral otitis media

BOW Bag of waters

BP Blood pressure

bpd Biparietal diameter

BPD Bronchopulmonary dysplasia

BPH Benign prostatic hypertrophy

BPM Beats per minute or breaths per minute

Br Bromide

br sounds Breath sounds

BRA Brow right anterior position

brady Bradycardia

BRJ Brachial radialis jerk

BRT Brow right transverse position

BS Bowel sounds or breath sounds

BSO Bilateral salpingo-oophorectomy

BSP Bromosulphalein

BT Bleeding time

BTBV Beat-to-beat variability

BTL Bilateral tubal ligation

BUE Both upper extremities

BUN Blood urea nitrogen

BUS Bartholin's glands, urethra, Skene's glands

BV Blood volume

Bx Biopsy

C

C & S Culture and sensitivity

Ca Calcium

CA Carcinoma, cancer

CABG Coronary artery bypass graft

cal Calorie, caloric

cap Capillary

CAPD Continuous ambulatory peritoneal dialysis

CARCO Consciousness, activity, respiration, circulation, oral mucosa color

CAT Computerized axial tomographic scan (syn. with CT) or cataract

Cath Catheter, catheterize

CBC Complete blood count

CBD Common bile duct

CBG Capillary blood gas

CBI Continuous bladder irrigation

CBR Complete bedrest

CBW Current body weight

C-C Cephalocaudad (x-ray view)

CC Chief complaint

cc Cubic centimeter

C/D Cup to disc ratio

CEA Carcinoembryonic antigen

ceph Cephalic (head)

CHB Complete heart block

CHD Congenital heart disease

CHF Congestive heart failure

CHO Carbohydrate

Chol Cholesterol

CI Cardiac index

CIE Counterimmuno-electrophoresis

CIN Cervical intraepithelial neoplasia

circ Circumcision

Cl Chloride

Clav Clavicle

cldy Cloudy

cm Centimeter

CM Costal margin

CMTS Circulation, motion, temperature, and sensation

CMV Cytomegalovirus

CN Cranial nerves

CNS Central nervous system

C/O Complains of

CO Cardiac output

CO₂ Carbon dioxide

comp Compound

conc Concentration

cont Continue, continuous

contr Contraction

CONV Convergence

COPD Chronic obstructive pulmonary disease

C-P Cerebellopontine

CP Cerebral palsy or chest pain

CPAP Continuous positive airway pressure

CPD Cephalopelvic disproportion

cpd Compound

CPK Creatinine phosphokinase

CPM Continuous passive motion

CPP Cerebral perfusion pressure

CPR Cardiopulmonary resuscitation

CPT Chest physiotherapy

CRF Chronic renal failure

CRP C-reactive protein

CS Cesarean section

CSF Cerebrospinal fluid

C-spine Cervical spine

CST Contraction stress test

ct Chest tube

CT Computerized tomographic scan (syn. with CAT)

CTA Clear to auscultation

Cu Copper

CVA Cerebrovascular accident or costovertebral angle

CVAT Costovertebral angle tenderness

CVP Central venous pressure

CVS Cardiovascular system

CWS Cotton wool spots

Cx Cervix

cysto Cystoscopy

D

D & C Dilatation and currettage

D & I Dry and intact

DAT Diet as tolerated

dc Discontinue

DD Disc diameter

decel Deceleration

decr Decrease

del Delivery

derm Dermatology

DES Diethylstilbestrol

DHEAS Dehydroepiandro-sterone sulfate

DHT Dihydrotestosterone

diag Diagnosis

DIC Disseminated intravascular coagulation

DIFF Differential

dil Dilatation

DIP Distal interphalangeal joint

disc Discontinue

disch Discharge

DISH Diffuse idiopathic systemic hyperostosis

DJD Degenerative joint disease

DNS Deviated nasal septum

DOA Date of admission *or* dead on arrival

DOE Dyspnea on exertion

DOS Day of surgery

DP pulse Dorsalis pedis pulse

dr Dram

DSA Digital subtraction angiography

dsg Dressing

DTR Deep tendon reflexes

DTs Delirium tremens

DVT Deep vein thrombosis

Dx Diagnosis

E

EAC External auditory canal

EBL Estimated blood loss

EBV Epstein-Barr virus

EC Enteric coated

ECG Electrocardiogram

ECMO Extracorporeal membrane oxygenator

ECT Electroconvulsive therapy

EDC Estimated date of confinement

EEG Electroencephalogram

EENT Eyes, ears, nose, and throat

eff Effacement

e.g. For example

EGD Esophagogastro-duodenoscopy

EIA Enzyme immunoassay

ELISA Enzyme-linked immunosorbent assay

Elix Elixir

EMG Electromyography

ENT Ears, nose, and throat

eom Extraocular movement

EOMI Extraocular movements intact

EOS Eosinophil

epid Epidural anesthesia

epis Episiotomy

epith Epithelial, epithelium

ERCP Endoscopic retrograde cholangiopancreatography

ERG Electroretinogram

ERT Estrogen replacement therapy

ESR Erythrocyte sedimentation rate

ESWL Extracorporeal shock wave lithotripsy

et And

ET Endotracheal tube

et al. And others

ETOH Ethyl alcohol

ETT Exercise tolerance treadmill

EU Etiology unknown

exam Examination

EXPIR Expiration or expiratory

Ext Extension

ext External

F

FA Fetal age

FB Finger breadth

fb Flow by

FBS Fasting blood sugar

Fe Iron

ff Force fluids

FF Fundus firm

FFC Fetal fat cell

FFP Fresh frozen plasma

FH Family history

FHR Fetal heart rate

FHT Fetal heart tone

fib Fibrillation

FIGLU Formiminoglutamic acid

FiO$_2$ Fraction of inspired oxygen

fl Fluids

FMI Fetal maturity indices

FN Finger-to-nose

FOC Fronto-occipital circumference

FOF Full of feces

FOV Field of view

fract Fracture

freq Frequent, frequency

FROM Full range of motion

FS Full strength

FSE fetal scalp electrode

FSH Follicle stimulating hormone

FSP Fibrin split products

FSS Fetal scalp sampling

FTA Fluorescent treponemal antibodies

FTT Failure to thrive

FUO Fever of unknown origin

FVC Forced vital capacity

FVEP Flash visual evoked potential

Fx Fracture

G

GB Gallbladder

GC Gonococcus

GDM Gestational diabetes mellitus

GE Gastro-esophageal

Gen General

gest Gestation

GGTP Gamma-glutamyl transpeptidase

GH Growth hormone

GI Gastrointestinal

gm Gram

GnRH Gonadotropin releasing hormone

GPT Glumatic pyruvic transaminase

gr Grain

GRASS Gradient recalled acquisition (in a) steady state

grav Gravida

gtt Drop

GTT Glucose tolerance test

G-tube Gastric tube

GU Genitourinary

gyn Gynecology

H

H & H Hemoglobin and hematocrit

H & P History and physical

HA Headache

HAA Hepatitis-associated antigen

HB$_s$Ag Hepatitis B surface antigen

HBD Hydroxybutyrate dehydrogenase

HCG Human chorionic gonadotropin

HCG RIA Human chorionic gonadotropin radioimmunoassay

Hct Hematocrit

HDL High density lipoprotein cholesterol

HEENT Head, ears, eyes, nose, and throat

Hg Mercury

Hgb Hemoglobin

HGH Human growth hormone

HHH syndrome Hypotonia-hypomentia-hypogonadism-obesity syndrome

hist History

HIV Human immunodeficiency virus

HJR Hepatojugular reflux

HK Heel-to-knee

HLA Human leukocyte antigen

HMD Hyaline membrane disease

HNP Herniated nucleus pulposus

H/O History of

H$_2$O Water

H$_2$O$_2$ Hydrogen peroxide

HOB Head of bed

HOH Hard of hearing

hpf High-powered field

HPI History present illness

HPL Human placental lactogen

HR Heart rate

hr Hour

HRCT High resolution computerized tomography

HS At bedtime

HSV Herpes simplex virus

ht Height

HTLV Human T-cell leukemia virus *or* human T-cell lymphotrophic virus

HVA Homovanillic acid

Hx History

hypo Hypodermic

hyst Hysterectomy

I

I^{131} Radioactive iodine

I & D Incision and drainage

I & O Intake and output

IABP Intra-aortic balloon pump

IAC Internal auditory canal

IBC Iron binding capacity

IBW Ideal body weight

ICD Isocitric dehydrogenase

ICP Intracranial pressure

ICS Intercostal space

ID Intradermal

i.e. That is

IEP Immunoelectrophoresis

IFM Internal fetal monitoring

Ig Immunoglobulin

IM Intramuscular

IMA Internal mammary artery

IMP Implants *or* impression

IMV Intermittent mandatory ventilation

incont Incontinent

incr Increase

ind of labor Induction of labor

inf Inferior

ING Inguinal

Inj Injection

INSPIR Inspiration or inspiratory

int Internal

invol Involuntary

IOP Intraocular pressure

IP Interphalangeal *or* intraperitoneal

IPPB Intermittent positive pressure breathing

IQ Intelligence quotient

IRDS Infant respiratory distress syndrome

IRR Irrigate, irrigation

IS Incentive spirometry

I-T Intertrochanteric

IUD Intrauterine device

IUFD Intrauterine fetal demise

IUGR Intrauterine growth retardation

IUP Intrauterine pregnancy

IV Intravenous

IVC Inferior vena cava

IVCD Intraventricular conduction defect

IVP Intravenous pyelogram

IVPB Intervenous piggyback

IVR Idioventricular rhythm

J

JEB Junctional escape beat

JF Joint fluid

Jnt Joint

JR Junctional rhythm

JT Junctional tachycardia

junc Junctional

JVD Jugular venous distension

K

K Potassium

KCl Potassium chloride

kg Kilogram

KJ Knee jerk

KO Keep open

KOR Keep open rate

KUB Kidneys, ureters, and bladder

KVO Keep vein open

KW Keith/Wagener (ophthalmoscopic findings, graded 1–4)

L

L2 Second lumbar vertebra

L & W Living and well

LA Left arm

LAA Left acromion anterior position

lac Laceration

LAL Left axillary line

LAO Left anterior oblique

lap Laparotomy

LAP Left acromion posterior position

laposc Laparoscopy

LAT Lateral

latex fix Latex fixation

LATS Long-acting thyroid stimulator

LB Low back

lb Pound

LBA Left brow anterior position

LBBB Left bundle branch block

LBP left brow posterior position

LBT left brow transverse position

LCM Left costal margin

LDH Lactic dehydrogenase

LDL Low density lipoprotein cholesterol

LE Lower extremities

LE test Lupus erythematosus test

LGA Large for gestational age

LH Luteinizing hormone

liq Liquid

LL Left leg

LL brace Long leg brace

LL cast Long leg cast

LLE Left lower extremity

LLL Left lower lobe

LLQ Left lower quadrant

LMA Left mentum anterior position

LMP Last menstrual period

LMT Left mentum transverse position

LNMP Last normal menstrual period

LOA Left occiput anterior position

LOC Level of consciousness *or* loss of consciousness

LOP Left occiput posterior position

LOT Left occiput transverse position

LP Lumbar puncture

lpf Low powered field

LPO Left posterior oblique

LR Lactated Ringer's solution

L/S ratio Lecithin-sphingomyelin ratio

LSA Left sacrum anterior position

LSO Left salpingo-oophorectomy

LSP Left sacrum posterior position

L-spine Lumbar spine

LST Left sacrum transverse position

LSW Left side weakness

LT Left

LTB Laryngotracheobronchitis

LUE Left upper extremity

LUL Left upper lobe

LUOQ Left upper outer quadrant

LUQ Left upper quadrant

L-V Left ventricular

L-VAD Left ventricular assist device

LVE Left ventricular enlargement

LVEF Left ventricular ejection fraction

LVG Left ventrogluteal *or* living

LVH Left ventricular hypertrophy

Lymphs Lymphocytes

M

M$_1$ Mitral first heart sound

MAE Moving all extremities

MAL Midaxillary line

MBC Minimal bacterial concentration

MCA Motorcycle accident

mcg Microgram

MCH Mean corpuscular hemoglobin

MCHC Mean corpuscular hemoglobin concentration

MCL Medial collateral ligament *or* midclavicular line

MCL Midclavicular line

MCP Metacarpophalangeal joint

MCV Mean corpuscular volume

mec Meconium

med Medicine

memb Membrane

mEq Milliequivalent

meta Metamyelocyte

MF Multi-focal

mg Milligram

MgSO$_4$ Magnesium sulfate

mHz Megahertz

MI Mitral insufficiency *or* myocardial infarction

MIC Minimal inhibitory concentration

mid Middle

min Minute

ML Midline

mL Milliliter

MLA Mentum left anterior position

MLC Mixed lymphocyte culture

MLE Midline episiotomy

MLP Mentum left posterior position

MLT Mentum left transverse position

mm Millimeter

MNSEP Median nerve somato-sensory evoked potential

mod Moderate

MOM Milk of magnesia

mono Monocytes

MPGR Multiplanar gradient recalled acquisition (in a) steady state scan

M-R Magnetic resonance

MR Mitral regurgitation

MRA Mentum right anterior position

MRI Magnetic resonance imaging (syn. with NMI and NMR)

MRP Mentum right posterior position

MRSA Methicillin resistant *Staphylococcus aureus*

MRT Mentum right transverse position

MS Multiple sclerosis

MSE Mental status exam

msec Millisecond

MSL Midsternal line

MTP Metatarsal phalangeal

MUGA Multiple-gated acquisition scanning

multip Multipara

MV Microvolt

mV Millivolt

MVA Motor vehicle accident

MVP Mitral valve prolapse

myelo Myelogram

N

N & T Nose and throat *or* numbness and tingling

N & V Nausea and vomiting

NA Not applicable

Na Sodium

NBT Nitroblue tetrazolium

NCV Nerve conduction velocity

neg Negative

NET Nasal endotracheal tube

Neuro Neurology

neutr Neutrophil

NG Nasogastric

NH₃ ammonia

NH$_3$ ammonia

NKA No known allergy

NMI Nuclear magnetic image or nuclear magnetic resonance (syn. with MRI)

NMR Nuclear magnetic imager or nuclear magnetic resonance (syn. with MRI)

no Number

Noc Night

Noct At night

NP Neuropsychiatric

NPhx Nasopharynx

NPO Nothing by mouth

NRBC Nucleated red blood cell

NROM Normal range of motion

NS Normal saline

NSE Normal saline enema

NSR Normal sinus rhythm

NST Non-stress test

NT Nasotracheal

NTG Nitroglycerine

Null Nullipara

NV Neurovascular

NWB No weight bearing

O

O & P Ova and parasites

O x 3 Oriented to person, place, and time

O x 4 Oriented to person, place, time, and situation

O₂ Oxygen

O₂ cap Oxygen capacity

O₂ sat Oxygen saturation

OA Occiput anterior position *or* osteoarthritis

occ Occasional

OCP Oral contraceptive pills

OCT Oxytocin challenge test

OD Right eye

ODD syndrome Oculodento-digital syndrome

O-G Orogastric

oint Ointment

oj Orange juice

OM Otitis media

OOB Out of bed

OP Occiput posterior position

op Operation, operative

Ophth Ophthalmic

ORA Occiput right anterior position

ORIF Open reduction, internal fixation

ORP Occiput right posterior position

ORT Occiput right transverse position

orth Orthopedic

ortho Orthopedic

OS Left eye *or* opening snap

os Mouth

osm Osmolality

OT Occupational therapy

OTC Over the counter medications

OU Both eyes *or* each eye

oz Ounce

P

P₂ Pulmonic second heart sound

PA Posterior-anterior *or* pulmonary artery

Pa line Pulmonary artery line

PAB Premature atrial beat

PAC Premature atrial contraction

pacer NC Pacer non-capture

pacer NS Pacer non-sensing

PAD Pulmonary artery diastolic

PAF Paroxysmal atrial fibrillation

palp palpable

PAP Papanicolaou smear

PARA Indicative of the number of children a woman has delivered

PAS Para-amniosalicylate

PAT Paroxysmal atrial tachycardia

path Pathology

PAW Pulmonary artery wedge

Pb Lead

PBG Phorphobilinogen

PBI Protein-bound iodine

PC After meals

PCA Patient-controlled analgesia

pCO₂ Partial pressure of carbon dioxide

PCV Packed cell volume

PD Peritoneal dialysis

PE Pulmonary embolism

ped Pediatric

PEEP Positive and expiratory pressure

peri Perineal

PERL Pupils equal, reactive to light

PERRLA Pupils, equal, round, reactive to light and accommodation

PET Preeclampsia

PFS Pulmonary function studies

pH Hydrogen ion concentration

PH Present history

phos Phosphatase

Phx Pharynx

PI Peripheral iridectomy *or* present illness

PICA Posterior inferior cerebellar artery

PID Pelvic inflammatory disease

PIE Pulmonary interstitial emphysema

PIF Prolactin-inhibiting factor

PIH Pregnancy induced hypertension

PIP Proximal interphalangeal joint

Pit Pitocin

PJC Premature junctional contraction

PJT Paroxysmal junctional tachycardia

PKU Phenylketonuria

PL Plantar *or* prolactin

PMN Polymorphonuclear leukocytes

PMP Previous menstrual period

PMS Premenstrual syndrome

PNC Premature nodal contraction

PND Paroxysmal nocturnal dyspnea *or* postnasal drip

PNP Postnasal pharyngeal

PNS Peripheral nervous system

PO By mouth

pO$_2$ Partial pressure of oxygen

PO$_4$ Phosphate

polys Polymorphonuclear leukocytes

pos Position

post Posterior, after

post op Postoperative

pp Pedal pulses

PP Postpartum *or* pin prick

P-PROM Preterm premature rupture of membranes

PP sugar Postprandial sugar

PPD Purified protein derivative

PPP Pedal pulses palpable

PRBC Packed red blood cells

premie Premature infant

preop Preoperative

prep Prepare for

pres Presentation

PRN Whenever necessary

procto Proctoscopy

PROM Passive range of motion *or* premature rupture of membranes

pros Progranulocytes

prot Protein

protime Prothrombin time

PRRE Pupils, round, reactive, equal

PRVEP Pattern reversal visual evoked potential

PS Posterior sacrum position

PSA Prostate specific antigen

PSP Phenolsulfonphthalein

PSVT Paroxysmal supraventricular tachycardia

psych Psychiatry, psychology

pt Patient

PT Prothrombin time, physical therapy

PT pulse posterior tibialis pulse

PTCA Percutaneous transluminal coronary angioplasty

PTL Preterm labor

PTM Penile tumescence monitor

PTSEP Posterior tibial somatosensory evoked potential

PTT Partial thromboplastin time

PUD Pudendal

Pul Pulmonary

PVB Premature ventricular beat

PVC Premature ventricular contraction

PVE Premature ventricular extrasystole

PVI Peripheral vascular insufficiency

PZI Protamine zinc insulin

Q

Q 2 hr, Q 3 hr, etc. Every 2 hours, every 3 hours, etc.

QD Every day

QID Four times per day

QOD Every other day

qs Quantity sufficient

qt Quart

quad Quadriplegic

quant Quantity

R

RA Rheumatoid arthritis *or* right arm

ra Right atrial *or* right atrium

RAA Right acromion anterior position

RAE Right atrial enlargement

RAI Radioactive iodine uptake

RAP Right acromion posterior position

RBA Right brow anterior position

RBBB Right bundle branch block

RBC Red blood cell *or* red blood count

RBP Right brow posterior position

RBT Right brow transverse position

RCM Right costal margin

RCV Red cell volume

RDS Respiratory distress syndrome

rect Rectal

REM sleep Rapid eye movement sleep

req Request, requisition

RESP Respiration

retic Reticulocyte

RF Rheumatoid factor

Rh factor Rhesus factor

RIA Radioimmunoassay

RL Right leg

RLE Right lower extremity

RLL Right lower lobe

RLQ Right lower quadrant

RMA Right mentum anterior position

RMCL Right Midclavicular Line

RML Right middle lobe

RMP Right mentum posterior position

RMT Right mentum transverse position

R/O Rule out

ROA Right occiput anterior position

ROM Range of motion

ROP Right occiput posterior position

ROT Right occiput transverse position

RPO Right posterior oblique

RPR Rapid plasma reagin

RR Respiratory rate

RRE Round, regular, equal

RRR Regular rhythm and rate

RSA Right sacrum anterior position

RSO Right salpingo-oophorectomy

RSP Right sacrum posterior position

RSR Regular sinus rhythm

RST Right sacrum transverse position

RSW Right-sided weakness

RT Right

RTC Return to clinic

RUE Right upper extremity

RUL Right upper lobe

RUOQ Right upper outer quadrant

RUQ Right upper quadrant

RV Right ventricle

RVAD Right ventricular assist device

RVE Right ventricle enlargement

RVG Right ventrogluteal

RVH Right ventricle hypertrophy

Rx Prescription

S

S$_1$ First heart sound

S$_2$ Second heart sound

SA Sacrum anterior position

sa Sinoatrial

S arrest Sinus arrest

S arrhy Sinus arrhythmia

SB Sinus bradycardia

sb Small bowel

SBA Saddle block anesthesia

SBE Subacute bacterial endocarditis

S blk Sinus block

SBP Systolic blood pressure

SC Subcutaneous

SE Spin echo

sec Second

sed rate Sedimentation rate

segs Segmented neutrophils

SEM Systolic ejection murmur

SEP Somatosensory evoked potential

SG cath Swan-Ganz catheter

SGA Small for gestational age

SGOT Serum glutamic-oxaloacetic transaminase

SGPT Serum glutamic pyruvic transaminase

SI Sacroiliac

SIDS Sudden infant death syndrome

sig Let it be labeled

SIJ Sacroiliac joint

sl Slight

SL Sublingual

SLA Sacrum left anterior position

SLC Short leg cast

SLE Slit lamp examination

SLP Sacrum left posterior position

SLR Straight leg raise

SLT Sacrum left posterior position

sm Small

SMA Sequential multiple (blood) analysis

SMD Senile macular degeneration

SO Salpingo-oophorectomy

SOAP Subjective, objective, assessment, plan

SOB Shortness of breath

sol Solution

S/P Status post

SP Sacrum posterior position

sp fl Spinal fluid

sp gr Specific gravity

spec Specimen

SPECT Single photon emission computed tomography

spon Spontaneous

SQ Subcutaneous

SR Sinus rhythm

SRA Sacrum right anterior position

SROM Spontaneous rupture of membranes

SRT Sacrum right transverse position

S/S Signs and symptoms

ss One-half

SSE Soap suds enema

ST Sinus tachycardia

ST↑ Elevation of the ST segment of an ECG tracing

ST↓ Depression of the ST segment of an ECG tracing

stab Bandform granulocyte

staph Staphylococcus

stat Immediately

str Straight

strep Streptococcus

STSG Split thickness skin graft

subling Sublingual

subq Subcutaneous

supp Suppository

surg Surgery

SVC Superior vena cava

SVE Sterile vaginal exam

SvO$_2$ Saturation of venous oxygen

SVR Systemic vascular resistance

SVT Supraventricular tachycardia

Sx Symptom

sym Symptom

symp Symptom

syn Syntocinon

T

T & C Type and crossmatch

T_1 Longitudinal relaxation time *or* MRI spin-lattice *or* tricuspid first sound

T_2 Transverse relaxation time *or* MRI spin-spin

T_3 Triiodothyronine

T_4 Thyroxine

TA Thyroglobulin autoprecipitin

TAB Tablet

tachy Tachycardia

TAH Transabdominal hysterectomy

TAH-BSO Transabdominal hysterectomy and bilateral salpingo-oophorectomy

TBG Thyroxin binding globulin

TBLC Term birth, living child

tbsp Tablespoon

TCDB Turn, cough, deep breathe

T-E Tracheo-esophageal

TE Time echo

TeBG Testosterone binding globulin

temp Temperature

TENS Transcutaneous electrical nerve stimulator

TF Tactile fremitus

th ab Threatened abortion

TIA Transient ischemic attack

TIA with RND Transient ischemic attack with residual neurologic deficits

Tib Tibia

TIBC Total iron binding capacity

TID Three times a day

tinct Tincture

TIUV Total intrauterine volume

TJ Triceps jerk

TKO To keep open

TLC Tender loving care

TM Tympanic membrane

TMJ Temporomandibular joint

TNT Nitroglycerine tablet

TO Telephone order

Toco Tocodynamometer

TOF Tetrology of Fallot

tol Tolerate *or* tolerance

TOS Thoracic outlet syndrome

TP Total protein

TPA Tissue plasminogen activator

TPN Total parenteral nutrition

TPR Temperature, pulse, respiration

TR MRI repetition time *or* tremor

tr Traction

trach Tracheostomy

trig Triglycerides

TRP Tubular reabsorption of phosphorus

TSH Thyroid stimulating hormone

tsp Teaspoon

TSP Total serum protein

T-spine Thoracic spine

TUR Transurethral resection

TURP Transurethral resection prostate

TV Tidal volume

TVH Transvaginal hysterectomy

TWE Tap water enema

Tx Treatment

U

UA Urinalysis

UA catheter Umbilico-arterial catheter

UAC Umbilico-arterial catheter

UBW Usual body weight

UC Uterine contraction

UCG Urinary chorionic gonadotropin

UCHD Usual childhood diseases

UE Upper extremity

UGI Upper gastrointestinal

UIBC Unsaturated iron binding capacity

ung Ointment

U/O Urine output

UP junction Ureteropelvic junction

UPJ Ureteropelvic junction

URI Upper respiratory infection

urol Urology *or* urological

US Ultrasound

ut dict As directed

UTI Urinary tract infection

UUN Urine urea nitrogen

UV Ultraviolet

UVC Umbilico-venous catheter

UVJ Ureterovesical junction

V

VA Visual acuity

V cap Vital capacity

v-fib Ventricular fibrillation

vag Vagina *or* vaginal

var Variable *or* variability

VD Venereal disease

Vd void

VDRL Venereal disease research laboratory

VER Visual evoked response

vert Vertex

VF Visual field *or* vocal fremitus

VH Vaginal hysterectomy

VI Ventricular index

vit Vitamin

VMA Vanillylmandelic acid

VO voice order

VOL volume

V-P Ventriculoperitoneal

V-paced Ventricular paced rhythm

VPB Ventricular premature beat

VPC Ventricular premature contraction

VS Vital signs

V-standstill Ventricular standstill

v-tach Ventricular tachycardia

vtx Vertex

VZV Varicella zoster virus (herpes zoster)

W

W/ With

WAP Wandering atrial pacemaker

WBC White blood cells *or* white blood count

WBCT Whole blood clot time (Lee-White)

WC Wheel chair

w/d Warm and dry

WD Well developed

WD/WN Well developed, well nourished

WD/WN in NAD Well developed, well nourished, in no acute distress

WNL Within normal limits

wt Weight

W/WO With and without

X

X-match Crossmatch

Z

Zn Zinc

Index

– Index –

- Index -